BIOMEDICAL ASPECTS
OF BOTULISM

Academic Press Rapid Manuscript Reproduction

The proceedings of an International Conference on the Biomedical Aspects of Botulism, convened at Fort Detrick, Frederick, Maryland, on March 16–18, 1981, sponsored by the U.S. Army Medical Research Institute of Infectious Diseases.

BIOMEDICAL ASPECTS OF BOTULISM

Edited by
GEORGE E. LEWIS, JR.
Department of Applied Toxin Research
Pathology Division
U. S. Army Medical Research Institute of Infectious Diseases
Fort Detrick
Frederick, Maryland

Assistant Editor

PHEBE SUMMERS ANGEL

U.S. Army Medical Research Institute of Infectious Diseases
Fort Detrick, Frederick, Maryland

1981

ACADEMIC PRESS
A Subsidiary of Harcourt Brace Jovanovich, Publishers
New York   London
Paris   San Diego   San Francisco   São Paulo
Sydney   Tokyo   Toronto

ACADEMIC PRESS, INC.
111 Fifth Avenue, New York, New York 10003

United Kingdom Edition published by
ACADEMIC PRESS, INC. (LONDON) LTD.
24/28 Oval Road, London NW1 7DX

Library of Congress Cataloging in Publication Data
Main entry under title:

Biomedical aspects of botulism.

"The proceedings of an International Conference on
the Biomedical Aspects of Botulism, convened at Fort
Detrick, Frederick, Maryland, on March 16-18, 1981,
sponsored by the U.S. Army Medical Research Institute
of Infectious Diseases"--P. ii.
    Includes index.
    1. Botulism--Congresses. 2. Botulinum toxin--
Congresses. I. Lewis, George E. II. International
Conference on the Biomedical Aspects of Bolulism (1981:
Fort Detrick, Frederick, Md.) III. United States Army
Medical Research Institute of Infectious Diseases.
[DNLM: 1. Botulinum toxins--Congresses. 2. Botulism--
Congresses. WC 268 B615 1981]
QR201.B7B56   615.9'52995   81-19119
ISBN 0-12-447180-3   AACR2

PRINTED IN THE UNITED STATES OF AMERICA

81 82 83 84   9 8 7 6 5 4 3 2 1

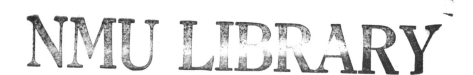

CONTENTS

IV. New Concepts

V. Detection, Isolation, and Identification

VI. Prophylaxis and Toxoid Production

CONTRIBUTORS

Numbers in parentheses indicate the pages on which the authors' contributions begin.

James H. Anderson, Jr.[1] (233), *Medical Division, U. S. Army Medical Research Institute of Infectious Diseases, Fort Detrick, Frederick, Maryland 21701*

Stephen S. Arnon (331), *Infant Botulism Research Project, California Department of Health Services, Berkeley, California 94704*

Nigel Bailey (247), *Vaccine Research and Production Laboratory, Center for Applied Microbiology and Research, Porton Down, Salisbury, Wiltshire SP4 OJG, England*

Thomas R. Bender (285), *Alaska Investigations Division, Center for Infectious Diseases, Centers for Disease Control, Anchorage, Alaska 99501*

J. D. Black (47), *Department of Biochemistry, Imperial College of Science and Technology, London, SW7 2AZ, England*

Lawrence W. Brown (347), *Department of Pediatrics and Neurology, Temple University School of Medicine, Philadelphia, Pennsylvania 19133*

Brian Capel (247), *Vaccine Research and Production Laboratory, Center for Applied Microbiology and Research, Porton Down, Salisbury, Wiltshire SP4 OJG, England*

M. Cherington (327), *Department of Neurology, University of Colorado Medical Center, Denver, Colorado 80262*

Alberto S. Ciccarelli (291), *Catedra de Microbiologia, Facultad de Ciencias Medicas, Universidad Nacional de Cuyo, 5500, Mendoza, Argentina*

Alan Crooks (247), *Vaccine Research and Production Laboratory, Center for Applied Microbiology and Research, Porton Down, Salisbury, Wiltshire SP4 OJG, England*

Bibhuti R. DasGupta (1), *Food Research Institute, University of Wisconsin, Madison, Wisconsin 53706*

M. Dezfulian[2] (205) *Bacteriology Division, Bureau of Laboratories, Centers for Disease Control, Atlanta, Georgia 30333*

[1]Present address: Department of Clinical Investigation, Brooke Army Medical Center, Fort Sam Houston, Texas 78234.

[2]Present address: Division of Infectious Diseases, School of Medicine, Johns Hopkins University, Baltimore, Maryland 21205.

J. Oliver Dolly (47, 247), *Department of Biochemistry, Imperial College of Science and Technology, London, SW7 2AZ, England*

V. R. Dowell, Jr. (205), *Bacteriology Division, Bureau of Laboratories, Centers for Disease Control, Atlanta, Georgia 30333*

M. W. Eklund (93), *Pacific Utilization Research Center, Northwest and Alaska Fisheries Center, Seattle, Washington 98112*

Roger A. Feldman (271), *Bacterial Diseases Division, Center for Infectious Diseases, Centers for Disease Control, Atlanta, Georgia 30333*

Domingo F. Giménez (291), *Laboratorio de Alimentos, Universidad Nacional de San Luis, San Luis, Argentina*

M. Gwilt (47), *Department of Pharmacology, Royal Free Hospital School of Medicine, London, England*

Ernst Habermann (129), *Rudolf Buchheim Institute of Pharmacology, Justus Liebig Universität, Giessen, West Germany*

Peter Hambleton (47, 247), *Vaccine Research and Production Laboratory, Center for Applied Microbiology and Research, Porton Down, Salisbury, Wiltshire SP4 0JG, England*

M. Carolyn Hardegree (217), *Division of Bacterial Products, Bureau of Biologics, Food and Drug Administration, Bethesda, Maryland 20205*

Charles L. Hatheway (165), *Bacteriology Division, Bureau of Laboratories, Centers for Disease Control, Atlanta, Georgia 30333*

Nicholas Heron (247), *Vaccine Research and Production Laboratory, Center for Applied Microbiology and Research, Porton Down, Salisbury, Wiltshire SP4 0JG, England*

William L. Heyward (285), *Alaska Investigations Division, Center for Infectious Diseases, Centers for Disease Control, Anchorage, Alaska 99501*

Hiroo Iida (109), *Department of Bacteriology, Hokkaido University School of Medicine, Sapporo, 060 Japan*

Katsuhiro Inoue (109), *Hokkaido Institute of Public Health, Sapporo 060, Japan*

Shunji Kozaki (21, 181), *Department of Veterinary Science, College of Agriculture, University of Osaka Prefecture, Sakai-shi, Osaka 591, Japan*

George E. Lewis, Jr. (233, 261), *Department of Applied Toxin Research, Pathology Division, U. S. Army Medical Research Institute of Infectious Diseases, Fort Detrick, Frederick, Maryland 21701*

Loretta M. McCroskey (165), *Bacteriology Division, Bureau of Laboratories, Centers for Disease Control, Atlanta, Georgia 30333*

Jack Melling (47, 247), *Vaccine Research and Production Laboratory, Center for Applied Microbiology and Research, Porton Down, Salisbury, Wiltshire SP4 0JG, England*

J. Glenn Morris, Jr. (271, 317), *Bacterial Diseases Division, Center for Infectious Diseases, Centers for Disease Control, Atlanta, Georgia 30333*

Servé Notermans (181), *Laboratory for Zoonoses and Food Microbiology, National Institute of Public Health, Bilthoven, The Netherlands*

Keiji Oguma (109), *Department of Bacteriology, Hokkaido University School of Medicine, Sapporo 060, Japan*

Iwao Ohishi (21), *Department of Veterinary Science, College of Agriculture, University of Osaka Prefecture, Sakai-shi, Osaka 591, Japan*

Robert A. Pollard (271), *Bacteriology Division, Bureau of Laboratories, Centers for Disease Control, Atlanta, Georgia 30333*

F. T. Poysky (93), *Pacific Utilization Research Center, Northwest and Alaska Fisheries Center, Seattle, Washington 98112*

Genji Sakaguchi (21), *Department of Veterinary Science, College of Agriculture, University of Osaka Prefecture, Sakai-shi, Osaka 591, Japan*

William Schaffner (359), *Departments of Medicine and Preventive Medicine, Vanderbilt University School of Medicine, Nashville, Tennessee 37232*

Edward J. Schantz (143), *Food Research Institute, Department of Food Microbiology and Toxicology, University of Wisconsin–Madison, Madison, Wisconsin 53706*

Alan B. Scott (143), *Smith–Kettlewell Institute of Visual Sciences, San Francisco, California 94115*

Lawrence C. Sellin (81), *Department of Applied Toxin Research, Pathology Division, U. S. Army Medical Research Institute of Infectious Diseases, Fort Detrick, Frederick, Maryland 21701*

Lynn S. Siegel (121), *Department of Applied Toxin Research, Pathology Division, U. S. Army Medical Research Institute of Infectious Diseases, Fort Detrick, Frederick, Maryland 21701*

Lance Simpson (35), *Department of Pharmacology, College of Physicians and Surgeons, Columbia University, New York, New York 10032*

Ortrud Sonnabend (191, 303), *Institute of Medial Microbiology, Kantonsspital St. Gallen, CH-9007 St. Gallen, Switzerland*

Wolfgang Sonnabend (191, 303), *Department of Pathology, Kantonsspital St. Gallen, CH-9007 St. Gallen, Switzerland*

Hiroshi Sugiyama (151), *Food Research Institute, Department of Bacteriology, University of Wisconsin–Madison, Madison, Wisconsin 53706*

Stephen Thesleff (65), *Department of Pharmacology, University of Lund, Lund, Sweden*

Chun-Kee Tse (47, 247), *Department of Biochemistry, Imperial College of Science and Technology, London SW7 2AZ, England*

R. S. Williams (47), *Department of Biochemistry, Imperial College of Science and Technology, London SW7 2AZ, England*

D. Wray (47), *Department of Pharmacology, Royal Free Hospital School of Medicine, London, England*

PREFACE

During the past five years there have been numerous developments, often in diverse and unrelated scientific disciplines, which have contributed substantially to both our understanding and awareness of botulism. The structure, actions, and effects of botulinal toxins have been described in much greater detail than ever before; methods for the laboratory identification, diagnosis, and conformation of botulism have improved considerably; *Clostridium botulinum* type G, once thought to be of little more than academic interest, has been recently associated with five sudden and unexpected human deaths; new chemotherapeutic approaches to the treatment of botulism have been explored in both laboratory animal models and in human patients; and probably the most significant of all recent developments have been the description and wide recognition of a toxicoinfectious form of botulism in infants. Thus, the time seemed appropriate to provide a forum for scientists and clinicians from all concerned disciplines to present, exchange, and discuss recent advances in our understanding of the biomedical aspects of botulism.

This volume is based on the proceedings of the first international conference devoted exclusively to the biomedical aspects of botulism. The text represents a melding of basic and applied works gathered from the disciplines of biochemistry, pharmacology, neurophysiology, microbiology, epidemiology, pathology, toxinology, and clinical medicine for the purpose of offering a complete and current reference text on botulism.

Section I provides the most complete and up-to-date information available on the structure, and structure–function relationships and oral toxicities of the various botulinal toxins. In Section II the current thinking about the cellular and subcellular effects of botulinal toxin are summarized along with the presentation of a model to account for toxin-induced blockage of transmitter release and a discussion of new approaches for dealing with and utilizing the botulinal toxins. The pre- and postsynaptic effects of botulinal toxin are examined in depth. The existence of two kinds of vesicular (quantal) transmitter release are proposed and the long-term alterations in the postsynaptic muscular membranes of botulinal toxin-poisoned preparations are examined.

Detailed evidence for the involvement of specific bacteriophages in the toxigenicity of *C. botulinum* types C and D is presented in the first two chapters of

Section III. Also included in this section is a discussion of the optimal fermentor conditions for toxin production by *C. botulinum* types A, B , and E.

Section IV provides the reader with a fascinating comparison of the many properties shared by, and the qualitative effects of, tetanus and botulinal toxins. Next the impressive use of botulinal toxin, "the most lethal substance known," to treat strabismus and thus employ this toxin to serve mankind is described. Data are presented which serve as the basis for understanding the etiology of infant botulism. The critical role of age of the host and the population of intestinal organisms in determining whether the gut of infant laboratory animal models is colonized by *C. botulinum* is convincingly presented in the last portion of this section.

Section V presents a compilation of available information on the laboratory investigation of human and animal botulism, to include infant botulism and shaker foal syndrome. The development of practical isolation and identification procedures are then reviewed in depth. The extremely thorough laboratory procedures utilized to document the association of clostridial organisms and toxins with sudden and/or unexpected human death are described in detail.

A review of selected aspects of the development of toxoids and an insight into the anticipated development of new bacterial products serve to introduce Section VI. A new generation of botulinal toxoids is initiated by the presentation of methodologies for the production, purification, and toxoiding of botulinal toxins. Recent clinical and serological data are presented from an evaluation of experimental botulinal toxoids in both laboratory animals and volunteers. An overview of approaches to prophylaxis, immunotherapy, and chemotherapy of botulism concludes this section.

Section VII begins with a comprehensive 30-year review of the epidemiologic characteristics of botulism in the United States, proceeds to a presentation of the epidemiologic and clinical findings of arctic botulism in Alaska, and continues with the detailing of botulism as it occurs in Argentina. The final chapter investigates the necropsy diagnosis of botulism in twelve patients who died unexpectedly and compares the epidemiology and pathology of these cases.

The text concludes with Section VIII in which the current trends in therapy of botulism are reviewed and two very detailed discussions on infant botulism are presented. The first chapter on infant botulism describes the pathogenesis and clinical aspects while the second chapter reviews controversies in management and treatment.

This volume should serve as a valuable reference to anyone disciplined in the fields of bacteriology, biochemistry, immunology, neurophysiology, pathology, pharmacology, and toxinology, as well as to both physicians and veterinarians interested in a single source for obtaining current information on the biomedical aspects of botulism.

I wish to thank all those who have contributed to this volume and to the very successful conference from which it was derived. Without the enthusiasm and responsible support of the staff of the U. S. Army Medical Research Institute of Infectious Diseases, these events would not have occurred.

I express my gratitude to my assistant, Phebe Summers Angel, and to Nancy Melching, Betty Magaha, Peggy Covert, Joyce King, Pat Baughman, Martin Hilt,

Carl Pederson, Michael Daley, Salvatore Kulinski, Barnard Streber, and Norman Covert. The assistance of Roger Feldman, Bud Dowell, Chuck Hatheway, Lynn Siegel, and Jack Melling in the selection of topics and participants was invaluable. The trust, support, and encouragement of Richard F. Barquist and Alexander DePaoli were everpresent.

STRUCTURE AND STRUCTURE FUNCTION RELATION
OF BOTULINUM NEUROTOXINS

Bibhuti R. DasGupta

Food Research Institute
University of Wisconsin
Madison, Wisconsin

This presentation has an ambitious title about a protein
made of nearly 1,500 amino acid residues. The report on our
current work, done with the help of Andrea Nicholas and
Stuart Rasmussen, is on a few amino acid residues of two
kinds. The presentation will show how much or how little we
know about the structure and structure-function relationship
of botulinum neurotoxin 35 years after its initial purification (see refs. in 1). It is appropriate that the conference
on Biomedical Aspects of Botulism is being held at Fort
Detrick where the pioneering work on botulinum neurotoxin
was initiated. The difficulty of studying the botulinum
neurotoxin has been reduced, from those pioneering days, by
a factor of six. As late as 1965 the most well characterized
botulinum toxin was thought to be of mol. wt. 900,000 (2).
Now we all recognize that the size of the neurotoxin is
1/6th of that huge size (2,3).
This presentation has four parts:
I. General considerations of the botulinum neurotoxin types;
II. Comparison of types A and B neurotoxins and location of
three 1/2 cystine residues in these two proteins; III. Study
of types A and E neurotoxins by selective modification of
amino groups; and IV. Discussion of activation and nicking
based on some old and new data.

[1]*This work was supported in part by the College of Agricultural and Life Sciences, University of Wisconsin-Madison;
by funds (DAMD 17-80-C-0100) from the U.S. Army Medical
Research and Development Command, Fort Detrick, Frederick;
and by the University of Wisconsin Food Research Institute.*

I. GENERAL CONSIDERATIONS OF THE BOTULINUM NEUROTOXIN TYPES

      The published information, from various laboratories,
about the neurotoxin types are summarized in Fig. 1. A, B,
C, D, E, and F represent antigenically distinguishable
types. One to 4 days and 4-7 days represent the number of
days the bacterial cultures were incubated before neurotoxin
purification steps were initiated. Note that in type A the
early culture has two molecular forms (4); the heavy solid
line represents the single chain polypeptide. Next to it is
the molecule made of two-chains, connected by a dashed line

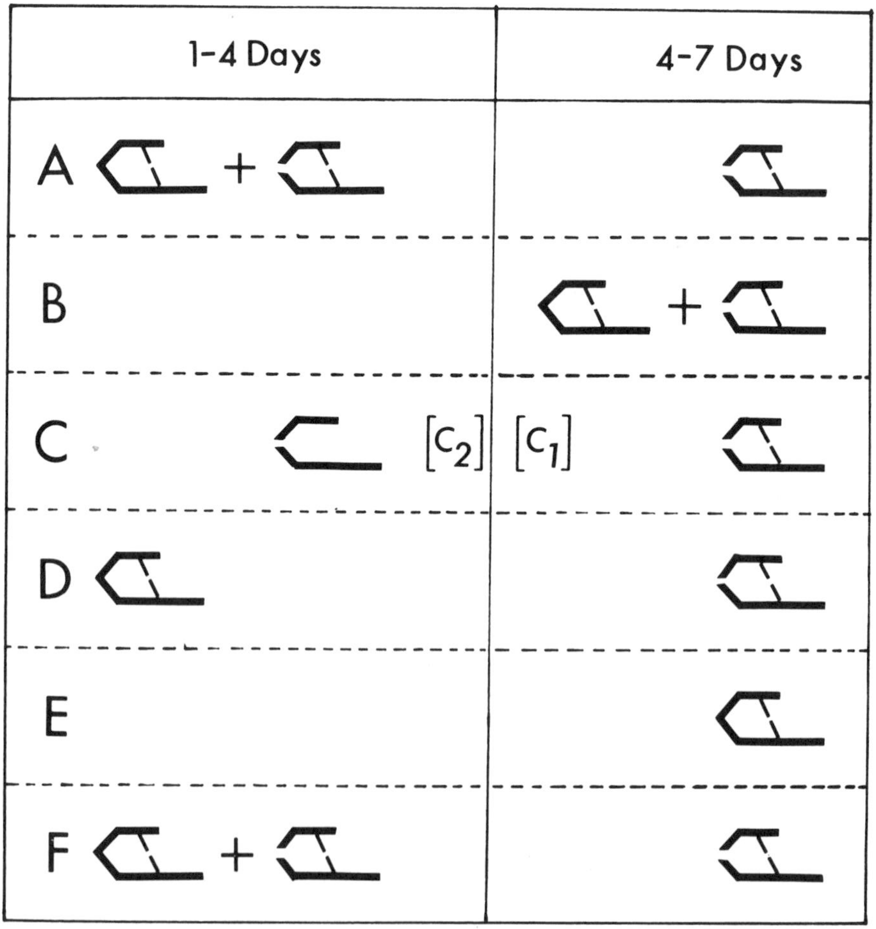

*Fig. 1. The neurotoxin polypeptide chains derived from
the bacterial cultures.*

which represents a disulfide bond. In the late culture only the two-chain structure is found (2,3). Exactly the same situation was found in type F cultures, i.e., two forms of neurotoxins in the early culture and only one form in the late culture (4,5). Types C (6,7) and D (8) in the late culture were found to have only the two-chain structure. Three-day-old cultures of type D yields single chain neurotoxin (9). All of these suggest that a proteolytic enzyme present in the culture clips a peptide bond of the single chain molecule, thus producing a dichain molecule. Type E cultures always yield single chain neurotoxin, the culture apparently lacks the enzyme that converts the single chain to the dichain form (2,3). The case of type B is a surprise. Studies in our (10) and Dr. Sakaguchi's (11) laboratories have independently demonstrated that late cultures contain mixtures of single and dichain neurotoxins. Presence of the dichain molecule suggests that the enzyme was present to produce it, but why is conversion of single chain to dichain incomplete? We don't know. Another important point in this illustration is that in each case the two chains are connected by a disulfide bond. The exception is C_2. The two chains are not connected by a disulfide bond (7). The structure with a disulfide bond in the 4 to 7 days column is C_1 (6).

The generalized structure of the neurotoxins, with some other features is presented in Fig. 2. Molecular weights of the two forms (i.e. the single chain and the dichain molecules) of any particular type are indistinguishable, they are ∿150,000 (2,9). The smaller chain is of mol. wt. ∿50,000, it is called light chain or fragment I. The bigger chain is of mol. wt. ∿100,000, it is called the heavy chain or fragment II. The two chains are connected by at least one disulfide bond (2,9), the exception is the type C_2 (7).

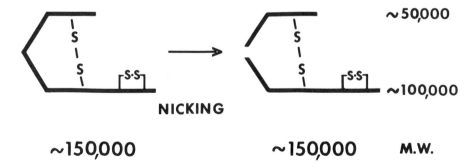

Fig. 2. Generalized structure of botulinum neurotoxin.

Another disulfide loop at one end of the heavy chain was
found in types A and B (12), other types have not been
examined yet. Size of type A neurotoxin, in terms of Stokes
radius is 48Å; the technique used was gel filtration (13).
For type E, a similar size, 90-100 Å diameter, was found
by electron microscopy (14). The 26% helix, 32% of β-sheet
and 44% of turns for type B were calculated by myself (following the technique in ref. 15) based on the amino acid
composition (16). The Q_{10} of 2.36 and activation energy for
neurotoxin-induced muscle paralysis of 1.55×10^4 cal/mol
were determined by Simpson (17).

Conversion of the single chain molecule to the dichain
form is called nicking. Nicking can be achieved with trypsin. The dichain molecules produced naturally, i.e. in the
bacterial culture, and produced artificially, i.e. with
trypsin, are indistinguishable (2).

Separation of the light and heavy chain of types B and
C_1 neurotoxins after reduction of the disulfide bond have
been reported (18,19). In the case of C_2 the two chains
were purified from the culture as separate entities (7).
The individual chains are not toxic; but when the two
chains are brought together, the combination becomes toxic
(7). This means that *in vivo* toxicity depends on the cooperative action of the complementary chains. The separated
chains of type B and C_1 neurotoxin are also nontoxic; the
reconstituted neurotoxins, after combining the constituent
chains, are toxic (18,19). The separated H and L chains of
type B (18), C_1 (19) and C_2 (7) were found to be distinct
antigens.

II. COMPARISON OF TYPES A AND B NEUROTOXINS

So far we have looked at the neurotoxin types at a gross
level. Let us now see what we can find at a higher resolution. For more precise comparison two neurotoxin types,
i.e. A and B and their respective heavy and light chains,
were studied. The two neurotoxins were mixed and then
subjected to coelectrophoresis in polyacrylamide gels containing SDS. The results are presented in Fig. 3. The
light chain of type A is of mol. wt. 53,000 and thus slightly
larger than type B. The heavy chain of type B is of mol.
wt. 104,000 and slightly larger than the heavy chain of type
A. The technique used to detect these small differences has
been published (20). The lengths of the straight lines are
drawn according to the scale of mol. wt. The vertical arrow
is the site of nicking. When A and B polypeptide chains are

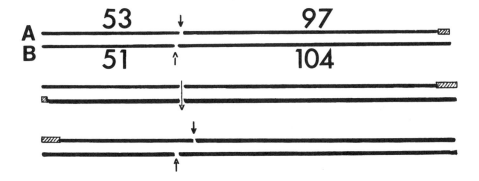

Fig. 3. Comparison of the polypeptide chains of types A and B neurotoxins.

paired in three different ways, at least three implications become apparent: i) In the top pair when the left ends of the two are aligned a small portion of type A, indicated by the hatched area, at the right, appears to be missing and the site of nicking on the two types appears at different positions. ii) In the middle pair when the nicking sites of the two are aligned we see that portions of type A and B are missing - represented by the hatched areas. iii) In the bottom pair, alignment at the right end shows that portion of type A is missing and the sites of nicking on the two types are different. The conjectural missing portions in these proteins could originate at the translational step and/or result from post-translational modification due to proteolytic degradation.

Let me now present some new and unpublished structural studies based on chemical cleavage of these two neurotoxin types. Half-cystine residues were chosen as sites of cleavage because there are only a few of them; 7 in type A and 11 in type B (see ref. 16 and 17 in 2). Hence the expected number of fragments would be 8 in A and 12 in B. The reaction mechanism (21) is presented in Fig. 4. The protein is incubated with the reagent 2-nitro-5-thiocyanobenzoate at pH 8.0 for 15 min at 37°C. This step converts the cysteine residues to S-cyanocysteine. In the next step at pH 9 for 12 hr at 37°C, cleavage of the amino peptide bond of the S-cyanocysteine residue is obtained. The newly formed N-terminal is blocked by a thiazolidine ring. The reaction products are then analyzed by polyacrylamide gel electrophoresis in the presence of SDS, to separate the fragments and to determine the mol. wt. of the fragments (22).

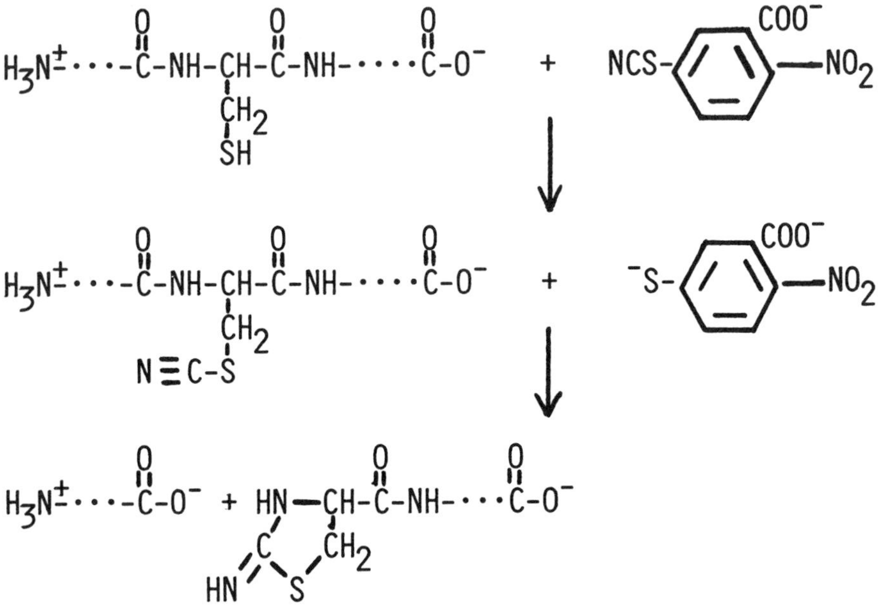

Fig. 4. Steps in the cleavage of a peptide bond formed by the amino group of a cysteine residue.

TABLE I. Fragmentation at 1/2 Cystine

	Type A (mol. wt.)		Type B (mol. wt.)	
			93.5×10^3	III
	91×10^3	VIII	89	VIII
			71.8	
	61.8	IV	65	IV
	37	VII	39	VII
	31	II & V		
			30	
			28	II
	26.9			
			24.9	V
	23.4	I	23.9	I
	21.5		21.8	
			16.6	
	13.8			

The fragments we found are listed in Table I. There are
8 fragments from type A neurotoxin with a range of mol. wt.
91,000 to 13,800. The Roman numerals, e.g. VIII next to 91,
are our designation of the fragments. The type B neurotoxin
yielded 11 fragments with a range of mol. wt. 93,500 to
16,600. The fragments listed here were identified in 5% and
10% polyacrylamide gels. A few other fragments were found
that produced faint bands and could not be obtained repeatedly hence are not listed. The intensity of a Coomassie
brilliant blue R-250 stained band in the polyacrylamide gel
was used as the relative measure of the amount of a fragment
generated. For example in type A, intensity of the band
corresponding to mol. wt. 31,000 was disproportionately high
suggesting that at least two fragments of mol. wt. 31,000,
or very similar size were comigrating. This is why fragment
No. II and V are next to 31,000. The fragments with the
Roman numerals were used to develop a probable model of the
intact molecule. The remaining fragments are yet to be
fitted in the jigsaw puzzle.
     The best fit is shown in Fig. 5. The thick horizontal
line at the top represents the type A molecule. The thick
line the middle is the type B molecule. The vertical dashed
line slightly to the left of the center is the site of

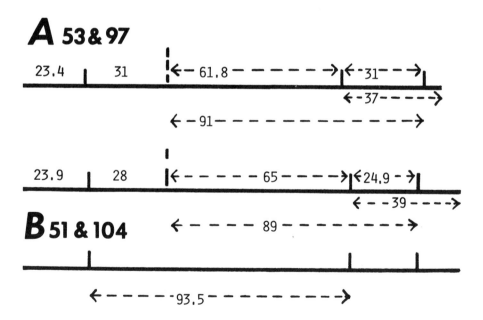

Fig. 5. Probable location of three 1/2 cystine residues
based on fragmentations at the 1/2 cystine residues.

nicking. The light chain is at the left of the nicking site, and the heavy chain is at the right. The thick horizontal line at the bottom is the unnicked type B neurotoxin (type B is a mixture of nicked and unnicked molecules). The numbers 53 and 97 in bold face next to A are the mol. wts. of the light and heavy chains. Similarly, 51 and 104 next to B are the mol. wts. of the light and heavy chains. The numbers in lighter type are the mol. wt. of the fragments listed in Table I. For example, in type A, 23.4 plus 31.0 adds up to 54.4; good agreement with the light chain. Therefore the site of a cleavage and location of a 1/2 cys residue is marked by the small vertical line. Another 1/2 cys is located 61.8 units away from the site of nicking and another one 31 units further to the right. With these two 1/2 cys on the heavy chain one also expects to find fragments of mol. wt. 37,000 and 91,000. Indeed they were found and they fit the model very well. There are two fragments of mol. wt. 31,000 in type A, one assigned to the light chain and one assigned to the heavy chain. This means that each mole of type A yielded two moles of 31,000 fragments. The basis for this consideration is the disproportionately intense band corresponding to the 31,000 fragment mentioned earlier. The expected small fragment of mol. wt. 6,000 located at the very right has not been found yet. Let us now examine type B represented in the middle. Sites of fragmentation or locations of the three 1/2 cys residues are approximately the same as in type A. To the unnicked B molecule, the bottom line, we have assigned the 93,500 fragment because we expect to find 28 plus 65, i.e. 93 from the unnicked molecule. Once again it should be emphasized that this is a probable model. The model shows a homology of at least three 1/2 cys residues between types A and B. We have yet to account for the other five 1/2 cys in type A and eight other 1/2 cys residues in type B.

III. SELECTIVE MODIFICATION OF AMINO GROUPS

Because trypsin nicks and also activates the neurotoxins one presumes that arginyl and/or lysyl bonds are somehow critical. We have previously reported that selective modification of arg residues prevents nicking of type E (23). This suggested that the site of nicking is an arginyl bond. The modification also detoxified types E and A neurotoxins. Currently we are studying the effect of selective modification of lysyl residues and the α-NH_2 group.

2-methoxy-5-nitrotropone selectively reacts with the ε-NH_2 group of lysine and the α-NH_2 group of a protein (24); see Fig. 6 (the letters PRO are for protein). The type E

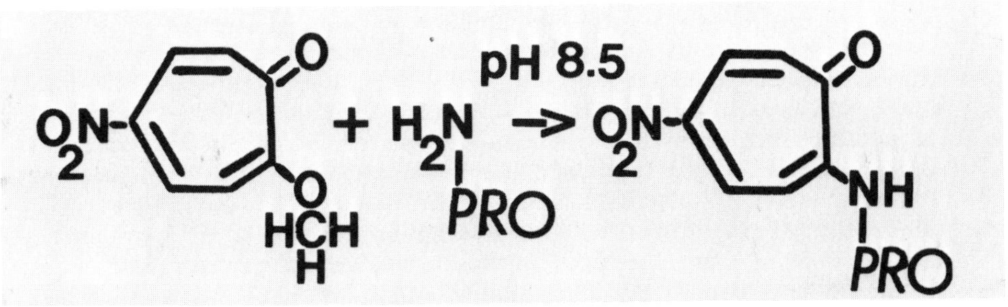

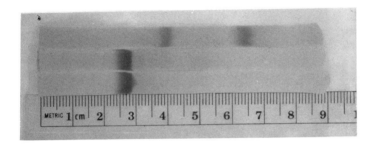

Fig. 6. Reaction of 2-methoxy-5-nitrotropone with a protein.

Fig. 7. Polyacrylamide gel electrophoresis (in presence of SDS) of type E neurotoxin modified with 2-methoxy-5-nitrotropone (molar ratio of reagent to protein 100:1). Migration of the bands was from left to right (positive). Bottom gel: neurotoxin not trypsinized and not reduced. Middle gel: neurotoxin not trypsinized and reduced. Top gel: neurotoxin trypsinized and reduced. The 5% gels, loaded with 200 μl samples of 0.184 A_{278}, were run for 6 hr at 8 mA/gel.

neurotoxin was modified with nitrotropone. After the reaction excess reagent was removed by dialysis, the modified protein was trypsinized at pH 6.0 for 30 min at 37°C. The modified neurotoxin was completely nicked, just like the unmodified neurotoxin (for a representative picture see Fig. 7). The neurotoxin modified at different reaction conditions (varying reagent to protein ratios and incubation times) was nicked by trypsin. How do we know that lysine residues were indeed modified? The modified protein (i) in solution after removing the excess reagent was yellow (absorption maxima at 420 nm, see ref. 24) and (ii) migrated in the polyacrylamide gels in presence of SDS as a yellow band which was subsequently stained with Coomassie brilliant blue R-250.

That the protein was substituted at several sites with nitrotropone groups was evident from the strong chromogenicity of the protein sample. One of these sites is possibly the α-NH_2 group, the rest being lysine residues. The number of substitutions on the protein is not presented here because the correct extinction coefficient of type E neurotoxin at 278 nm (based on accurate dry weight) is not known. A reagent to protein ratio of 1000:1 (incubated for 3 hr) is about 10X more than the amount of reagent needed to completely detoxify the neurotoxin (see Table II). Even this extensively modified neurotoxin was completely nicked. We therefore conclude that it is highly probable that lysine is not at the site of nicking. This conclusion is in agreement with the previous finding (23) that an arginyl residue is probably at the site of nicking.

We studied the effect of modification with nitrotropone on three other parameters: 1) toxicities and 2) serological reactivities of types E and A neurotoxins; and 3) the effect

TABLE II. Toxicity of Type E and A Neurotoxins Modified with 2-methoxy-5-nitrotropone[a]

	Reagent: protein	Control LD_{50}/ml	Percent loss of toxicity (duration of modification reaction)			
			1/2	1	2	3 hr
	25:1	2.9×10^4 T[b]		18		T
	50:1	2.9×10^4 T	55	72	79	T
	100:1	1.8×10^5 T			>99	T
E	100:1	1.3×10^3 NT			100[c]	NT
	120:1	2.1×10^5 T			100[c]	T & NT
	300:1	1.3×10^4 NT			100[c]	NT
	360:1	7.2×10^4 T			100[c]	T & NT
	100:1	1.9×10^5 (62 min)[d]		89 (116 min)[d]		
A	300:1	1.1×10^5 (72 min)[d]		>90 (274 min)[d]		

[a] Each test mouse was injected (i.v.) with 0.1 ml sample.

[b] T = trypsinized before toxicity assay; NT = not trypsinized before toxicity assay.

[c] mice survived beyond 4 days.

[d] mean survival time of mice after injection.

of lysine modification on activation due to trypsin.   The
effect on toxicity is presented in Table II.   The type E
neurotoxin could be completely detoxified at 120X molar
excess of the reagent.   The type A neurotoxin appeared to be
more resistant to complete detoxification.   Even at a 300X
molar excess of the reagent it was not detoxified completely.

For the effect on serological reactivity the completely
detoxified type E and over 90% detoxified type A were tested.
Type A neurotoxin not modified (control) produced one precipitin band in Ouchterlony plate (Fig. 8); the incompletely
detoxified type A (300X molar excess of the reagent) barely
reacted with the antiserum.   In contrast, the completely
detoxified type E neurotoxin (300X molar excess of the
reagent) produced precipitin bands just the same as the
control (Fig. 9a).   The similarity between the precipitin
bands produced by the unmodified (toxic) and detoxified type
E neurotoxin was further examined by changing the distance
between the wells and concentrations of the antigens (Fig.
9b).   The completely detoxified (120X molar excess of the
reagent) type E neurotoxin reacted with the antiserum just
like the unmodified protein.

The complete detoxification of type E neurotoxin does
not appear to be associated with a detectable damage of

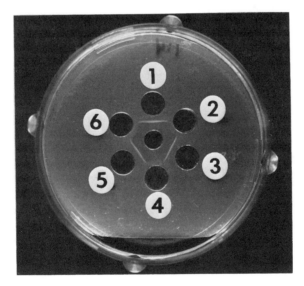

Fig. 8. Ouchterlony gel diffusion of type A neurotoxin
not modified (wells 1, 3, 5) and modified (wells 2, 4, 6)
with 2-methoxy-5-nitrotropone; molar ratio of reagent to
protein 300:1. Central well (4 mm diam): rabbit type A
antiserum, 1:4 diluted. Peripheral wells (5 mm diam) were
loaded with 35 μl antigen of 0.76 A_{278}.

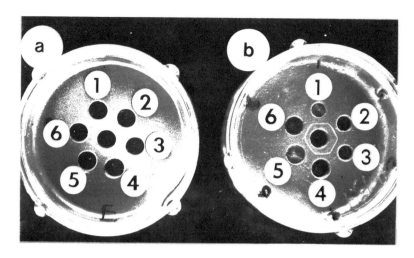

Fig. 9. Ouchterlony gel diffusion of type E neurotoxin not modified (wells 1, 3, 5) and modified (wells 2, 4, 6) with 2-methoxy-5-nitrotropone; molar ratio of reagent to protein for samples in (a) 300:1, in (b) 120:1. Central well: rabbit type E antiserum. Fig. 3a: well 6 was blank; all wells were of 5 mm diam; peripheral wells were loaded with 35 µl antigen of 0.82 A_{278}. Fig. 3b: wells 1, 2 and 3 were of 4 mm diam; all other wells were of 5 mm diam. Antigen load: well 1 = 22 µl of 1.2 A_{278}; well 2 = 22 µl of 1.2 A_{278}; well 3 = 22 µl of 0.6 A_{278}; well 4 = 35 µl of 0.6 A_{278}; well 5 = 35 µl of 1.2 A_{278}; well 6 = 35 µl of 1.2 A_{278}.

serological reactivity, while *incomplete* detoxification of type A is associated with extensive damage of its serological reactivity. The lysine residue(s) and/or the α-NH_2 group therefore appears to have different roles in the biological activities of the two neurotoxins.

Results of selective modification of amino groups have expanded our knowledge of the structure-function relationship further: We also know from previous work that modification of i) tryptophan residues of type A crystalline toxin (other types have not been tested) with 2-hydroxy-5-nitrobenzyl bromide results in the loss of toxicity, immunogenicity and serological reactivity (25); and ii) modification of arginine residues detoxifies types A and E neurotoxins and damages the serological reactivity of at least one antigenic determinant of type A (other types have not been tested) (23). Although detoxification of crystalline type A toxin achieved with HNO_2 or Ketene (see ref. 50 and 51 in 2) may suggest importance of the ϵ-NH_2 and α-NH_2 group, their

role(s) remained ambiguous because of the nonspecific nature
of the two reagents (2). The type E neurotoxin completely
detoxified as a result of selective modification of the NH_2
groups is serologically reactive to the antiserum prepared
against the native neurotoxin. This suggests that the
immunogenicity of the modified protein would be intact or
nearly so and therefore the modified neurotoxin could be
useful as an immunogen.

   The effect of modification on activation: What does the
modification do to the activation of type E neurotoxin?
Stated in another way does a lysyl residue have any role in
the mechanism of activation? We found that modified neurotoxin (not trypsinized) that often appeared completely
detoxified (injected mice survived for 4 days) was toxic if
the sample was trypsinized. Such low levels of toxicities
could not be quantified reliably. However partial detoxification experiments provided a clearer picture (see Fig. 10).
For example toxicity of the neurotoxin incubated without 2-
methoxy-5-nitrotropone (i.e., control) for 2 hr was 1.3 x
10^3 LD_{50}/ml. Modification with 50X molar excess of the
reagent brought the toxicity down to 1.5 x 10^2 LD_{50}/ml, i.e.
88% loss. Trypsinization of the control produced 142 fold
activation (1.85 x 10^5 LD_{50}/ml). Trypsinization of the 88%

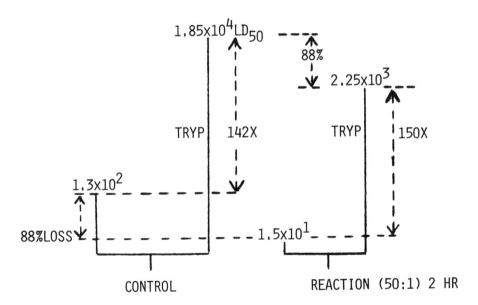

Fig. 10. Effect of 2-methoxy-5-nitrotropone on the
toxicity and activation of type E neurotoxin. Each test
mouse was injected (i.v.) with 0.1 ml sample.

detoxified neurotoxin produced 150 fold activation (2.25 x 10^4 LD_{50}/ml) which is similar to that of the control. Clearly, modification caused 88% detoxification but did not damage the activation. Does this mean that in this case 88% of the population of molecules were detoxified completely which could not be activated and the rest of the unmodified molecules were then fully activated? Or each of the molecules was detoxified 88% and then activated to their maximum potential toxicity? In the latter case it would be reasonable to think that lysine modification does not affect the activation mechanism. The argument can be confined to lysine residue(s) and not include the α-NH_2 group because trypsin is an endopeptidase and does not act on the α-NH_2 group.

IV. ACTIVATION AND NICKING

Let me now take up the last part of this presentation by asking one question in two different ways. Is nicking responsible for activation? The answer seems to be no. Are nicking and activation different events? The answer seems to be yes.

The story on activation began in 1955 with Sakaguchi and Tohyama's discovery of activation of type E toxin (26), thanks to a contaminating proteolytic culture that supplied the proteolytic enzymes to the non-proteolytic type E culture. One year later investigators at Fort Detrick reported activation of type E toxin with trypsin under controlled conditions (27). Thereafter, investigators from several laboratories reported activation of other neurotoxin types (see discussions in ref. 2). The general picture that developed is as follows: The neurotoxin molecule is synthesized having low toxicity. It is then activated by the endogenous enzyme in the culture; when the culture lacks such an enzyme the neurotoxin remains unactivated. Such molecules can be activated by trypsin. The mechanism of activation remained unknown.

In 1970 I reported isolation of a proteolytic enzyme from the type B culture (28). The enzyme activated the toxin from the young, but not old cultures of the same strain. Substrate specificity of this enzyme is restricted only to arg and lys bonds, and it is an -SH dependent enzyme (29). Hence it was named TLE for trypsin-like-enzyme. TLE also activated the type E neurotoxin but not as much as activated by trypsin (30). In 1972 we proposed that at least two bonds are cleaved by trypsin during activation of type E, and natural activation in the bacterial culture may also involve cleavage of more than one bond (30). These proposals were made a few months before we discovered that during activation trypsin nicks the single chain type E (31). So, the concept of nicking entered the picture at this point. Then in 1976 we found that the bonds attacked by TLE and trypsin are different, but the two enzymes also appeared to clip at least one common bond; because while trypsin caused activation and nicking TLE produced only partial activation without nicking (10). This implied that the cultures that produced nicked and activated neurotoxin have two enzymes, one for nicking and one for activation (2,10,30). Why these proposals were made would be clearer with the next illustration in Fig. 11. At the left is the single chain molecule that is not activated, it has a small tail at the end of the heavy chain near the position 2. On the right side is the nicked (dichain) and activated neurotoxin. Let the fragmented small tail represent the molecular change responsible for activation. During trypsinization, going from left to right, two events take place, bonds at positions 1 and 2 are clipped. We can go from left to right

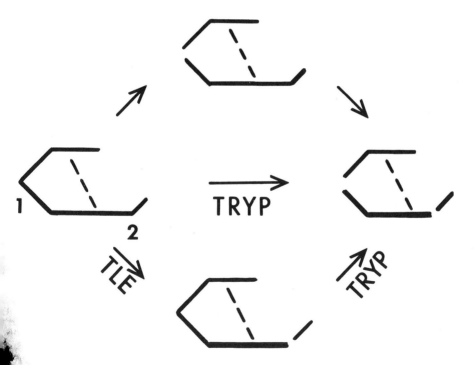

Fig. 11. Probable pathways of nicking and activation of botulinum neurotoxin.

in two ways. In the upper route the first event is nicking, cleavage at position 1. In the lower route nicking is the second event.

When we treated type E neurotoxin with TLE it was not nicked but it was activated partially (10,30). TLE must have broken a covalent bond during this activation. The nature and location of this bond is still unknown. The small tail piece split off from the heavy chain represents that event. When this unnicked but partially activated molecule was trypsinized it was nicked and further activated. If trypsin acts in two steps one would expect that the rate of the two events would be different. A notable attempt was made by Ohishi and Sakaguchi in 1977 to dissociate the activation and nicking steps by slowing down the action of trypsin at pH 4.5 (4). They found that maximum activation of type B neurotoxin occurred without complete nicking. They were probably following the lower route of Fig. 11.

For experimental proof of this model, two enzymes are needed from the cultures of *Clostridium botulinum*. One responsible only for nicking and the other responsible only for activation. The nicking enzyme has not been isolated yet. The second enzyme has perhaps been identified. Enzymes similar to the TLE have been isolated in different labora- tories (32,33). These enzymes activate type B and/or E toxin to various degrees, often as much as trypsin does. One enzyme was reported to activate type A toxin (34). But whether any of these enzymes also nick the neurotoxin was not reported.

The most recent discovery of the structure and activation of C_2 neurotoxin by Ohishi, Iwasaki and Sakaguchi (7) argues strongly for the upper route as the normal sequence of events. They isolated the C_2 neurotoxin as two separate chains. When this nicked molecule, i.e. combination of the two chains, was trypsinized, it was activated. More inter- estingly if the light chain was separately trypsinized and then combined with the heavy chain there was no activation. But if the heavy chain was trypsinized and then combined with the light chain there was activation. The small tail piece fragmented off the heavy chain, in Fig. 11, therefore represents the effect of trypsinization associated with activation.

These ideas are put together in Fig. 12. The hatched vertical bar is the ribosome complex. The top horizontal row of structures shows that the neurotoxin is synthesized as a single chain and then it undergoes two post-transla- tional modifications; one cleavage is nicking (step N), and then another cleavage produces activation (step A). The middle row shows that type C_2 is probably also synthesized

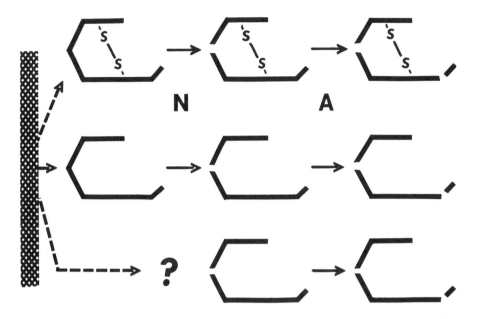

Fig. 12. Probable sequence of nicking and activation of botulinum neurotoxins.

as a single chain molecule which has not been isolated yet. The molecule is then nicked but remains unactivated. Trypsinization activates it in step A. The sequential order of nicking and activation depicted here is tentative and is not to be taken as a generalized scheme for all neurotoxin types that undergo activation and nicking in the bacterial culture. Type D neurotoxin appears to attain the maximum potential toxicity in the culture without undergoing nicking; trypsinization nicks the single chain molecule with none or very little activation (9).

The familiar disulfide bond between the light and heavy chains of type C_2 neurotoxin may not be there for two reasons: i) one or both of the 1/2 cys residues are missing in the amino acid sequence because they were not coded for, or ii) the 1/2 cys residues are there, but the disulfide could not form due to a unique 3-D structure of the growing nascent protein. In the bottom row, the question mark asks; is it possible that the two chains are translated separately, i.e., not as a continuous long chain of 1,500 amino acid residues?

REFERENCES

1. Lamanna, C., *Science 130*, 763 (1959).
2. DasGupta, B. R., and Sugiyama, H., *in* "Perspectives in Toxinology" (A. W. Bernheimer, ed.), p. 87. John Wiley & Sons, New York, (1977).
3. Sugiyama, H., *Microbiol. Rev. 44*, 419 (1980).
4. Ohishi, I., and Sakaguchi, G., *Infect. Immun. 17*, 402 (1977).
5. DasGupta, B. R., and Sugiyama, H., *Toxicon 15*, 466 (1977).
6. Syuto, B., and Kubo, S., *Appl. Environ. Microbiol. 33*, 400 (1977).
7. Ohishi, I., Iwasaki, M., and Sakaguchi, G., *Infect. Immun. 30*, 668 (1980).
8. Boroff, D. A., and Shu-Chen, G., *Annu. Meet. Am. Soc. Microbiol. Abst.*, p. 19 (1973).
9. Miyazaki, S., Iwasaki, M., and Sakaguchi, G., *Infect. Immun. 17*, 395 (1977).
10. DasGupta, B. R., and Sugiyama, H., *Infect. Immun. 14*, 680 (1976).
11. Kozaki, S., and Sakaguchi, G., *Infect. Immun. 11*, 932 (1975).
12. DasGupta, B. R., and Sugiyama, H., *Annu. Meet. Am. Soc. Microbiol. Abst.*, p. 25 (1978).
13. DasGupta, B. R., and Boroff, D. A., *J. Biol. Chem. 243*, 1065 (1968).
14. Kitamura, M., and Sakaguchi, G., *Biochim. Biophys. Acta 194*, 564 (1969).
15. Singleton, R., Jr., Middaugh, C. R., and MacElroy, R. D., *Int. J. Peptide Protein Res. 10*, 39 (1977).
16. Beers, W. H., and Reich, E., *J. Biol. Chem. 244*, 4473 (1969).
17. Simpson, L. L., *Neuropharmacology 10*, 673 (1971).
18. Kozaki, S., Miyazaki, S., and Sakaguchi, G., *Infect. Immun. 18*, 761 (1977).
19. Syuto, B., and Kubo, S., *Jap. J. Med. Sci. Biol. 32*, 132 (1979).
20. DasGupta, B. R., and Sugiyama, H., *Toxicon 15,* 357 (1977).
21. Jacobson, G. R., Schaffer, M. H., Stark, G. R., and Venamau, T. C., *J. Biol. Chem. 248*, 6583 (1973).
22. Weber, K., and Osborn, M., *J. Biol. Chem. 244*, 4406 (1969).
23. DasGupta, B. R., and Sugiyama, H., *Biochem. Biophys. Res. Commun. 93*, 369 (1980).
24. Tamaoki, H., Murase, Y., Minato, S., and Nakanishi, K., *J. Biochem. (Japan) 62*, 7 (1967).

25. Boroff, D. A., and DasGupta, B. R., *Biochim. Biophys. Acta 117*, 289 (1966).
26. Sakaguchi, G., and Tohyama, Y., *Jap. J. Med. Sci. Biol. 8*, 255 (1955).
27. Duff, J. T., Wright, G. G., and Yarinsky, A., *J. Bacteriol. 72*, 455 (1956).
28. DasGupta, B. R., *J. Bacteriol. 108*, 1051 (1971).
29. DasGupta, B. R., and Sugiyama, H., *Biochim. Biophys. Acta 268*, 719 (1972).
30. DasGupta, B. R., and Sugiyama, H., *Infect. Immun. 6*, 587 (1972).
31. DasGupta, B. R., and Sugiyama, H., *Biochem. Biophys. Res. Commun. 48*, 108 (1972).
32. Miura, T., *Jap. J. Med. Sci. Biol. 27*, 285 (1974).
33. Ohishi, I., Okada, T., and Sakaguchi, G., *Jap. J. Med. Sci. Biol. 28*, 157 (1975).
34. Inukai, Y., *Jap. J. Vet. Res. 11*, 143 (1963).

PURIFICATION AND ORAL TOXICITIES OF
CLOSTRIDIUM BOTULINUM PROGENITOR TOXINS

Genji Sakaguchi
Iwao Ohishi
Shunji Kozaki

Department of Veterinary Science
College of Agriculture
University of Osaka Prefecture
Sakai-shi, Osaka, Japan

I. INTRODUCTION

Clostridium botulinum is classified into seven types, A
through G. With a few exceptions, one strain of the organism
produces an immunologically single toxin, but type C and D
strains produce multiple toxic factors. Type Cα strains
produce C1, C2, and D; type Cβ strains C2 only; and type D
strains C1 and D (1). The species, *C. botulinum,* involves at
least four biologically different groups (2). Group I comprises all type A and some type B and F strains, that are
strongly proteolytic. Group II comprises all type E and some
type B and F strains, that are nonproteolytic but strongly
saccharolytic. The toxin of Group II strains requires tryptic
activation for its full toxicity. Group III comprises all
type C and D strains, that are nonproteolytic but gelatino-
lytic. Group IV comprises only one strain of type G that is
proteolytic but nonsaccharolytic.
The present communication deals with the methods for purification of progenitor toxins, implying the natural toxin
produced in food and culture, of types A through F with a
brief review of the previous methods for purification, the
molecular structure of the progenitor toxins, and the oral
toxicities and the intestinal absorption of botulinum toxin in
relation to the molecular structure.

II.   PROCEDURES FOR PURIFICATION OF *C. BOTULINUM* PROGENITOR
      TOXINS

A. *Historical Aspects*

    C. botulinum type A toxin was obtained in a crystalline
form for the first time among bacterial toxins (3, 4). The
methods for purification involved acid precipitation, treatment with chloroform, and salting out with ammonium sulfate.
The crystalline toxin had a molecular weight of 900,000 and
an $S_{20,w}$ of 17.4 (5), being composed of neurotoxic and hemagglutinating protein components (6). It behaved as a homogeneous protein in ultracentrifugation, but the hemagglutinin
was separable from the neurotoxic component by absorption with
erythrocytes (7).   Type B toxin was purified in the following
year (8), principally by acid precipitation. The molecular
weight of type B toxin was reported to be 60,000, but later
to be 500,000 (9).
    Until 1960, the purification procedures were principally
the initial concentration of the toxin by acid precipitation,
followed by ammonium sulfate and/or alcohol precipitation (10,
11, 12, 13, 14, 15). By such classical methods, type A, B,
and D toxins were purified to 90% or higher purity.
    After 1960, such modern techniques as ion exchange chro-
matography and molecular sieving were introduced. Gerwing and
her associates applied diethylaminoethyl (DEAE)-cellulose
chromatography at pH 4.5 or 5.6 to purify type A, B and E
toxins. The toxins they purified had such low molecular
weights as 12,200 for type A (16), 9,000-10,000 for type B
(17), and 18,600 for type E (18). They claimed that acid precipitation and other harsh method might have caused aggregation of the toxin. This explanation seems irrelevant, since
Schantz and Spero (19) estimated the sedimentation constants
$(S_{20,w})$ of type A through F toxins in cultures at 14 or larger.
The molecular sizes of type A and B toxins produced may change
depending upon food constituents, but they have molecular di-
mensions of at least 12S; those of type E and F toxins are
always 12S (20, 21).
    The toxins larger than 12S were proved to be complexes
of a toxic component of 7S and a nontoxic component of different molecular sizes with or without hemagglutinin activity.
The term "progenitor toxin" was proposed to designate such a
toxic complex appearing in food or culture (22). The toxic
component is released when the progenitor toxin is exposed to
a slightly alkaline condition or an anion exchanger even at a
low pH value. The term "derivative toxin" was proposed to
designate the released toxic component (22). Type E toxin is
produced in a weakly toxic form, that is activated upon tryp-

sinization. Type E progenitor toxin is such activable toxin initially produced in food and culture and the trypsinized toxin is called not derivative toxin but "activated progenitor toxin", since trypsinization does not accompany any molecular dissociation. The dissociated type E toxic component, no matter whether it is activable or already activated, is called derivative toxin. It is the derivative toxin that is detected in the blood serum or lymph of the man and animals given progenitor toxin perorally or intravenously (23, 24, 25).

Chromatography of type A (26) and B toxins (27, 28) on acidified DEAE-cellulose or DEAE-Sephadex was re-examined. The toxins obtained had molecular weights of about 150,000, being free from hemagglutinin, and considered to be the derivative toxins.

It appeared that acid precipitation would not cause molecular aggregation, but anion exchange chromatography, even if the matrix is acidified, would cause molecular dissociation. Therefore, such cation exchangers as carboxymethyl(CM)- and sulphopropyl(SP)-Sephadex were adopted by the author's group to purify type A through F progenitor toxins. The procedures may be summarized as follows:

B. Purification of Progenitor Toxin of Group I Organisms

The medium consisted of glucose 0.5%, peptone 2.0%, yeast extract 0.5% (PYG), and sodium thioglycolate 0.05% (pH 7.0). A spore suspension of each type was inoculated and the culture was incubated for 4 days at 30 C, when 3 N sulfuric acid was added to pH 4.0. The precipitate formed was collected by centrifugation, and extracted with 0.2 M phosphate buffer, pH 6.0. The toxin in the extract was precipitated at 50% saturation of ammonium sulfate, and the precipitate was dissolved in a small amount of an appropriate buffer. The extract contained a large amount of RNA and other acidic substances, which did not seem to be bound to the toxin molecule. Such acidic substances were removed by treating the extract with protamine at pH 4.5. Without the protamine treatment, the toxin would be precipitated when dialyzed against a buffer at pH 4.5. The toxin was chromatographed on SP-Sephadex at pH 4.5 by elution with linear NaCl gradient. The eluted toxin, usually in a single fraction but occasionally in two fractions, was concentrated by salting out or ultrafiltration and subjected to gel filtration on Sephadex G-200. Type A (29) and B toxins (30) were eluted in two separate fractions and type F toxin in a single fraction (31). The toxin of a type B strain of Group II was purified by the same procedures (32).

C. *Purification of Progenitor Toxin of Group II Organisms*

The medium was PYG containing sodium thioglycolate at
0.025%, with pH 6.2. Such a low pH was chosen so as to mini-
mize the toxin release from the bacterial cells. A spore suspension was inoculated and the culture was incubated for 2
days at 30 C, when it was centrifuged to collect the bacterial
cells. Prolonged incubation would result in releasing more
toxin. The precipitate, containing most toxin, was extracted
with 0.2 M phosphate buffer, pH 6.0. The extract was dialyzed
against 0.01 M phosphate buffer, pH 6.0, and chromatographed
on CM-Sephadex equilibrated with the same buffer. No toxin
was adsorbed, since it was in a form of complex with RNA (33).
Unlike type E toxin, type B toxin of Group II organisms was
not bound to RNA. The pass-through fraction was treated with
ribonuclease, and the toxin freed of RNA was chromatographed
on CM-Sephadex under the same conditions as the preceding
chromatography. The toxin was adsorbed onto the column this
time, and eluted with a linear NaCl gradient in the same
buffer. The toxin eluted was concentrated by salting out and
subjected to gel filtration on Sephadex G-200 to obtain a
single peak near the void volume (34).
Type F toxin of Group II strains has not been purified.

D. *Purification of Progenitor Toxin of Group III Organisms*

The spores were inoculated into PYG medium containing
cysteine at 0.1%, with pH 7.2, for 3 days at 30 C. Sodium
thioglycolate seemed to be inhibitory upon group III organisms.
The RNA contents of whole cultures of group III organisms are
usually lower than those of group I and II organisms. Therefore, acid precipitation of C1 and D toxins usually requires
addition of yeast RNA (0.4 mg/ml) as a precipitation aid (31).
The precipitate was extracted with 0.2 M phosphate buffer, pH
6.0, concentrated by salting out, and treated with protamine
at pH 4.0 to remove the endogenous and exogenous RNA and other
acidic substances. The toxin was subjected to SP-Sephadex
chromatography with 0.05 M acetate buffer, pH 4.0 with NaCl
gradient, followed by concentration with ammonium sulfate and
gel filtration on Sephadex G-200. C1 (35) and D toxins (36)
were each eluted in two fractions.
For C2 toxin production, cooked meat medium fortified with
calcium carbonate 0.5%, ammonium sulfate 1.0%, glucose 0.8%,
yeast extract 1.0%, and cysteine 0.1% (pH 7.6) was used. Cultures were incubated for 2 days at 37 C, when spore population
reached the highest (37). C2 toxin was purified by ammonium
sulfate precipitation from the culture supernatant, chromatography on DEAE-Sephadex at pH 7.5, followed by chromatography

on CM-Sephadex at pH 6.0, by which components I and II were separated (38). Components I and II were each subjected to gel filtration on Sephadex G-100. Components I and II were each virtually nontoxic, but when they were mixed together and trypsinized at pH 8.0, the highest toxicity, being 12.5-25×10^4 mouse ip LD_{50}/mg N, was obtained (39).

III. MOLECULAR STRUCTURE OF *C. BOTULINUM* PROGENITOR TOXINS

The molecular structures of *C. botulinum* progenitor toxins type A through F are shown in *Fig. 1*.

Type A progenitor toxin involves three different molecular forms, 19S, 16S and 12S (29), type B (30), C, and D (36) two forms, 16S and 12S, and type E (34) and F (40) a single form, 12 or 10S. The 12S toxin was named "medium-sized" or "M toxin", the 16S toxin "large-sized" or "L toxin", and the 19S toxin "extra large-sized" or "LL toxin". The presence of toxins of all these forms in cultures was proved. All the progenitor toxins, when subjected to DEAE-Sephadex chromatography or sucrose density gradient ultracentrifugation at pH

Toxin Type		S value	Mouse ip LD_{50}/mg N $(\times 10^{-6})$
A	LL	19	240
	L	16	300
	M	12	500
B	L	16	300
	M	12	550
C	L	16	57
	M	12	97
D	L	16	240
	M	12	500
E		11.6	50
F		10.3	120

Fig. 1. Molecular structure of C. botulinum progenitor toxins. Black area: toxic component; blank area: nontoxic component; hatched area: activable toxic component; dotted area: hemagglutinin activity.

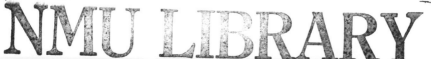

7.5-8.0, are separated into toxic and nontoxic components. The toxic component is uniform in the molecular size, being 7S (5.6S for type F), regardless of the molecular size of the parental progenitor toxin. The dissociated 7S toxic component was named "small-sized" or "S toxin". The molecule of the progenitor toxin, therefore, is a complex of one molecule each of the 7S toxic component and the 7S or larger molecular-sized nontoxic component combined together with a noncovalent bond(s). Hemagglutinin activity is shown only with the nontoxic component of the 16S or larger progenitor toxin. The type A crystalline toxin may correspond to LL toxin.

C. botulinum type A produced L and LL toxins when grown in boiled string beans, whereas it produced M toxin only when grown in the same medium supplemented with 5 mM ferrous sulfate. It produced also M toxin only in PYG medium, whereas L toxin was induced when the culture supernatant was dialyzed against 0.05 M phosphate buffer, pH 6.0. M toxin, therefore, may be the real progenitor toxin, to which another nontoxic protein containing hemagglutinin is bound forming L and LL toxin molecules. It was also found that iron or manganese ion inhibits the binding between M toxin and the second nontoxic protein (20).

The molecular dissociation of the progenitor toxin is reversible. When the toxic and nontoxic components at an equimolar ratio are mixed together and the mixture is dialyzed against 0.05 M phosphate buffer, pH 6.0, molecular reassociation occurs forming molecules indistinguishable from the parental progenitor toxin.

Type E progenitor toxin forms a single boundary at the 12S position when centrifuged below pH 6.8, and also a single boundary at the 7S position when centrifuged above pH 7.2. When centrifuged at pH 7.0, it forms a single boundary at the 10S position. This was interpreted as a molecular unfolding taking place at pH 7.0 (41). Hence, the toxic and the nontoxic components are bound together with two qualitatively different bonds; one is susceptible to pH 7.0, whereas the other is resistant to pH 7 but susceptible to pH 7.2 or higher.

Type E progenitor toxin extracted from young cultured bacterial cells is a complex with RNA of various molecular sizes. The RNA molecules are bound with only the toxic component (41).

C2 toxin has a molecular structure entirely different from those of progenitor and derivative toxins of other types. C2 toxicity is elicited by two distinct protein components, component I with a molecular weight of 55,000 and component II with a molecular weight of 105,000, that are present without binding together (39). When components I and II are injected simultaneously or one after the other, C2 toxicity is demonst-

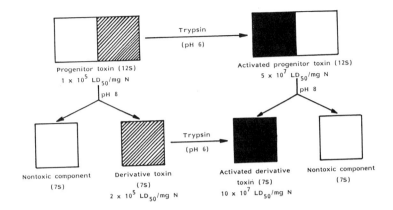

*Fig. 2. Activation and molecular structure of C. botuli-
num type E toxin. Black area: activated toxic component;
blank area: nontoxic component: hatched area: activable
toxic component.*

rated.

Tryptic activation accompanies removal of RNA from the
type E toxin molecule (33). The removal of RNA with ribonuclease, however, does not increase the toxicity. Type E
progenitor toxin free from RNA (1 x 10^5 mouse ip LD_{50}/mg N)
and the activated progenitor toxin (5 x 10^7 LD_{50}/mg N) are
indistinguishable each other physicochemically and immunologically. Toxicities in conjunction with activation and
molecular dissociation of type E toxin are shown in *Fig. 2*.

The optimum pH for tryptic activation is about 6. If
type B progenitor toxin is trypsinized at pH 6, complete
activation occurs; SDS electrophoresis of the reduced, pH 6-
activated derivative toxin showed complete nicking. If it is
trypsinized at pH 4.5, the toxicity increases to the same
level as that attained at pH 6, but SDS electrophoresis of
the reduced, pH 4.5-activated derivative toxin demonstrated
only a partial nicking. Therefore, "nicking" in the toxic
component may not be the basis for the increased toxicity
(42). From the fact that trypsinization of the RNA-progenitor
toxin complex accompanies an increased toxicity and the release of RNA (33), it seems possible that the increased
toxicity results from hydrolysis of an ester bond formed
between carboxyl group of the C-terminal basic amino acid,
perhaps lysine (43) and a hydroxyl group of ribose in RNA.

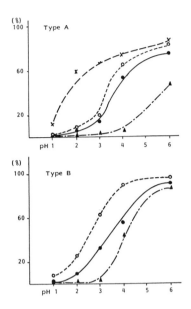

Fig. 3. *Resistance of differently molecular-sized toxins of types A and B to exposure to different pH values for 30 min at 35°C. The toxicity of each toxin in 0.05 M acetate buffer, pH 6.0 was taken as 100.*x— — —x; *type A crystalline toxin;*o-----o: *L toxin;*●———● : *M toxin;*▲—··—··—▲ : *derivative toxin.*

IV.   ORAL TOXICITIES OF BOTULINUM TOXINS: STABILITIES IN THE
       DIGESTIVE TRACT AND THE INTESTINAL ABSORPTION IN RELATION
       TO THE MOLECULAR SIZE

We, using mice, tried to correlate the molecular structures of botulinum toxins to their oral toxicities *(TABLE I)*
(44, 45, 46).
The derivative toxin (S toxin) showed an oral LD_{50} several
tens of million ip LD_{50}. It seems impossible for it to cause
food-borne human botulism (44, 45). The M toxin showed an
oral LD_{50} 95,000-3,600,000 times and L toxin 1,500-2,200,000
times ip LD_{50} of the respective toxin. The oral toxicity of
progenitor toxin is much higher than that of derivative toxin
and that of L toxin is apparently higher than that of M toxin
of the same type. If the same toxicities in mouse ip LD_{50}
were ingested, L toxin would be more toxic than M toxin, or if
the same levels of toxin were produced and the same quantities
of the foodstuffs were ingested, such foodstuffs that would

TABLE I. *Molecular Structures and Oral Toxicities of Clostridium botulinum Toxins*

Toxin		Mouse oral LD_{50} in equivalent number of ip LD_{50} x 10^{-3}	Reference
Type	Molecular size		
A	LL	120	
	L	2,200	
	M	3,600	
	S	43,000	(45)
B	L	1.5	
	M	1,100	
	S	24,000	(45)
C	L	2.7 to 6.7	
	M	95 to 270	(46)
D	L	35 to 76	
	M	96 to 880	(46)
E	M	220	
	S	>750	(44)
F	M	1,100	
	S	>6,000	(45)

support production of L toxin are more fatal than those supporting production of M toxin. Vegetables (string beans and mushrooms) were shown to support production of L and LL toxins, while meat (pork and tuna fish) to support production of M toxin by type A and B organisms (20).

Type A crystalline toxin and type E progenitor toxin are more stable than their derivative toxins and such higher stability is more profound at pH lower than 4 and 5, respectively (25). The stabilities were compared among type A-S, M, L (a mixture of L and LL toxins), and crystalline toxins and among type B-S, M and L toxins in buffers at pH 1-6 *(Fig. 3)* (47). It was demonstrated that the larger the molecular size of the toxin, the more stable at any pH value.

The in vitro destruction curves of type A and B toxins of different molecular sizes when exposed to pepsin at pH 2.0 are shown in *Fig. 4,* which shows that the larger the molecular size of the toxin, the more resistant to pepsin and/or pH 2.0. Similar results were obtained when type B toxins of different molecular sizes were exposed in vitro to rat gastric juice (pH 1.4) at 35 C *(Fig. 5)* (47).

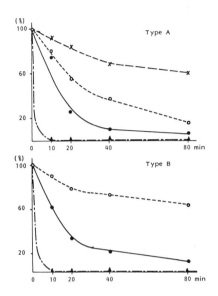

Fig. 4. Resistance of differently molecular-sized toxins of types A and B to pepsin at pH 2.0 and 35°C. The toxicity of each toxin in 0.2 M sodium acetate-hydrochloride buffer, pH 2.0, was taken as 100. ×————×: *type A crystalline toxin;* o----o: *L toxin;* o———●: *M toxin;* ▲—·—·—▲: *derivative toxin.*

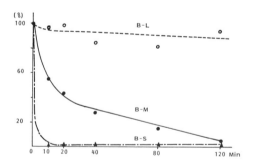

Fig. 5. Resistance of type B toxins to in vitro exposure to rat gastric juice (pH 1.4) at 35°C. The toxicity of each toxin in gastric juice at zero time was taken as 100. o----o: *L toxin;* ●———●: *M toxin;* ▲—·—·—▲: *derivative toxin.*

The rates of absorption of B-L, B-M, and B-S toxins from the rat ligated duodenal loops are shown in *Fig. 6.* Type A

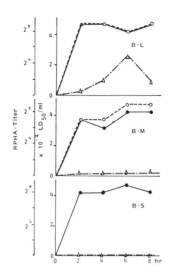

Fig. 6.   Absorption of B-L, B-M, and B-S toxins from the
rat ligated duodenum.   A 0.5-ml dose of each toxin containing
8 x 10⁷ LD₅₀ was injected into a 5-cm segment of the duodenum.
●————●: RPHA titer of toxic component;o------o : RPHA titer of
nontoxic component; ▲—·—··▲ : mouse lethal activity.

toxin appears in the lymphatics after intestinal absorption
and that the toxin appearing in lymph is the derivative toxin
(23, 25). The lymph collected by cannulation of the thoracic
duct was titrated for both the toxic and nontoxic components
by reversed passive hemagglutination with sheep red blood cells
coupled with anti-toxic component and those coupled with anti-
nontoxic component (of B-M toxin) immunoglobulins. The lethal
activity of the lymph was determined by the mouse ip injection
test. The rates of absorption of the antigens of type B toxins
of different molecular sizes were nearly the same. The lymph of
the animals given L toxin became highly lethal, that of those
given M toxin became slightly lethal, and that of those given
S toxin did not become lethal. The results showed also that
compatible quantities of the toxic and the nontoxic components
were absorbed in the animals given either L or M toxin (48).
    In ultracentrifugation of B-L and B-M toxins in sucrose
density gradient (5-20%) prepared in rat intestinal juices
pH 7.0, no molecular dissociation was indicated (48). The
progenitor toxin, therefore, would not dissociate in the
duodenum; the whole molecule without dissociation would be
absorbed through the intestinal wall. After the toxin reaches

the lymphatics, molecular dissociation would immediately occur (24, 25).

In summary, it is the progenitor toxin that causes food-borne botulism. The molecular sizes of type A and B (and perhaps type C and D) progenitor toxins change depending upon the constituents of the foodstuff. The larger the molecular size of the toxin, the higher the oral toxicity, due to the higher stability in the stomach.

The whole toxin molecules, no matter whether 19S, 16S, or 12S, seem to be absorbed at the same rates without molecular dissociation in the intestines. Only the toxicity surviving after absorption differs depending upon the molecular structure of the toxin.

REFERENCES

1. Jansen, B. C., *Onderstepoort J. Vet. Res. 38,* 93 (1971).
2. Smith, L. DS., "Botulism--the organism, its toxins, the disease" Charles C. Thomas, Springfield, Ill. (1977).
3. Abrams, A., Kegeles, G., and Hottle, G. A., *J. Biol. Chem. 164,* 63 (1946).
4. Lamanna, C., MacElroy, O. E., and Eklund, H. W., *Science 103,* 613 (1946).
5. Putnam, F. W., Lamanna, C., and Sharp, D. G., *J. Biol. Chem. 165,* 735 (1947).
6. Lamanna, C., *Proc. Soc. Exp. Biol. Med. 69,* 332 (1948).
7. Lowenthal, J. P., and Lamanna, C., *Amer. J. Hyg. 57,* 46 (1953).
8. Lamanna, C., and Glassman, H. N., *J. Bacteriol. 54,* 575 (1947).
9. Wagman, J., and Bateman, J. B., *Arch. Biochem. Biophys. 31,* 424 (1951).
10. Duff, J. T., Wright, G. G., Klerer, J., Moore, D. E. and Bibler, R. H., *J. Bacteriol. 73,* 42 (1957).
11. Duff, J. T., Klerer, J., Bibler, R. H., Moore, D. E., Gottfried, C., and Wright, G. G., *J. Bacteriol. 73,* 597 (1957).
12. Cardella, M. A., Duff, J. T., Gottfried, C., and Begel, J. S., *J. Bacteriol. 75,* 360 (1958).
13. Cardella, M. A., Duff, J. T., Wingfield, B. H., and Gottfried, C., *J. Bacteriol. 79,* 372 (1960).
14. Gordon, M., Fiock, M. A., Yarinsky, A., and Duff, J. T. *J. Bacteriol. 74,* 533 (1957).
15. Fiock, M. A., Yarinsky, A., and Duff, J. T., *J. Bacteriol. 82,* 66 (1961).
16. Gerwing, J., Dolman, C. E., and Bains, H. S., *J. Bact-*

eriol. 89, 1383 (1965).

17. Gerwing, J., Dolman, C. E., Kason, D. V., and Tremaine, J. H. *J. Bacteriol. 91,* 484 (1966).

18. Gerwing, J., Dolman, C. E., and Ko, A., *J. Bacteriol. 89,* 1176 (1965).

19. Schantz, E. J., and Spero, L., *in* "Botulism 1966" (M. Ingram and T. A. Roberts, eds.), p. 296. Chapman and Hall, London (1967).

20. Sugii, S., and Sakaguchi, G., *J. Food Safety 1,* 53 (1977).

21. Sakaguchi, G., Sakaguchi, S. and Karashimada, T., *Japan. J. Med. Sci. Biol. 19,* 201 (1966).

22. Lamanna, C., and Sakaguchi, G., *Bacteriol Rev. 32,* 242 (1971).

23. Heckly, R. J., Hildebrand, G. J., and Lamanna, C., *J. Exp. Med. 111,* 745 (1960).

24. Hildebrand, G. J., Lamanna, C., and Heckly, B. J., *Proc. Soc. Exp. Biol. Med. 107,* 284 (1961).

25. Kitamura, M., Sakaguchi, S., and Sakaguchi, G., *J. Bacteriol. 98,* 1173 (1969).

26. DasGupta, B. R., Berry, L. J., and Boroff, D. A., *Biochim. Biophys. Acta 214,* 343 (1970).

27. Beers, W. H., and Reich, E., *J. Biol. Chem. 244,* 4473 (1969).

28. DasGupta, B. R., Boroff, D. A., and Cheong, K., *Biochem. Biophys. Res. Commun. 32,* 1057 (1968).

29. Sugii, S., and Sakaguchi, G., *Infec. Immunity 12,* 1262 (1975).

30. Kozaki, S., Sakaguchi, S., and Sakaguchi, G., *Infec. Immunity 10,* 750 (1974).

31. Ohishi, I., and Sakaguchi, G., *Appl. Microbiol. 28,* 923 (1974).

32. Miyazaki, S., Kozaki, S., Sakaguchi, S., and Sakaguchi, G., *Infec. Immunity 13,* 987 (1975).

33. Sakaguchi, G., and Sakaguchi, S., *J. Bacteriol. 78,* 1 (1959).

34. Kitamura, M., Sakaguchi, S., and Sakaguchi, G., *Biochim. Biophys. Acta 168,* 207 (1968).

35. Iwasaki, M., and Sakaguchi, G., *Infec. Immunity 19,* 749 (1978).

36. Miyazaki, S., Iwasaki, M., and Sakaguchi, G., *Infec. Immunity 17,* 395 (1977).

37. Nakamura, S., Serikawa, T., Yamakawa, K., Nishida, S., Kozaki, S., and Sakaguchi, G., *Microbiol. Immunol. 22,* 591 (1978).

38. Iwasaki, M., Ohishi, I., and Sakaguchi, G., *Infec. Immunity 29,* 390 (1980).

39. Ohishi, I., Iwasaki, M., and Sakaguchi, G., *Infec. Immunity 30,* 668 (1980).

40. Ohishi, I., and Sakaguchi, G., *Appl. Microbiol. 29,* 444 (1975).

41. Kitamura, M., and Sakaguchi, G., *Biochim. Biophys. Acta 194,* 564 (1969).

42. Ohishi, I., and Sakaguchi, G., *Infec. Immunity 17,* 402 (1977).

43. Ohishi, I., and Sakaguchi, G., *Japan. J. Med. Sci. Biol. 30,* 179 (1977).

44. Sakaguchi, G., and Sakaguchi, S., *Japan. J. Med. Sci. Biol. 27,* 241 (1974).

45. Ohishi, I., Sugii, S., and Sakaguchi, G., *Infec. Immunity 16,* 107 (1977).

46. Ohishi, I., and Sakaguchi, G., *Infec. Immunity 28,* 303 (1980).

47. Sugii, S., Ohishi, I., and Sakaguchi, G., *Infec. Immunity 16,* 910 (1977).

48. Sugii, S., Ohishi, I., and Sakaguchi, G., *Infec. Immunity 17,* 491 (1977).

PHARMACOLOGICAL STUDIES ON THE CELLULAR AND SUBCELLULAR
EFFECTS OF BOTULINUM TOXIN

Lance Simpson[1]

Department of Pharmacology
College of Physicians & Surgeons
Columbia University
New York, New York

I. INTRODUCTION

Botulinum toxin is a generic term that refers to at least
eight biological substances. Although each of these substances is antigenically distinct, the group as a whole shares
a number of common features. For example, all eight substances are synthesized by the same species of bacterium,
Clostridium botulinum. In addition, the various toxins possess similar molecular weights and probably a similar structure. Most importantly, all of the toxins exert the same
pharmacological effect; they block the release of acetylcholine from cholinergic nerve endings (1-5). Apparently the
eight different botulinum toxins have a common origin, structure and pharmacological activity.

Both the origin and the structure of botulinum toxin have
been described in preceding chapters. The present chapter
will concern itself with studies on the mechanism of action
of the toxin. In particular, several earlier studies are reviewed and some new data are presented that help in developing
a model to account for toxin-induced blockade of cholinergic
transmission. This information is discussed in a way that,
hopefully, will achieve three goals: (i) summarize current
thinking about the cellular and subcellular effects of botulinum toxin, (ii) relate the actions of botulinum toxin to the

[1]*Supported in part by grants NS-15409 and HL-12738.*

actions of other bacterial toxins, such as cholera toxin and
diphtheria toxin, and (iii) suggest some new approaches, both
research and conceptual, for dealing with botulinum toxin.

II. A SPECIFIC MODEL FOR NEUROMUSCULAR BLOCKADE

In the intact mammalian preparation, botulinum toxin exerts it's effects at four different sites: the neuromuscular
junction, autonomic ganglia, postganglionic parasympathetic
nerve endings and postganglionic sympathetic nerve endings
that release acetylcholine. The toxin also affects nonmamma-
lian preparations that contain these structures (e.g., frog
neuromuscular junction) or the anatomical equivalent of these
structures (e.g., the electric organ of Electrophorus electri-
cus). In dismembered preparations, the toxin can affect central nervous tissue (e.g., tissue slices and synaptosomes) and
tissue cultures. In all cases, the primary action of the
toxin is to block neurogenic release of acetylcholine.

In spite of the fact that numerous tissues are vulnerable
to the poisoning effects of botulinum toxin, almost all pharmacological and physiological studies dealing with mechanism
of action have focused on the neuromuscular junction. In
1923, several different groups demonstrated that the neuromuscular junction was a principal site of toxin action (6-8).
They showed that the toxin did not block nerve transmission,
muscle transmission, or muscle responses to agonists. Their
collective findings indicated that the toxin acted at the
point of transmission between nerve and muscle. Several decades later, Burgen et al. (9) and Brooks (10) confirmed that
transmission was blocked, and furthermore, showed that the de-
fect was one in which neurogenic release of acetylcholine was
diminished.

The study by Burgen et al. (9) is especially noteworthy.
Aside from their findings on transmitter release, these workers made two invaluable contributions to the field. The first
of these was the introduction of the isolated neuromuscular
preparation (rat phrenic nerve-hemidiaphragm preparation) as a
suitable tissue on which to do toxin studies. Virtually all
previous work had been done on in vivo or in situ preparations. A second contribution was the observation that the
binding of botulinum toxin to the neuromuscular junction could
be distinguished, at least in part, from paralysis of the neuromuscular junction. They found that tissues bound the toxin
irreversibly long before there was onset of transmission
blockade. Although not fully appreciated at the time, the
work by Burgen et al. (9) was among the first to show that a

bacterial toxin could bind to a cell surface receptor, and that this binding per se was not toxic.

Several years later, Hughes and Whaler (11) studied the effects of several drugs and experimental manipulations on the rate of onset of toxin-induced neuromuscular blockade. Of their observations, the one pertaining to nerve stimulation has proved to be the most important. They found that the rate of development of neuromuscular blockade was related to the rate of nerve stimulation. More precisely, nerves that were stimulated rapidly became paralyzed more quickly than unstimulated or slowly stimulated nerves. In response to these data, Hughes and Whaler suggested that the action of the toxin was dependent upon one of two phenomena, the nerve depolarization-repolarization cycle or the process of excitation-secretion coupling.

These two possibilities were examined in a series of studies (12-14), out of which emerged several findings that tended to link the previous work by Burgen et al. (9) and Hughes and Whaler (11). In particular, it was confirmed that toxin-induced neuromuscular blockade could be divided into a binding phase and a paralytic phase; it was established that excitation-secretion coupling was integral to toxin activity; and it was demonstrated that the role of excitation-secretion coupling was manifested during the paralytic phase and not during the binding phase. The fact that a particular experimental manipulation would exert different effects on the binding and paralytic phases prompted an effort to find other procedures that would also exert differing effects, and thus to characterize the two phases. It was shown that the binding phase was relatively rapid, had a low Q_{10}, did not require calcium and was not influenced by nerve stimulation. By contrast, the paralytic phase was relatively slow, had a high Q_{10} and was markedly influenced by nerve stimulation. Additionally, calcium seemed to have a dual effect; initially, it promoted the action of the toxin, but later acted to antagonize it.

Experiments with antitoxin produced a result that had not been anticipated, but one that was very revealing (15). In agreement with earlier work (9), it was found that antitoxin could neutralize toxin before its addition to tissue preparations, but had no effect on toxin that had caused paralysis. The unexpected finding was that the antitoxin produced a partial neutralizing effect on toxin that was bound to tissue, but had not yet caused paralysis. The fact that the antitoxin could produce this effect on tissue-bound toxin made it possible to pose two interrelated questions. Firstly, when did the toxin disappear from accessibility to antitoxin? And secondly, was the rate at which the toxin disappeared from accessibility to antitoxin equivalent to the rate of onset of paralysis? Experiments designed to answer these questions

showed that the toxin disappeared rather quickly; its disap-
pearance was much more rapid than onset of paralysis (15).
These findings suggested that there was at least one step or
process that intervened between binding and paralysis.

Taken together, the foregoing data seem to support the
following model. The first step in the interaction between
the toxin and the cholinergic nerve ending involves the binding of the toxin to a cell surface receptor. This step is
essential to the development of paralysis, but in itself
causes no toxic effects. The next step is a translocation
process, during which the externally bound toxin, or some
fragment of it, is internalized. This step too is essential,
but like the binding step produces no ill effects. Finally,
the internalized toxin evokes some lytic effect, the outcome
of which is blockade of transmitter release.

III. A GENERAL MODEL FOR TOXICITY

Claims about the mechanism by which botulinum toxin blocks
transmitter release are based on a narrow range of experiments. They involve only one species of animal (rat), only
one tissue preparation from that species (the phrenic nerve-
hemidiaphragm), and only one type of toxin (crystalline type
A). To achieve some generalizations for the model, studies
have been done that include three species (rat, mouse and
guinea pig), two nerve preparations (phrenic nerve-hemidiaphragm and vagus nerve-sinoatrial node) and four toxins (crystalline type A toxin and types A, B and E neurotoxins). In
addition, some of the actions of botulinum toxin have been
compared to those of tetanus toxin, another bacterial toxin,
and contrasted with those of β-bungarotoxin, a component of
snake venom (16).

The most obvious thing that studies such as these reveal
is that there are marked species and tissue differences in
susceptibility to botulinum and tetanus toxins (see also ref.
9). For instance, the rat is quite resistant to type B neurotoxin, both in vivo and in vitro. Also, the rat and the guinea pig are both relatively resistant to the in vitro actions
of tetanus toxin. And finally, as a general rule, the autonomic nervous system of any particular species is more resistant
to botulinum and tetanus toxins than is the α-motorneuron system in the same species.

Of particular interest, all preparations that are respon-
sive to either botulinum toxin or tetanus toxin behave in accordance with the model proposed above. The toxins invariably
go through a complex sequence of events before their pharmacological actions are fully expressed. This sequence involves

a binding step, a translocation step and a lytic step. The characteristics that were alluded to earlier seem to have wide applicability. For both toxins, the binding and translocation steps are rapid compared to the paralytic step. The binding step is relatively little influenced by temperature (27-37°C), but the translocation and lytic steps are notably influenced. The binding step does not vary with nerve stimulation, while the paralytic step does, and the effect that stimulation has on translocation is not fully resolved.

These data form the basis for arguing that a generalized model to account for botulinum and tetanus toxin-induced blockade of cholinergic transmission has been established. Beyond this, they make clear that the behavior of these two toxins in relation to their target cells is somewhat similar to the behavior of numerous bacterial toxins that attack eukaryotic cells (17, 18). The best examples of these might be cholera and diphtheria toxins. In both cases, the toxins are composed of two major components, one of which governs cell-surface binding and one which evokes a lytic effect. The latter component requires the former to poison intact cells, but does not need it -- or may even be inhibited by it -- in broken cell preparations. In other words, the lytic component is tissue-targeted and perhaps even internalized by the binding component, but targeting and internalization are not required when a vulnerable tissue system is exposed in a broken cell preparation.

At the moment, one can reasonably assume that a host of bacterial cytotoxins, including botulinum and tetanus toxins, share a common mechanism in poisoning their respective target cells (17). For all of them, there is the sequence of binding, translocation and lytic steps. One must wonder to what extent the various receptors and processes attacked by these several toxins are alike or even identical.

IV.   CELLULAR AND SUBCELLULAR EVENTS IN PARALYSIS

A. *Binding Step*

    The desired goal in studying the interaction between botulinum toxin and the nerve membrane is to isolate and characterize the receptor. This goal is far from being realized. At the moment, most research merely examines the binding of botulinum toxin in the presence of drugs or under experimental conditions that might inhibit binding. Research such as this has revealed the properties of binding that were discussed in the last section (e.g., rapid, low Q_{10}, etc.). It has also revealed that the actions of botulinum toxin are inhibited by gangliosides, with the trisialoganglioside designated GT_{1b} being most effective (19, 20). The fact that a naturally oc- curring ganglioside can inhibit the actions of botulinum toxin certainly does not prove that the ganglioside in question is a receptor. More realistically, such findings only indicate that sialic acid-containing molecules should be considered as possible candidates for a receptor role.

In the recent past, a series of studies has been done that help clarify the nature of the toxin receptor. These studies demonstrate at least four features of the toxin-receptor in- teraction: (i) the receptor mediating the action of phospho- lipase A_2 neurotoxins (e.g., β-bungarotoxin) is different from the receptor(s) mediating the actions of botulinum and tetanus toxins, (ii) the initial stage of botulinum toxin and tetanus toxin binding to the neuromuscular junction is, in some spe- cies, easily and extensively reversible, (iii) a variety of lectins, sugars and hormones do not antagonize the actions of botulinum and tetanus toxins, and (iv) the in situ receptors for these two toxins are not very susceptible to the actions of trypsin or collagenase.

The experiments that support the conclusions just present- ed can be summarized as follows. A distinction between phos- pholipase A_2 neurotoxin receptors and clostridial neurotoxin receptors can be made by taking advantage of the cation stron- tium. On the one hand, this ion antagonizes the catalytic, but not the binding, properties of phospholipase A (21). On the other hand, strontium can act as a substitute for calcium in neuromuscular transmission, and can do so without impairing either the binding or lytic actions of clostridial toxins (16). Therefore, neuromuscular preparations bathed in stron- tium-containing medium were exposed to a large molar excess of β-bungarotoxin for a length of time adequate to permit bind- ing. The preparations were then exposed to botulinum or teta- nus toxin. It was found that large excesses of bound, but catalytically inactive, β-bungarotoxin did not antagonize the paralytic actions of either toxin. That β-bungarotoxin was actually bound was demonstrated by incubating tissues in strontium-containing medium with toxin for extensive periods of time, and then washing the preparations free of the metal. When such preparations were re-immersed in normal medium with- out strontium, the paralytic action of bound β-bungarotoxin was expressed.

Two studies have found that the binding of botulinum toxin to the rat neuromuscular junction is rapid and poorly revers- ible (9, 15). Experiments on the mouse neuromuscular junction produced a somewhat different outcome (16). If preparations were exposed to botulinum or tetanus toxin for an amount of time adequate to produce substantial binding and then washed extensively in toxin-free medium, the resulting toxicity was strikingly diminished. The extent to which binding was reversible hinged upon the amount of time that tissues were exposed to toxin. For short incubation times, binding was almost completely reversible; as incubation time was extended, reversibility became less apparent and then was absent.

A variety of lectins, sugars and hormones were tested for their abilities to antagonize botulinum toxin and tetanus toxin-induced neuromuscular blockade. When tested at concentrations of 1-30 μg/ml, and when exposed to tissues for 30 minutes prior to the addition of toxins, none of the following lectins or lectin sources antagonized onset of paralysis: concanavalin A (substrates, d-glucose and d-mannose), Lens culinaris (substrate, N-acetyl-d-glucosamine), Arachis hypogaea (substrate, d-galactose) or Glycine max (substrate, N-acetyl-d-galactosamine). Presumably the toxin receptors do not contain the lectin substrates in a terminal position, or if the substrates are present, their accessibility to lectins is hindered. Negative findings were also obtained in experiments that involved sugars (d-glucose, N-acetyl-d-glucosamine, d-galactose, N-acetyl-d-galactosamine; 0.1 M) and hormones (human chorionic gonadotropin, 750 units/ml; thyrotropic hormone, 1 unit/ml; luteinizing hormone, 800 units/ml).

Finally, limited enzymatic treatment of neuromuscular preparations with collagenase or trypsin did not alter clostridial neurotoxin binding and activity. Collagenase is customarily used to release nonintegral proteins from the membrane, and trypsin is used to digest exposed amide linkages (e.g., arginine). The data suggest that the toxin receptors are not loosely integrated or fully exposed proteins.

There is one additional finding that resulted from these studies. There are numerous techniques that can be used to inactivate botulinum toxin. A question naturally arises as to whether inactivation means loss of binding activity, loss of lytic activity or both. If the toxin were to lose binding activity, then the inactivated molecule would not fix to receptors and would not occlude the actions of native toxin. Conversely, if the toxin were to retain binding activity and lose lytic activity, then it would fix to the receptor and in so doing antagonize native toxin. Interestingly, every procedure that has been tested (alkaline, formalin and heat treatments and chemical denaturation) causes loss of binding activity. As yet, no procedure has been found for inactivating the intact neurotoxin without abolishing binding.

B. *Translocation Step*

There is good reason to believe that the externally bound clostridial neurotoxins, or some fragments obtained from them, are internalized. Unfortunately, there are virtually no data that permit one to decide how a clostridial neurotoxin penetrates the nerve membrane. At most, one can only speculate about broad categories of mechanisms. The most likely choices are adsorptive pinocytosis or a protein carrier (17, 18). Insofar as the latter possibility is concerned, the toxin molecule itself may play an essential role in membrane penetration. Conceivably, one portion of the molecule, acting alone or in concert with the membrane, creates a channel or carrier mechanism. It is worth noting that the translocation process that mediates membrane penetration for all of the potent bacterial toxins remains undetermined.

C. Lytic Step

Botulinum toxin is believed to act directly or indirectly to block excitation-secretion coupling. Several tentative models have been proposed to account for paralysis [e.g, blockade of a calcium gate (22), blockade of a transmitter gate (23)], but none is supported by firm evidence. The only point upon which all investigators agree is that botulinum toxin antagonizes the transmitter-releasing effects of calcium. The literature that bears on this point is reviewed more fully in later chapters.

In the recent past, the author and his colleagues have been examining certain quantitative aspects of the interaction between botulinum toxin and the neuromuscular junction. Within the scope of this work is one project aimed at determining the smallest concentration of toxin that will paralyze a mouse phrenic nerve-hemidiaphragm. It has been possible to show that 1 ml of a toxin solution that is 1×10^{-14} M will reproducibly cause paralysis. This was demonstrated by using conventional techniques for isolating and bathing tissues. However, unconventional techniques are now being used that permit lengthy survival of control tissues (e.g., a fluorocarbon medium); these techniques may permit the detection of toxicity at even lower concentrations.

The rationale behind this work can best be understood in quantitative terms. Assume that 1 ml of a 10^{-15} M solution will cause paralysis. Using Avagadro's number, one can calculate that this solution contains 10^{-18} moles or 6×10^5 molecules. The mouse diaphragm contains between 10^3 and 10^4 nerve endings. Therefore, the maximal number of molecules that could interact with each nerve ending would be in the range of 10^2 to 10^3. This means that even if every molecule binds and is successfully internalized and exerts a toxic effect, the toxin need attack only 10^2 to 10^3 sites to cause poisoning.

There is an especially important point that is inherent in these calculations. To date, no one has identified a molecule or a structure that is involved in transmitter release and that exists in quantities of only several hundred per nerve ending. Therefore, if the toxin does cause paralysis at a nerve-ending to toxin-molecule ratio of $\simeq 10^2$ or less, that would have profound implications for understanding the lytic event. Such findings would virtually assure that the toxin acts in a multiplicative fashion, and as such is an enzyme or enzyme inhibitor. Although botulinum toxin has never been shown to be an enzyme, or a modifier of an enzyme, such possibilities are well worth considering. In view of the importance of these possibilities, experiments are being done to determine the least number of toxin molecules necessary to cause paralysis.

V. FUTURE DIRECTIONS

Botulinum toxin is often viewed as a "mystery" toxin. The explanation for this may reveal more about the secularization of science than it does about the nature of botulinum toxin. Microbiologists and molecular biologists who study bacterial toxins tend to think of botulinum toxin as being foreign, mainly because of its target organ. Such workers are not ordinarily familiar with the cholinergic nerve ending; consequently, they tend to segregate botulinum toxin from other microbial substances like cholera and diphtheria toxins. At the same time, neuropharmacologists and neurophysiologists customarily regard bacterial toxins like diphtheria and cholera toxins as being somewhat foreign. This attitude stems from the fact that these, and almost all other, bacterial toxins act on tissues with which the neuroscientists are not familiar. Regrettably, this secularization has probably retarded efforts to unravel the mechanism of action of botulinum toxin. It has diminished the ease with which ideas and research tactics can cross the boundaries of different disciplines. Not surprisingly, investigators have rationalized this by calling botulinum toxin a "mystery" toxin.

It may be that the time has come to abandon secular views. As information on the clostridial neurotoxins accumulates, the likelihood that these substances share common features with other microbial toxins increases. At the very least, the sequence of binding, translocation and lytic steps appear to be shared features. If the clostridial neurotoxins are found to be enzymes, the similarities among potent bacterial toxins would be undeniable.

It may be instructive to consider what might be some of
the implications of finding that the clostridial neurotoxins
are like other bacterial toxins. The implications of such
findings are arguably among the most important considerations
to be borne in mind in shaping the direction that future botulinum toxin work will take. Some specific examples may illustrate the point.

If botulinum toxin (and/or tetanus toxin) is a typical
binding fragment-lytic fragment toxin, then the ability of the
toxin to paralyze cholinergic transmission may be a function
of the binding fragment. This portion of the molecule may
tissue target the toxin, and only after tissue binding has
occurred will the lytic effect be expressed. This in turn
raises the possibility that by changing the binding fragment,
one could direct the toxin to a different target organ. In
the terminology of immunopharmacology, one could create "edu-
cated cytotoxins" (24). Merely by choosing the appropriate
binding (viz., targeting) moiety and by linking this to the
lytic fragment, one could direct the latter to poison cells of
choice. If the lytic effect is specific to excitation-secretion coupling, then linking the lytic fragment to the proper
binding fragment would result in nerve toxins that block
transmitter release from any desired type of targeted cell.
Hence, modified relatives of botulinum toxin could be potent
blockers of the release of norepinephrine, serotonin, neuro-
peptide, etc. Even if the lytic effect is of a generalized
nature, such as inhibition of protein synthesis, the modified
toxins could still be directed to poison only those nerves of
a particular transmitter type.

The obverse of these experiments might also prove highly
fruitful. For example, the binding fragment could be used to
direct a variety of pharmacologically active substances to,
and into, cholinergic nerve endings. This technique could become one of the most powerful ever developed for dissecting
and analyzing the function of the nerve ending. If an investigator were interested in knowing whether a particular molecule was present in a nerve ending and was playing an essential role in nerve function, then antibodies to that molecule
could be developed and linked to the binding fragment. This
complex could then be applied to a suitable nerve preparation,
and the effects on transmitter release or other processes
could be studied. The technique has the added advantage that
the antibodies could be localized histologically. This means
that the binding fragment-antibody complex could be used not
only to determine whether particular molecules were involved
in nerve function, but also to determine the site or region in
which the molecules exerted their effects.

The technique just mentioned may have applications that
extend beyond the research laboratory and into the clinic.

The antibody that is complexed to the binding fragment need not necessarily be directed against an endogenous molecule. The antibody could be one that interacts with an exogenous substance, such as a bacterial toxin. It is entirely plausible that the binding fragment of botulinum toxin could be complexed to an antibody directed against the lytic fragment from botulinum toxin. This complex could be used to counteract the effects of botulinum toxin, even after it has entered the nerve terminal. This strategy might offer advantages over traditional antibody therapy, because traditional antibodies are not tissue targeted and do not penetrate the nerve membrane. It would be truly exciting if a portion of the botulinum toxin molecule could be modified to make it part of a useful therapeutic approach to the treatment of botulism.

VI. CONCLUDING REMARKS

It must be candidly admitted that the precise mechanism of action of botulinum toxin remains unknown. Nevertheless, a model that may explain certain aspects of poisoning has been proposed, and the model has been generalized to include tetanus toxin. This model may provide a useful context in which to do studies aimed at further defining the cellular and subcellular actions of clostridial neurotoxins.

Without doubt, the subcellular action of botulinum toxin that is of greatest concern is that which culminates in blockade of transmitter release. To date, no specific mechanism has been proposed that is supported by rigorous evidence. However, quantitative data seem to point to the possibility that botulinum toxin is an enzyme. If so, botulinum toxin would join a host of other bacterial toxins that cause cytotoxicity through an enzymatic mechanism.

REFERENCES

1. DasGupta, B. R., and Sugiyama, H., in "Perspectives in Toxinology" (A. W. Bernheimer, ed.), p. 87. Wiley, New York, (1977).
2. Lamanna, C., *Science 130,* 764 (1959).
3. Lamanna, C., and Carr, C. J., *J. Clin. Pharmacol. Therap. 8,* 286 (1967).
4. Sugiyama, H., *Microbiol. Rev. 44,* 419 (1980).
5. Wright, G. P., *Pharmacol. Rev. 7,* 413 (1955).
6. Dickson, E. C., and Shevky, R., *J. Exp. Med. 38,* 327 (1923).

7. Edmunds, C. W., and Long, P. H., *JAMA 81*, 542 (1923).
8. Schübel, K., *Pathol. Pharmacol. 96*, 193 (1923).
9. Burgen, A. S., V., Dickens, F., and Zatman, L. J., *J. Physiol. (London) 109*, 10 (1949).
10. Brooks, V. B., *J. Physiol. (London) 134*, 264 (1956).
11. Hughes, R., and Whaler, B. C., *J. Physiol. (London) 160*, 221 (1962).
12. Simpson, L. L., *Neuropharmacology 10*, 673 (1971).
13. Simpson, L. L., *Neuropharmacology 12*, 165 (1973).
14. Simpson, L. L., *Neuropharmacology 13*, 683 (1974).
15. Simpson, L. L., *J. Pharmacol. Exp. Ther. 212*, 16 (1980).
16. Simpson, L. L., *J. Pharmacol. Exp. Ther.* in press (1981).
17. Gill, D. M., *in* "Bacterial Toxins and Cell Membranes" (J. Jeljaszewicz and T. Wadström, eds.), p. 291. Academic Press, New York, (1978).
18. Neville, D. M., and Chang, T.-M., *Curr. Top. Memb. Transport 10*, 65 (1978).
19. Kitamura, M., Iwamori, M., and Nagai, Y., *Biochim. Biophys. Acta 628*, 328 (1980).
20. Simpson, L. L., and Rapport, M. M., *J. Neurochem. 18*, 1751 (1971).
21. Chang, C. C., Su, M. J., Lee, J. D., and Eaker, D., *Naunyn Schmiedeberg's Arch. Pharmacol. 299*, 155 (1977).
22. Hirokawa, N., and Heuser, J. E., *J. Cell Biol. 88*, 160 (1980).
23. Hanig, J. P., and Lamanna, C., *J. Theor. Biol. 77*, 107 (1979).
24. Parker, C. W., *Pharmacol. Rev. 25*, 325 (1973).

BOTULINUM NEUROTOXIN TYPE A AS A PROBE
FOR STUDYING NEUROTRANSMITTER RELEASE

J. O. Dolly, C. K. Tse, J. D. Black, and R. S. Williams

Department of Biochemistry
Imperial College
London

D. Wray and M. Gwilt

Department of Pharmacology
Royal Free Hospital School of Medicine
London

P. Hambleton and J. Melling

Vaccine Research and Production Laboratory
C.A.M.R.
Porton Down, Wiltshire

I. INTRODUCTION

Little is known about the molecular mechanism(s) of neurotransmitter release or the membrane components responsible for
this process. Availability of probes, such as neurotoxins,
that specifically interfere with release of transmitter(s)
from nerve terminals and whose actions are well characterised
by electrophysiological and biochemical techniques, should
prove invaluable in gaining information on this important system. Such an approach is based partly on the successful
application of snake α-neurotoxins and cholera toxin to extensive studies on nicotinic acetylcholine receptors (1) and an
effector for certain hormones (2), respectively. Already, a
number of presynaptically-acting neurotoxins have been purified and are proving helpful for investigations on the uptake,

47

synthesis and release of transmitters (3). Of all these neurotoxic proteins, botulinum toxin, produced by a number of
different strains of *Clostridium botulinum*, is the most potent
neuroparalytic agent when injected into animals, and appears
to be the most promising biochemical tool for investigations
on nerve membrane components concerned with transmitter release. It is known to specifically and irreversibly inhibit
spontaneous and evoked release of acetylcholine at the verte-
brate neuromuscular junction both *in vitro* (4) and *in vivo*
(5); also, it is effective in blocking evoked release at certain other peripheral and central synapses though with varying
potency [discussed in (6) and other chapters in this volume].

Until very recently, practically all studies on the action
of botulinum toxin employed crude or, in some cases, purified
preparations of neurotoxin-haemagglutinin complex(es), due to
the unavailability of adequate quantities of the pure neurotoxin. In initial studies in our laboratories, a crystalline
preparation of type A neurotoxin-haemagglutinin complex (molecular weight of about 10^6) kindly provided by Professor E.
Schantz (see chapter by him in this volume) was tritiated by
propionylation with N-succinimidyl $[2,3-^3H]$propionate. This
novel reagent (7), which is available commercially at relatively high specific radioactivity (> 50 Ci/mmol), can triti-
ate proteins under very mild conditions and thereby often
avoid loss of biological activity. In this case, the preparation of ^3H-propionylated toxin conjugate retained its neuro-
toxcity. It was found to bind with high affinity to membranes
of rat cerebrocortical synaptosomes (C. K. Tse, J. O. Dolly,
P. Hambleton and J. Melling, unpublished data). The observation that the majority of this binding was prevented by galac-
tose (an inhibitor of haemagglutinin), together with its ability to interact with erythrocytes, indicates the dominant
role of the much more abundant (relative to the neurotoxin
portion of the protein complex) haemagglutinin components.
Although the neurotoxin-haemagglutinin complex can be used for
certain studies, it is clearly unsuitable for biochemical experiments. Hence, sufficient quantities of haemagglutinin-
free botulinum neurotoxin type A (BoNT) were purified to homogeneity [(8), also chapter by Hambleton *et al.* in this volume]
from a preparation of the complex by sequential affinity
chromatography on p-aminophenyl-β-D-thiogalactopyranoside
coupled to Sepharose 4B and ion-exchange chromatography on
DEAE-Sephacel.

In this chapter, evidence is presented that this stable
and highly neurotoxic protein (8.3 x 10^7 mouse LD$_{50}$ units/mg
of protein) is a useful probe for studying neurotransmitter
release at the mammalian neuromuscular junction and at synapses in the central nervous system. Also, successful preparation of a biologically active ^{125}I-BoNT preparation enabled

its binding sites to be located at synaptic regions in rat
diaphragm and a saturable neurotoxin binding component to be
detected on brain synaptosomal membranes.

II.   INTERACTION OF BOTULINUM NEUROTOXIN WITH NERVE TERMINALS

A.   *Inhibitory Effects of Botulinisation on Acetylcholine Re-*
     lease at the Rat Neuromuscular Junction as Demonstrated by
     Electrophysiological Techniques

The ability of the purified BoNT to produce blockade of
neuromuscular transmission *in vitro* was first tested by apply-
ing the toxin in the bathing solution (0.40 nM) to a frog sar-
torius muscle while its nerve was stimulated. Within 15 min
of adding the toxin, a slight increase in tension occurred
lasting for around 20 min; eventual blockade was seen after a
further 90 min. Direct electrical stimulation of the muscle
or bath application of carbachol continued to produce contraction, implicating a presynaptic action of the neurotoxin, as
also shown for a different preparation of neurotoxin (9).
   To investigate further the action of the neurotoxin, BoNT
was injected (60 pg, 5 mouse LD_{50} units) subcutaneously into
rat hind-leg and the extensor digitorum longus (EDL) muscle
examined *in vitro* 1-3 days later. Intracellular recordings
were made at end-plates with microelectrodes in the standard
way at 22-25°C (10). Leg muscles became paralysed within 24
hr of injection. When the nerve innervating the muscle was
stimulated, end-plate potentials of small amplitude (0.5-2.0
mV) were produced, with a large number of failures of the
nerve impulse to release transmitter (see chapter by Thesleff
in this volume). The effect of BoNT on miniature end-plate
potentials (m.e.p.p.s) is shown in Figure 1. It can be seen
that the neurotoxin causes a marked, significant, fall in frequency of m.e.p.p.s when compared to controls. The mean
m.e.p.p. amplitude progressively decreased up to 2 days after
poisoning, while at 3 days control values were restored. However, the distribution of m.e.p.p. amplitudes in botulinised
muscle was no longer symmetrical and "bell shaped," as found
for normal muscle (Fig. 2A); instead, the distribution was
skewed towards lower amplitudes (Fig. 2C). When the degree of
skewness is quantitated (Fig. 1), it can be seen that the
neurotoxin caused m.e.p.p. amplitude distributions to become
significantly skewed at all the periods tested. Associated
with the skew distribution, there was also a greater spread in
amplitudes, and this was reflected in a significantly increased coefficient of variation of the distribution, compared

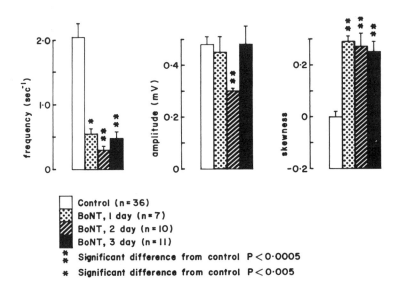

*FIGURE 1. Effect of BoNT on miniature end-plate poten-
tials in rat EDL muscle. Intracellular recordings were made
at end-plates, located by finding m.e.p.p.s with fast rise
time (< 1 msec). In botulinised muscle, there is wide scatter
in rise times, so recordings were made only if at least some
m.e.p.p.s had fast rise times. Mean values (+ S.E.M.; n end-
plates) are given for m.e.p.p. frequency, amplitude and skewness (mean-median/SD) of the amplitudes for control and botu-
linized (rats injected in the leg with BoNT 1-3 days previously) muscles.*

with controls. These results are in agreement with published
observations using partially purified haemagglutinin-neurotoxin complex (11). Botulinum toxin appears to block transmitter release without seeming to affect calcium entry into
nerve terminals or altering the filling of vesicles with
acetylcholine (5, 12). This suggests that it is the calcium-
triggered exocytosis step that is blocked by the toxin. Experimental observations show that botulinisation alters the normal release sites at the active zones, thereby accounting for
the decreased frequency of m.e.p.p.s. Possibly a limited release occurs from these perturbed sites leading to a skew distribution in m.e.p.p. amplitudes; alternatively, release may
continue to occur less readily away from the active zones, and
the skew distribution could then be explained by large and
variable diffusion paths for the released acetylcholine.
    Another neurotoxin with presynaptic actions, β-bungaro-
toxin (β-BuTX), is known to cause an increase in frequency of
m.e.p.p.s prior to eventual blockade (13). This transient

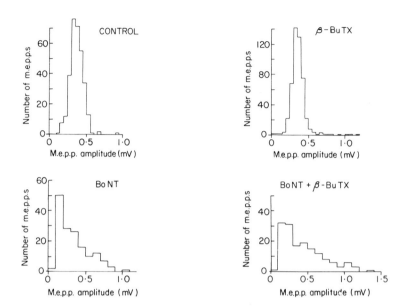

FIGURE 2. Distributions of m.e.p.p. amplitudes: effect of β-bungarotoxin (β-BuTX) and BoNT. Recordings from different end-plates: (A) control, (B) 20-21 min after addition in vitro of 0.14 µM β-BuTX, (C) muscles of rat injected 2 days previously with 60 pg BoNT, (D) as in (C), 41-45 min after addition in vitro of 0.14 µM β-BuTX.

effect of bath application of β-BuTX (0.14 µM) to normal muscle is shown in Figure 3 (upper curve). After such treatment, the amplitude of m.e.p.p.s does not change from normal values during the phase of increased transmitter release (e.g., Fig. 2B) and the amplitude distribution remains "bell shaped." The toxin is thought to act by specifically binding to presynaptic nerve membrane and through the subsequent expression of its phospholipase A_2 activity (13). It was therefore of interest to investigate if botulinisation affects the action of β-BuTX. It was found that botulinisation prevented the large increase in the frequency produced by a homogeneous preparation (14) of β-BuTX (Fig. 3), but did however cause a much smaller, sustained increase from the starting value. The m.e.p.p. amplitude was increased slightly by β-BuTX, when applied to poisoned muscles (e.g., Fig. 3). These small increases in frequency and amplitude of m.e.p.p.s produced by β-BuTX were confirmed in recordings at numerous end-plates of muscles botulinised for 1-3 days; the increase in frequency reached statistical significance (P < 0.05) for animals

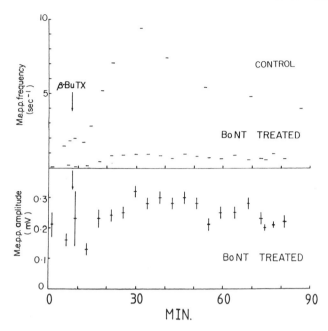

FIGURE 3. Time course of the effect of β–BuTX on m.e.p.p.s in muscle from normal and botulinised rats. Continuous recordings of frequency and amplitude of m.e.p.p.s were made at an end-plate of a control and a botulinised muscle (60 pg, 3 days previously). The arrow indicates the time of addition of 0.14 μM β–BuTX. The length of the longitudinal bars represents period of analysis; vertical bars are S.E.M.

botulinised for 3 days, while the increase in amplitude reached statistical significance (P < 0.0005) for 2-day botulinised animals.

The increase in m.e.p.p. amplitude produced by β–BuTX contrasts markedly with the action of this drug on control muscle where amplitudes are not affected, so it was of interest to investigate further how this came about. As shown (Fig. 2C), the m.e.p.p. amplitude distribution is skewed for botulinised muscle. If the two toxins act independently, one might expect β–BuTX to cause the addition to the skew distribution of a second "bell shaped" peak at larger normal amplitudes, as shown schematically in Figure 4. However, no clear sign of such a peak was seen (e.g., Fig. 2D), the distributions remaining skewed. To test this quantitatively, the skewness and coefficient of variation were calculated for botulinised end-plates before and after addition of β–BuTX. Both these parameters would be decreased if β–BuTX caused the addition of a second peak to the distribution pattern. However, as shown in

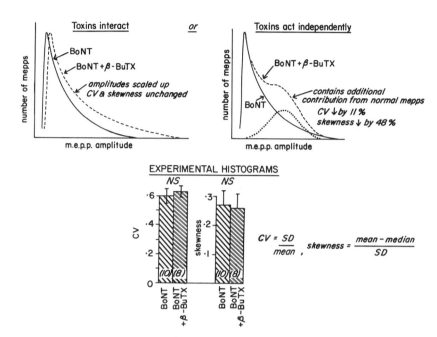

FIGURE 4.   Action of β-BuTX on botulinised muscle.   Top:
Schematic drawing of m.e.p.p. amplitude distribution for bo-
tulinised muscle in the presence and absence of β-BuTX.
Below: mean values (± S.E.M.) are shown for coefficient of
variation (CV) and the skewness of observed m.e.p.p. ampli-
tudes for rat muscle injected 2 days previously with 60 pg
BoNT, before and after the addition of 0.14 µM β-BuTX.   The
number of end-plates measured is shown in parentheses.

Figure 4, there was no significant change in these parameters,
so that β-BuTX does not simply cause the addition of normal
"bell shaped" m.e.p.p.s.   Instead, the m.e.p.p. amplitude
distributions are simply scaled up to larger values, as shown
schematically in Figure 4.

One possible explanation for the action of β-BuTX on
botulinised muscle is that, following its specific binding to
the nerve in the vicinity of the release sites, its subsequent
phospholipase A_2 action aids membrane vesicle fusion/emptying.
One might expect that such an effect would lead to a small increase in all m.e.p.p. amplitudes, thus scaling up the amplitude distribution, as well as increasing the m.e.p.p. frequency slightly.   This suggestion is in accord with results
using β-BuTX with its phospholipase activity removed by modification of a histidine residue in the active site by p-bromo-
phenacyl bromide (13); this modified toxin did not alter

m.e.p.p. frequency in botulinised muscle (data not shown). To
summarize, the action of native β-BuTX on the abnormal spontaneous release observed in botulinised muscle, contrasts
markedly with its action on normal nerve endings.

B. *Effects of Botulinum Neurotoxin on other Peripheral
    Synapses*

    With respect to the specificity of the pure neurotoxin for
different types of peripheral synapses, it is notable that
relatively high concentrations ($\simeq$ 5 nM) irreversibly inhibit
neurotransmission at postganglionic cholinergic junctions
in guinea pig ileum (15); this is similar to observations made
with haemagglutinin-neurotoxin preparations (16, 17). The
motor response of the rat anococcygeus muscle following sympathetic nerve field stimulation can be only partially antagonised *in vitro* by a similar dose of this pure preparation of
type A neurotoxin (15). This may concur with a report (17)
that a longer incubation time with type D botulinum toxin is
required to impair adrenergic transmission than that needed
for intoxication of autonomic cholinergic neurones. Interestingly, BoNT failed to affect the nonadrenergic, noncholinergic
inhibitor response of the guinea pig taenia çoli, elicited by
field stimulation but did block atrophine-resistant excitation
of bladder (15).

C. *Demonstration of Botulinum Neurotoxin Binding at Motor
    End-plates*

    To facilitate biochemical studies on a possible specific
binding component for this neurotoxin, it was necessary to
prepare a radioactive derivative that retained neurotoxicity.
In view of the unique potency of this protein (12 pg represents one mouse LD_{50} dose), it is envisaged that occupancy of
few sites is required to produce fatal, neuromuscular paralysis. Hence, a radiolabelled preparation of very high specific
radioactivity would be needed for detection of such minute
quantities of binding component. ^{125}I-Iodination of the
neurotoxin ($\simeq$ 200 μg) was therefore performed to high specific
radioactivity (400-5000 Ci/mmol) using 5 mCi ^{125}I and a modification of the Chloramine T method (18). Gel filtration was
used to remove the free iodine. The resultant labelled material exhibited 30-80% of the toxicity of unlabelled neurotoxin,
as determined by lethality tests (8) in mice. Complete separation of the iodinated species from unlabelled neurotoxin was
achieved by gel isoelectric focussing, followed by elution
with buffer. This radiolabelled material was shown to be
biologically active by lethality tests in mice; it produced

paralysis of rat leg muscle following local administration and
reduced the frequency of m.e.p.p.s. Due to the low recoveries
of neurotoxin obtained from the focussing gel, this separation
was not routinely employed. On dodecyl sulphate polyacrylamide gel electrophoresis, under non-reducing conditions, the
iodinated neurotoxin gave a single peak with a molecular weight
of 140,000 (Fig. 5), as observed with the unlabelled protein
(8). After reduction, two polypeptides with molecular weights
of 99,000 and 55,000 were detected, again as expected. This
iodinated neurotoxin preparation was stable for 2 weeks, when
stored at 5°C in 0.1 M phosphate buffer, pH 7.5/0.15 M
NaCl/0.25% gelatin.

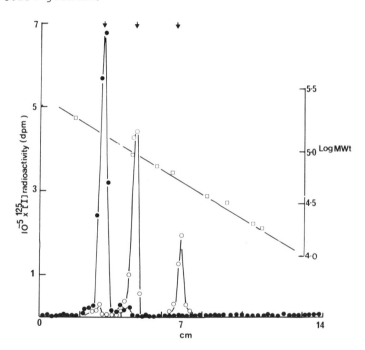

*FIGURE 5. Dodecyl sulphate polyacrylamide gel electropho-
resis of labelled* ^{125}*I-BoNT. This was performed on a 4-30%
gradient pore polyacrylamide gel in a Tris-acetate system, pH
7.4 containing 40 mM Tris, 20 mM sodium acetate, 2 mM EDTA and
0.2% SDS in the absence (●) or presence (O) of 5% β-mercaptoethanol. The molecular weights of the native and labelled
neurotoxins were determined by comparing their electrophoretic
mobility with those of known molecular weight standards. The
gel was then cut into slices (1.1-mm) and their radioactive
contents were determined. Arrows indicate the positions of
the native neurotoxin and its subunits.*

For location of neurotoxin binding sites, mouse diaphragm
muscle was incubated with 2 x 10^{-10} M ^{125}I-neurotoxin in
Krebs-Ringer solution at 25°C for 2-3 hr, followed by extensive washing before fixation with 2% glutaraldehyde. Controls
were treated similarly, except that an excess of unlabelled
toxin was included. One hemidiaphragm from each sample was
stained for acetylcholine esterase (19). After fixation in
OsO_4 and embedding, sections were processed for light microscope autoradiography (20). In the test samples silver grains
were present in localised regions, with few grains visible
elsewhere (Fig. 6). Absence of such deposition of silver
grains in control samples indicated that the binding of ^{125}I-
neurotoxin was saturable. Furthermore, the areas in test
samples containing silver grains were identified as end-plate
regions by staining for acetylcholine esterase, known to be
located therein (Fig. 6). Acetylcholine receptors can also be
localised in these areas by the binding of radiolabelled α-
bungarotoxin. These studies show that there are saturable
binding sites for BoNT at the synaptic region; the specificity
of these sites is being further elucidated by ultrastructural

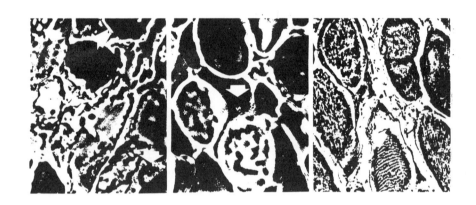

FIGURE 6. *Localisation of ^{125}I-BoNT binding sites in*
mouse diaphragm muscle by light microscope autoradiography.
Diaphragm was incubated with 0.2 nM ^{125}I-BoNT in Krebs-Ringer,
pH 7.4 for 3 hr at 25°C; control sample (right) was treated
similarly, except a 100-fold molar excess of unlabelled neuro-
toxin was included. After washing, the specimens were fixed,
embedded, sectioned and processed for light microscope auto-
radiography. One test hemidiaphragm (centre) was also stained
for acetylcholine esterase. Silver grains were clearly seen
at synaptic regions (arrows) of test specimens after 3 weeks
exposure; no grains were visible in these areas in controls.

localisation studies using electron microscope autoradiography
and immunocytochemistry. Such experiments should help to
establish the functional significance of these binding sites,
which are labelled with toxin concentrations known to produce
inhibition of acetylcholine release.

III. INTERACTION OF BOTULINUM NEUROTOXIN WITH SYNAPSES IN
      MAMMALIAN CENTRAL NERVOUS SYSTEM

A. *Effects of the Neurotoxin on Choline Uptake and Acetyl-*
    choline Release by Rat Synaptosomes

     Apart from changes induced in encephalogram recording of
monkeys injected with impure botulinum toxin (21), no electrophysiological evidence is available that the neurotoxin acts
at central synapses. However, biochemical experiments *in
vitro* have shown that preparations of haemagglutinin-neurotoxin complex can perturb both choline uptake (3) and release
of acetylcholine (22) by certain brain tissue preparations.
As the presence of haemagglutinin in the toxin sample could
conceivably contribute in some way to these actions, in the
present investigation, these same parameters were examined by
using pure BoNT and brain synaptosomes. This preparation
facilitates the aforementioned biochemical measurements and
also kinetic studies on the binding component for BoNT; such
experiments are not feasible at the neuromuscular junction.
     Synaptosomes purified from rat brain cortex (14) were pre-
incubated for various times at 37°C in the absence or presence
of 4 nM BoNT, before the addition of ^{3}H-choline. Accumulation
of radioactivity by the synaptosomes over the subsequent 1-hr
period was quantified by a filtration assay (14). Exposure to
BoNT decreased by a small degree the amount of ^{3}H-choline taken
up by the synaptosomes relative to the untreated sample (Fig.
7). Impairment of choline uptake by synaptosomes has been
reported for high concentration of neurotoxin-haemagglutinin
conjugate (22). It is of interest that synaptosomes
prepared from brain slices that were pretreated with the
latter, also show a somewhat diminished ability to accumulate
choline, but direct treatment of isolated synaptosomes with
toxin failed to show an effect (3). As the diminution in
choline uptake observed in these studies is minimal, it may
be that this is not a primary effect, but rather a consequence (3) of the inhibition of acetylcholine release (see
following) produced by the toxin. In view of the evidence
presented earlier that β-BuTX can bind to botulinised neuromuscular junctions, it was of interest to establish if β-BuTX
interacts with BoNT-treated synaptosomes. β-BuTX alone

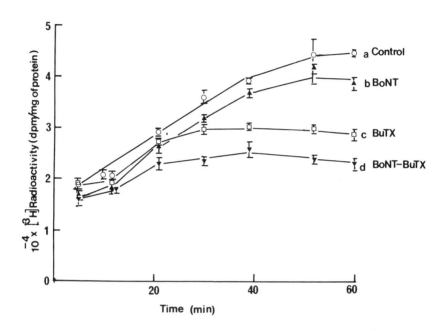

FIGURE 7.   Effect of BoNT on the accumulation of ^3H-cho-line by cerebrocortical synaptosomes. Suspensions (4-5 mg protein/ml) were incubated with or without 4 nM BoNT for 75 min at 37°C with continuous gassing (95% O_2/5% CO_2) before the addition of ^3H-choline (final concentration of 0.22 µM; 6.4 Ci/mmol). These suspensions were separated into aliquots followed by the addition of β-BuTX (0.8 µM) or an equal volume of buffer as control. The time course of accumulation of radioactivity (± S.D.) was measured by a filtration assay.

produced an apparent decrease in choline uptake by synapto-somes (Fig. 7), as previously reported for this pure prepara-tion of toxin; it was then suggested this may be an indirect effect (14). It is noteworthy that pretreatment of synapto-somes with BoNT did not prevent the inhibitory action of β-BuTX on choline uptake (Fig. 7); in fact, the effects of BoNT and β-BuTX appeared additive. It seems, therefore, that these two neurotoxins do not display antagonism, at least in their effects on choline accumulation by synaptosomes.

With respect to acetylcholine release it was notable that incubation of synaptosomes at 37°C with 4 nM BoNT for about 2 hr (^3H-choline was present for the last 25 min) reduced sig-nificantly the resting (in 5 mM K^+) and K^+-stimulated efflux of ^3H-acetylcholine (Table I). This observation is consistent with the neurotoxin's ability to reduce resting total efflux

TABLE I. Effect of BoNT on Release of Neurotransmitters from Cerebrocortical Synaptosomes

Treatments	% Inhibition[a] by 4.3 nM BoNT	
	^{3}H-ACh	^{14}C-GABA
Control (5 mM K$^+$)	57.4 ± 6.6 (4)	13.4 ± 2.0 (4)
27 mM K$^+$	26.8 ± 2.8 (4)	–
55 mM K$^+$	52.3 ± 3.2 (4)	5.2 ± 0.6 (4)
0.9 μM β-BuTX	4.2 ± 0.7 (4)	–

[a]*Difference in radioactive content after 20 min (minus* the value in 5 mM K$^+$) of untreated and BoNT-treated samples ÷ Radioactive content (minus* the value in 5 mM K$^+$) of untreated sample after 20 min; 0 time value was subtracted from all readings. Assays were performed as described previously (14; number of determinations are shown in parentheses).*
* Except for the control samples.

(23), spontaneous and evoked release of acetylcholine (as shown above) at the neuromuscular junction. The difficulties in measuring resting release and also in distinguishing this from leakage of transmitter from damaged synaptosomes may explain the reported inability of botulinum-haemagglutinin complex to reduce resting efflux of acetylcholine (3, 22); also, the high molecular weight toxin complex might behave differently from the pure neurotoxin in this respect. Interestingly, the ability of β-BuTX to induce a large efflux of acetylcholine from synaptosomes (14) was not antagonised by BoNT, consistent with similar observations on choline uptake. Regarding the specificity of action of BoNT on the central nervous system, it should be emphasised that the same concentration of neurotoxin displayed a much lesser effect on release of γ-aminobutyrate. This agrees with the observation of Habermann and colleagues (chapter in this volume) that the toxin inhibits release from synaptosomes of several transmitters but, generally, with lower efficiency relative to the effect on acetylcholine efflux. In the context of a possible mechanism for this inhibitory action of BoNT on transmitter release, it should be noted that the apparent ability of synaptosomes to synthesize ^{3}H-choline is unaffected by the concentrations of BoNT shown herein to cause blockade of release of the transmitter. Likewise the rate of ^{45}Ca^{2+} influx (in 5 mM and 55 mM K$^+$) into synaptosomes was not retarded by 4 nM BoNT (Fig. 8). This accords with results of electrophysiological measurements at the neuromuscular junction, but the heterogeneity of synaptosomes in terms of different types of synapses, possibly varying greatly in their sensitivity to BoNT, makes it difficult to draw firm conclusions from these experiments.

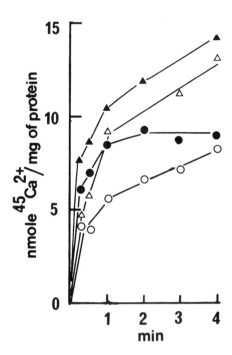

FIGURE 8. Accumulation of $^{45}Ca^{2+}$ by synaptosomes in absence and presence of BoNT. Synaptosome suspensions (2 mg/ml) were incubated with (closed symbols) and without (open symbols) BoNT (4 nM) at 37°C for 60 min; synaptosomes were washed and resuspended in toxin-free buffer containing 1 mM $CaCl_2$. At 0 time, $^{45}Ca^{2+}$-containing buffer was added; the amount of radiolabelled Ca^{2+} accumulated was determined by passing the synaptosomes down a cation exchange Dowex AG W50 X-8 column and measurement of radioactivity in the void volume. The amount of $^{45}Ca^{2+}$ accumulated by synaptosomes (mean values of 4 determinations) in low (5 mM; O or ●) and high (55 mM; Δ or ▲) K^+ concentrations are presented.

B. *Detection of a Binding Component for Botulinum Neurotoxin on Rat Brain Synaptosomes*

Insight into the mechanism of action of BoNT should be obtained by studies of its binding sites on synaptosomal membrane which ought to be located specifically on the presynaptic membrane. It is obviously of great interest and importance to characterize such a component which could well be concerned either directly or indirectly with transmitter release.

Binding of ^{125}I-BoNT to synaptosomes was determined with a standard centrifugation assay; non-specific binding was measured with the same amount of radiolabelled BoNT, but in the presence of an excess of the unlabelled protein. With a fixed incubation time of 1 hr and variable ^{125}I-BoNT concentrations, the amount of specific binding reached a plateau of about 150 fmol/mg of synaptosomal protein (Fig. 9). Saturability of this binding was confirmed by the observed reduction in the amount of ^{125}I-BoNT binding produced by unlabelled BoNT (Fig. 10). More importantly, the efficacy of two neurotoxin preparations in competing with ^{125}I-BoNT for binding sites was related to their specific neurotoxicities, suggesting that the binding component is of functional significance. Preliminary experiments have shown that β-BuTX does not competitively inhibit the binding of ^{125}I-BoNT to synaptosomes. This

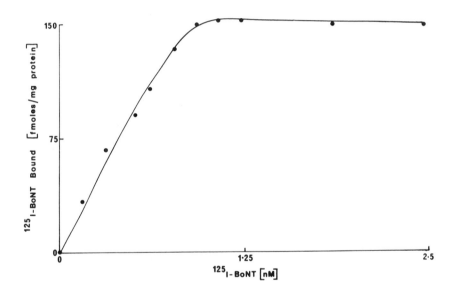

FIGURE 9. *Saturable binding of ^{125}I-BoNT to rat cerebrocortical synaptosomes. Synaptosomes were incubated for 1 hr at 37°C in Krebs-phosphate medium, pH 7.4, containing 2 mg/ml bovine serum albumin with different concentrations of ^{125}I-BoNT. The amount of toxin binding was measured by centrifugation assay. Specific binding was calculated by subtracting non-specific binding (determined in the presence of 200-fold excess of native BoNT) from total binding. Each point is the average of 2 or more determinations. Heat-treated or trypsinized samples failed to specifically bind toxin.*

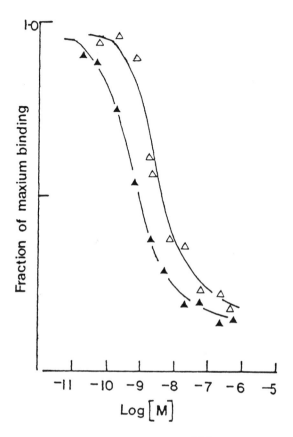

FIGURE 10. *Competitive binding of* ^{125}I-*BoNT and unlabelled*
BoNT. Synaptosomes (0.5 mg/ml) were incubated with 8.4 x
10^{-10} *M* ^{125}I-*BoNT at 37°C for 30 min in the absence and pre-*
sence of increasing concentrations of two different prepara-
tions of pure neurotoxin having specific toxicity of 8.3 x
10^7 *(* ▲ *) and 3.6 x* 10^7 *(* △ *) mouse* LD_{50} *units/mg, respec-*
tively. The amount of ^{125}I-*BoNT binding in each sample is*
expressed relative to that observed in the absence of unla-
belled neurotoxin. Binding was measured as described in
legend to Figure 9. Heat-inactivation of ^{125}I-*BoNT destroyed*
its ability to show specific binding.

confirms that β-BuTX and BoNT have distinct binding sites on
synaptosomes. Measurement of the association rate of ^{125}I-
BoNT with its binding site at 5°C showed that only one class
of sites was distinguishable; in contrast, plots of dissociation rates were biphasic with the slower dissociating component representing greater than 55% of the total specific

binding. It has not been established yet if this biphasic plot is due to heterogeneity in the binding component or ^{125}I-BoNT preparation. Using the single observed association rate constant and the rate constant for the slowly dissociating species, a dissociation constant, $K_D = 2 \times 10^{-10}$ M, was calculated.

Inadequate information is available to establish if the BoNT binding sites are similar in the central and peripheral nervous system. Judging by the unique toxicity of BoNT when injected subcutaneously into rat leg, it would appear that the neurotoxin is more potent at the neuromuscular junction. Unfortunately, no information is available on the degree of occupancy of sites by BoNT needed to produce blockade of neurotransmission. In this context, it is worthy of mention that concentrations less than 10^{-10} M toxin are known to take a few hours to inhibit transmission at the neuromuscular junction (24), although lower amounts cause paralysis, but after much longer incubation periods (chapter by Simpson in this volume). Hence, it would be informative to determine the K_D for the binding of BoNT to neuromuscular junction, but such information cannot be obtained readily. Although BoNT cannot apparently abolish binding of β-BuTX at motor end-plates or synaptosomes, it minimizes the effects of β-BuTX at the neuromuscular junction; in contrast, the two toxins appear to act independently at central synapses. The interpretation of these experimental results is difficult, due to certain differences that may exist in the action of β-BuTX and/or BoNT in the periphery and the brain; also quantal and total efflux of acetylcholine was measured in these two areas, respectively.

ACKNOWLEDGMENTS

This work was supported by studentships from the Medical Research Council (J.B.) and the Science Research Council (R.W. and M.G.). J. O. Dolly is grateful for a grant from the University of London Central Research Fund. We thank D. Green for performing the injections of BoNT according to a protocol approved by the Home Office. C. K. Tse is thankful to the Public Health Laboratory Service for financial support and the laboratory facilities provided at Porton Down. Sincere thanks are offered to Mrs. E. Ashton for efficiently typing this manuscript.

REFERENCES

1. Dolly, J. O., *Int. Rev. Biochem. 26,* 257 (1979).
2. Moss, J., and Vaughan, M., *Annu. Rev. Biochem. 48,* 581 (1979).
3. Howard, B. D., and Gunderson, C. B., *Annu. Rev. Pharmacol. Toxicol. 20,* 307 (1980).
4. Harris, A. J., and Miledi, R., *J. Physiol. 217,* 497 (1971).
5. Cull-Candy, S. G., Lundh, H., and Thesleff, S., *J. Physiol. 260,* 177 (1976).
6. Simpson, L. L., *Adv. Cytopharmacol. 3,* 27 (1979).
7. Dolly, J. O., Nockles, E. A. V., Lo., M. S., and Barnard, E. A., *Biochem. J. 193,* 919 (1981).
8. Hambleton, P., Tse, C. K., Capel, B. J., Dolly, J. O., and Melling J., *in* "Proceedings of the World Congress on Food-borne Infections and Intoxications," Paul Parley, West Berlin (1981) in press.
9. Boroff, D. A., del Castillo, J., Evoy, W. H., and Steinhardt, R. A., *J. Physiol. 240,* 227 (1974).
10. Wray, D., *J. Physiol. 310,* 37 (1981).
11. Thesleff, S., and Lundh, H., *Adv. Cytopharmacol. 3,* 35 (1979).
12. Simpson, L. L., *J. Pharmacol. Exp. Ther. 206,* 661 (1978).
13. Abe, T., Alema, S., and Miledi, R., *Eur. J. Biochem. 80,* 1 (1977).
14. Spokes, J., and Dolly, J. O., *Biochim. Biophys. Acta 596,* 81 (1980).
15. MacKenzie, I., Burnstock, G., and Dolly, J. O., *Neuroscience* (in press).
16. Bigalke, H., and Habermann, E., *Naunyn-Schmiedeberg's Arch. Pharmacol. 312,* 255 (1980).
17. Westwood, D. A., and Whaler, B. C., *Br. J. Pharmacol. Chemother. 33,* 21 (1968).
18. Greenwood, F. C., Hunter, W. M., and Glover, J. S., *Biochem. J. 89,* 114 (1963).
19. Tsuji, S., *Histochemistry 42,* 99 (1974).
20. Barnard, E. A., *in* "The Receptors - A Comprehensive Treatise" (R. D. O'Brien, ed.), vol. 1, p. 247. Plenum Press, New York (1979).
21. Poley, E. H., Vick, J. A., Ciuchta, H. P., Fischetti, D. A., Macchitelli, F. J., and Montranarelli, N., *Science 147,* 1036 (1965).
22. Wonnacott, S., *J. Neurochem. 34,* 1567 (1980).
23. Gunderson, C. B., *Prog. Neurobiology 14,* 99 (1980).
24. Simpson, L. L., *J. Pharmacol. Exp. Ther. 212,* 16 (1980).

NEUROPHYSIOLOGIC ASPECTS OF BOTULINUM POISONING

Stephen Thesleff

Department of Pharmacology
University of Lund
Lund, Sweden

I. INTRODUCTION

The neurotoxic component of botulinum toxin (BoTx) blocks
selectively cholinergic synaptic transmission, the death of
the animal resulting from respiratory paralysis. Most experimental studies on the mode of action of this toxin have been
made on neuromuscular cholinergic transmission and in this
chapter, I will describe some of the results which we have obtained in electrophysiological studies with BoTx type A in the
rat.

II. MATERIALS AND METHODS

BoTx type A, either as a crude powdered preparation or as
the isolated and purified neurotoxic component (obtained by
the courtesy of Dr. J. O. Dolly, Dept. of Biochemistry, Imperial College, London) was dissolved in buffer solution as described by Ambache (1). A single injection of the toxin solution (about 5 mouse LD_{50}) subcutaneously into the anterolate-
ral region of the hind leg of adult rats (150-200 g body
weight) produced complete paralysis which persisted for several weeks. The local effect of this amount of toxin was probably maximal since increasing the dose 20 times did not further affect neuromuscular transmission as observed in studies
on dying rats (2). At various times after poisoning, the extensor digitorum longus nerve-muscle preparation of the injected leg was removed and examined by conventional

intracellular recording techniques in an oxygenated Krebs-
Ringer solution at a constant temperature of 29 or 37°C.

III.   RESULTS

A.   *Spontaneous Quantal Transmitter Release*

As shown by Figure 1, BoTx reduces, but does not totally
abolish, spontaneous miniature endplate potentials (mepps).
Initially the mepp frequency is reduced to about 1% of normal,
but subsequently, as paralysis persists, the frequency is

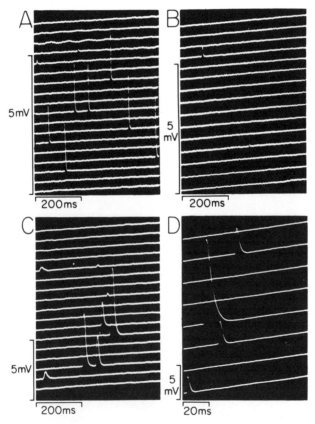

FIGURE 1. *Examples of mepps recorded in A, normal muscle;*
B, 1 day after BoTx poisoning; C, 9 days after BoTx; and D,
14 days after poisoning. Temperature 37°C. (Reproduced by
permission J. Physiol., ref, 2).

somewhat increased (Table I). During the first day after paralysis, mepp amplitude histograms show a skewed distribution
with a predominance of small mepps (Fig. 2). Three or more
days after paralysis, a population of mepps with larger than
normal amplitude appears as shown by the amplitude histograms
in Figures 2 and 3. When mepp rise-time and rate of rise are
determined, it is obvious that the shift towards larger sized
mepps is accompanied by an increase in mean rise time and a
fall in the mean rate of rise of mepps, as shown by the values
in Table I and by the histograms in Figure 3. However, an
examination of mepp amplitude and rise time distribution in
unpoisoned muscles also reveals a small portion of large and
small amplitude mepps, as seen in the histograms of Figures 2
and 3. Similarly, the rise-time and rate of rise of a small
portion of mepps at an unpoisoned junction are respectively
prolonged and reduced (Fig. 3). At the normal junction, the
portion of sub- or giant mepps is much smaller than in BoTx
poisoned muscles due to a predominance of intermediate sized
mepps.
     An interpretation for the amplitude and rise-time histo-
grams for mepps in BoTx poisoned muscles is that the toxin

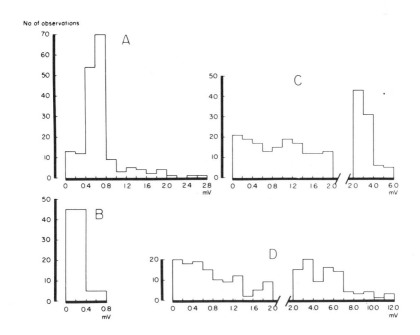

FIGURE 2.   Amplitude distribution of mepps at single end-
plates.   A, control muscle; B, 1 day after BoTx poisoning; C,
6 days after poisoning; D, 14 days after BoTx.   Temperature
37°C.   (Reproduced by permission J. Physiol., ref. 2).

TABLE I. Characteristics of mepps Recorded at Control and BoTx Poisoned Endplates. Sampling Time Indicates the Total Time Period of Recording. Temperature 29°C.

Treatment	Frequency (Hz)	Amplitude (mV[a])	Rise time (msec[a])	Rate of rise (V/sec[a])	Number	Sampling time (min)
Control	5.5	0.5 ± 0.26	0.6 ± 0.42	1.1 ± 0.56	2785	8.4
BoTx, 3 days	< 0.05	0.8 ± 0.57	0.9 ± 0.58	0.9 ± 0.59	83	–
BoTx, 5 days	≈ 0.05	1.1 ± 1.27	2.0 ± 1.09	0.6 ± 0.49	314	–
BoTx, 7 days	0.2	1.5 ± 1.29	2.0 ± 0.97	0.8 ± 0.53	328	27.3

[a] Mean ± SD.

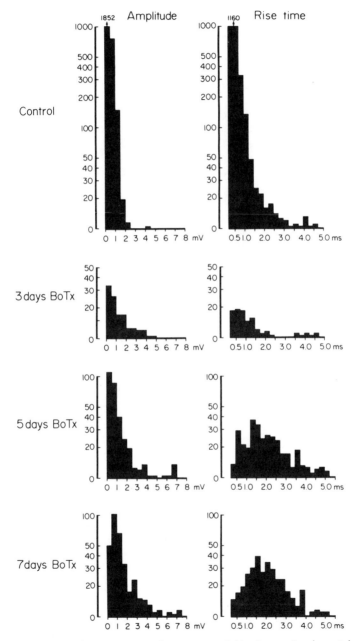

FIGURE 3. Histograms of mepp amplitude and rise-time. Temperature 29ºC.

selectively blocks the release of intermediate sized and fast-
rising mepps, but leaves the release of sub-mepps and giant
and slow-rising mepps intact. In fact, it appears from the
histograms that the frequency of sub-mepps and particularly
that of giant and slow-rising mepps may increase with time of
BoTx poisoning.

B. Evoked Quantal Transmitter Release

Depolarization of unpoisoned normal neuromuscular junctions by high extracellular potassium concentrations causes a
drastic increase of mepp frequency but fails to affect the
frequency of sub- and giant mepps (3, 4).
In BoTx poisoned preparations, raising the extracellular
potassium concentration has little or no effect on the frequency of mepps (5). Thus, maintenance of depolarization of
nerve terminals only accelerates the frequency of intermediate
sized mepps in normal muscle and has no effect on the frequency of mepps in BoTx poisoned ones.

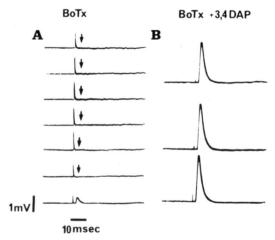

BoTx   **BoTx +3,4 DAP**

1mV

10 msec

*FIGURE 4. Records of consecutive epps obtained in a BoTx
treated endplate 24 h after poisoning. Frequency of stimulation, 0.5 Hz. In A, no drug was present, arrows indicate
failures of release. In B, 3,4-diaminopyridine (4 μM) was
added, abolishing all failures of transmitter release and
greatly increasing epp amplitude. Temperature 29°C. (Reproduced by permission Eur. J. Pharmacol., ref. 13).*

Following BoTx treatment, nerve impulses give rise to end-plate potentials (epps) of small amplitude (0.5-1 mV) at most endplates. However, when the nerve is stimulated at a low frequency (0.5 Hz), more than 50% of all nerve impulses fail to release any transmitter (Fig. 4A).

When nerve stimulus-evoked transmitter release from unpoisoned terminals is blocked by high extracellular magnesium so that more than 50% of the nerve impulses fail to release transmitter, most of the epps are made up of single quanta, and amplitude histograms of the epps and mepps are almost coincident (6).

Figure 5 shows amplitude histograms of epps and mepps from BoTx poisoned junctions, 1, 5 and 14 days after treatment. In these junctions, amplitude distributions of mepps and epps fail to coincide, showing that the transmitter quanta released by nerve stimuli are different from those spontaneously released. The amplitude distribution of the epps seems to coincide with that of mepps in unpoisoned muscles, but to have no relation to mepps at BoTx poisoned endplates. The difference between epps and mepps is further emphasized in Figure 6, which illustrates examples of mepps and epps recorded at the same junction in a muscle 8 days after BoTx poisoning. In addition to a difference in amplitude distribution, it is evident that the epps have a shorter and a more uniform rise-time than the epps.

It appears that in BoTx poisoning, nerve impulses fail to release the transmitter quanta which give rise to the majority of the mepps at these junctions. Instead the nerve impulse causes the release, but with low probability, of quanta which are similar to those responsible for intermediate sized, fast-rising mepps at unpoisoned normal junctions.

C. Calcium and Transmitter Release

Spontaneous and evoked quantal transmitter release is a calcium-requiring process. This is illustrated by the graphs in Figure 7, which show the dependence of mepp frequency on extracellular calcium concentration. Normal muscle shows increased mepp frequencies with elevation of extracellular calcium, while in BoTx treated mucles there is no increase in the rate of mepps. However, if calcium is introduced into the axoplasm of nerve terminals in poisoned muscles by the use of calcium ionophore A 23187 (Fig. 8) or by black widow spider venom a massive release of mepps occurs (2) and the mepp amplitude distribution is altered from a skew or bimodal distribution toward a normal bell-shaped distribution, as shown by the histograms in Figure 8.

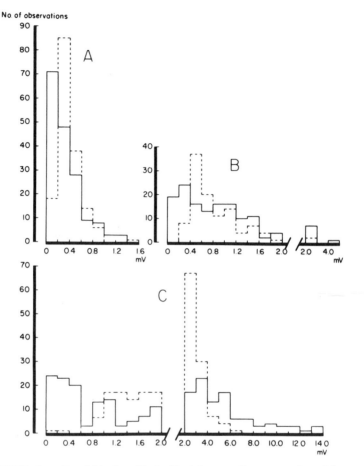

FIGURE 5. Amplitude distributions of mepps (continuous line) and epps (interrupted line). Graphs A, B and C from muscles 1, 5 and 14 days after BoTx, respectively. Amplitudes of epp were obtained from endplates where the number of fail- ures to release transmitter was higher than 50%. Temperature 37°C. (Reproduced by permission J. Physiol., ref. 2).

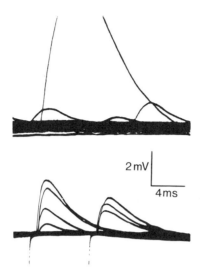

FIGURE 6. Examples of mepps (upper record) and epps (lower record) at the same endplate in a muscle poisoned 8 days previously by BoTx. Superimposed oscilloscope sweeps. Temperature 29°C.

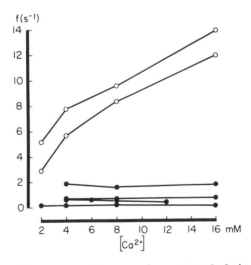

FIGURE 7. Mean mepp frequencies recorded in different extracellular calcium concentrations (abscissa) at two end-plates in normal muscle (open circles), and at four endplates in muscles 2-4 days after BoTx poisoning (filled circles). Temperature 37°C. (Reproduced by permission J. Physiol., ref. 2).

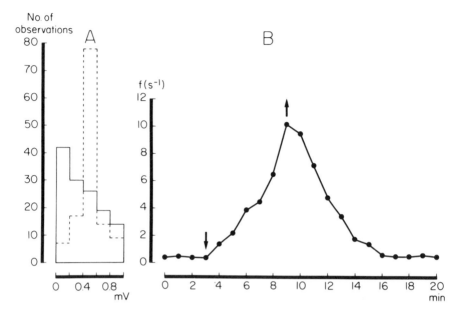

FIGURE 8. A, amplitude distributions of mepps in a 3-day
BoTx poisoned muscle before (continuous line) and in the presence of the calcium ionophore A 23187 and 10 mM extracellular
calcium (interrupted line). B, frequency of mepps at a BoTx
poisoned endplate in the presence of the calcium ionophore and
4 mM calcium. Between the arrows the endplate was superfused
with 20 mM calcium from a pipette. Temperature 37°C. (Reproduced by permission J. Physiol., ref. 2).

Thus, it seems that the frequency of mepps in BoTx poisoned muscles is uninfluenced by alterations in the extracellular calcium concentration, but if the intracellular calcium
concentration is sufficiently raised, mepp frequency is increased by the appearance of a new population of mepps with an
amplitide distribution corresponding to mepps at normal unpoisoned junctions.

Nerve impulse-evoked transmitter release in BoTx poisoned
muscles is enhanced by elevating the extracellular calcium
concentration. However, the calcium dependence of transmitter
release seems to be lower, about one-half of that at normal
junctions blocked by a high magnesium concentration, as shown
in Figure 9. When large amounts of calcium enter the nerve
terminal by the use of drugs (e.g., aminopyridines), which
prolong the duration of the preterminal action potential (14),
normal amounts of transmitter are released also from BoTx

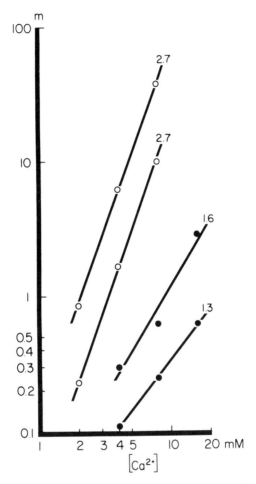

FIGURE 9. Mean quantum content, m, at various extracellular calcium concentrations at two normal endplates (open circles) and at two BoTx poisoned endplates (filled circles) 2 and 4 days after poisoning. The values from normal muscles were obtained in the presence of 20 mM magnesium. The slope of each line is shown by the adjacent number. Temperature 37°C. (Reproduced by permission J. Physiol., ref. 2).

poisoned nerve terminals and neuromuscular transmission is restored. This is illustrated in Figure 4B, which shows that 3,4-diaminopyridine (4 µM) causes a marked increase in the amount of transmitter released by each nerve impulse as shown, the abolishment of all failures of transmitter release by nerve impulses and by an increased amplitude of epps. Note

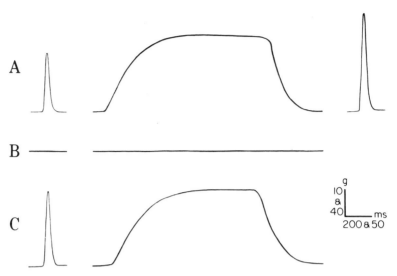

FIGURE 10. Records of indirectly elicited isometric twitch and tetanic (100 Hz) contractions of rat extensor digitorum longus muscles in vivo. (A) From a normal unpoisoned rat. The last record was obtained after the i.v. administration of 4 mg/kg body weight of 4-aminopyridine. (B) From a BoTx poisoned muscle, showing a complete block to single and tetanic stimulation. (C) From the same poisoned muscle, but following the administration of 5 mg/kg 4-aminopyridine. (Reproduced by permission J. Neurol. Sci., ref. 14).

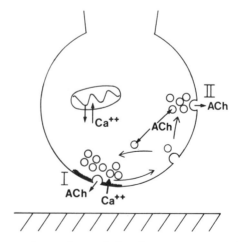

FIGURE 11. Schematic model of a nerve terminal illustrating the two kinds of proposed vesicular transmitter release, I and II.

also that the epps have a uniform and fast rise-time. Figure 10 shows that 4-aminopyridine (5 mg/kg body weight) is able to restore to normal neuromuscular transmission in a rat paralyzed by BoTx.

IV. DISCUSSION AND CONCLUSIONS

Figure 11 is a schematic model of a nerve terminal for which I propose the existence of two kinds of vesicular (quantal) transmitter release. One (I) occurs from specialized areas in the nerve terminal, the "active zones," initially described by Couteaux and Pécot-Dechavassine (7). These transmitter quanta are responsible for the bell-shaped, monomodal amplitude distribution of mepps in normal muscle. At this site, synaptic vesicle exocytosis and thereby transmitter release are quantitatively related to the intracellular calcium concentration and influx of calcium into the terminal enormously enhances the probability of vesicle fusion, as proposed by del Castillo and Katz (6). Vesicular transmitter release from this site is enhanced during nerve terminal depolarization and synchronized by calcium entry during a nerve terminal action potential. The mepps and epps resulting from this type of quantal release have a rapid and uniform rise-time, since the release sites ("active zones") are in close proximity to the highest postsynaptic density of acetylcholine receptors, i.e., opposite the crests of endplate folds (8).

I propose that a second kind of vesicular, quantal transmitter release also occurs from the nerve terminal, as depicted by II in Figure 11. This second type of release is independent of the intracellular calcium concentration and of transmembrane calcium fluxes and therefore uninfluenced by nerve terminal depolarization and by nerve stimuli. The release sites for these transmitter quanta are probably highly dispersed in the terminal, some being closer and some more distant from the acetylcholine receptors at the crests of the postsynaptic folds. Quantal release will therefore produce mepps with variable, generally prolonged rise-times. Depending upon whether single or clusters of vesicles are released from these sites, the amplitude of resulting mepps will be small or large. I suggest that quantal release from these sites is responsible for the small population of sub- and giant mepps seen at normal endplates. The characteristics of mepps caused by the proposed type II release are similar to those previously reported for spontaneous potentials at denervated motor endplates of the frog where quantal release of acetylcholine has been shown to occur from the Schwann cell

(9). In BoTx poisoning, the release, however, seems to originate from the nerve terminal, since no mepps are present after surgical denervation (2).

Furthermore, I propose that BoTx blocks type I release, but leaves type II intact. This would explain why the large population of fast-rising mepps with a bell-shaped amplitude distribution is abolished by BoTx and why only mepps with a low frequency, long rise-time and skew or bimodal amplitude distribution are left. Similarly, it would account for the block of depolarization-evoked transmitter release by BoTx.

It appears that after about 5 days of BoTx poisoning, a genuine increase occurs in the frequency of spontaneous mepps, resulting from type II release. An explanation for this might be that in poisoned nerves, the amount of acetylcholine is increased compared to normal (10) and that this might enhance spontaneous vesicular exocytosis. Another possibility is that nerve sprouting, which has been reported to start at about this time (11), accelerates type II synaptic vesicle exocytosis.

The block of type I release by BoTx is not absolute, since occasional quanta are released by nerve stimuli. Furthermore, it may be overcome by high intracellular calcium concentrations, as shown when a calcium ionophore or drugs like the aminopyridines are used. It suggests that BoTx interferes with, but does not irreversibly block, a calcium-sensitive step essential for this type of transmitter release. It is of interest that a calcium-binding protein recently has been extracted from synaptic membranes and that the incorporation of this protein into artificial lipid membranes enormously increases the fusion rate of phospholipid vesicles, but only in the presence of low concentrations of calcium (12). A selective interaction of the BoTx molecule with a protein regulating synaptic vesicle fusion and present only at "active zones" in nerve terminals might explain the high potency and specificity of the toxin for type I transmitter release.

BoTx probably blocks transmitter release following its internalization into the nerve terminal by endocytic uptake. In favour of internalization and an intracellular site of action are the kinetic studies of BoTx binding and block described by Simpson at this symposium. Furthermore, Habermann's presentation showing that tetanus toxin blocks neuromuscular transmission by a mode of action similar to BoTx suggests an intracellular site of action, since it is well-known that tetanus toxin is rapidly internalized in nerve terminals.

REFERENCES

1. Ambache, N., *J. Physiol. 198,* 121 (1949).
2. Cull-Candy, S. G., Lundh, H., and Thesleff, S., *J. Physiol. 260,* 177 (1976).
3. Bevan, S., *J. Physiol. 258,* 145 (1976).
4. Liley, A. W., *J. Physiol. 136,* 595 (1957).
5. Harris, A. J., and Miledi, R., *J. Physiol. 124,* 497 (1971).
6. del Castillo, J., and Katz, B., *J. Physiol. 124,* 560 (1954).
7. Couteaux, R., and Pécot-Dechavassine, M., *C. R. Acad. Sci. (Paris) D 271,* 2346 (1970).
8. Heuser, J. E., Reese, T. S., and Landis, D. M. D., *J. Neurocytol. 3,* 109 (1974).
9. Bevan, S., Grampp, W., and Miledi, R., *Proc. R. Soc. Lond. B 194,* 195 (1976).
10. Polak, R. L., Sellin, L. C., and Thesleff, S., *J. Physiol.* in press (1981).
11. Duchen, L. W., and Strich, S. J., *Q. J. Exp. Physiol. 53,* 84 (1968).
12. Zimmerberg, J., Cohen, F. S., and Finkelstein, A., *Science 210,* 906 (1980).
13. Molgo, J., Lundh, H., and Thesleff, S., *Eur. J. Pharmacol. 61,* 25 (1980).
14. Lundh, H., Leander, S., and Thesleff, S., *J. Neurol. Sci. 32,* 29 (1977).

POSTSYNAPTIC EFFECTS OF BOTULINUM TOXIN
AT THE NEUROMUSCULAR JUNCTION

Lawrence C. Sellin

Pathology Division
U. S. Army Medical Research
Institute of Infectious Diseases
Fort Detrick, Frederick, Maryland

INTRODUCTION

The action of botulinum toxin (BoTx) at the neuromuscular junction can be divided into presynaptic and postsynaptic effects. The toxin acts directly on the presynaptic nerve terminal where it inhibits the release of acetylcholine. Nonlethal doses of the toxin applied locally produce "denervation-like" effects on the postsynaptic junctional end-plate region and the extrajunctional muscle membrane, the sarcolemma. This results from the toxin's ability to interfere in an indirect way with the neurotrophic effect which the nerve normally exerts on the muscle (1). Neurotrophic effects may be defined as those functions of the nerve which regulate the biochemical, physiological, and morphological properties of the muscle fiber. The possible neurotrophic influences may be: nerve-induced muscle activity, the release of acetylcholine, the release of a yet unknown biochemical neurotrophic substance, or a combination of all of these (Fig. 1).

Denervation of mammalian skeletal muscle produces alterations in the electrical and chemosensitive properties of the muscle membrane. This paper presents data suggesting that nonlethal doses of BoTx produce a condition of partial denervation.

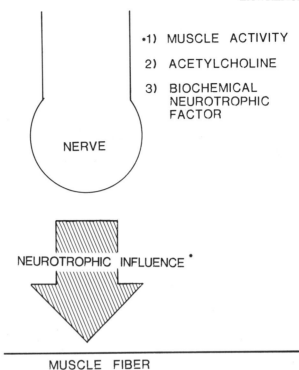

*1) MUSCLE ACTIVITY

2) ACETYLCHOLINE

3) BIOCHEMICAL
   NEUROTROPHIC
   FACTOR

NERVE

NEUROTROPHIC INFLUENCE *

MUSCLE FIBER

FIGURE 1.   BoTx acts indirectly on the postsynaptic muscle fiber by blocking neurotrophic influences. Since BoTx simultaneously inhibits the release of acetylcholine or another
neurotrophic substance and causes muscle paralysis; the specific neurotrophic influence affected remains to be elucidated.

MUSCLE ATROPHY

      The first postsynaptic effect reported after toxin injec-
tion, in addition to paralysis, was muscle atrophy (2). This
type of atrophy was shown to be similar in degree to that observed after surgical denervation (3). Between 2 weeks and 2
months after toxin injection into rats, muscle weight and
muscle fiber diameter decreased by 40%. The soleus muscle
showed a decrease in total fiber number due to some degeneration. However, the nerves innervating the affected muscles
were unchanged and the muscle spindles and intrafusal muscle
fibers were not significantly affected by the toxin. It is
interesting to note that, although fast-twitch and slow-twitch
muscles were paralyzed at the same time after toxin injection,
the soleus muscles became atrophic faster than the gastroc-
nemius (4).

RESTING MEMBRANE POTENTIAL

Surgical denervation of mammalian skeletal muscle produces
a 15-20 mV depolarization of the resting membrane potential
(E_m) within 1 week after nerve section (5, 6). Locally injected nonlethal doses of BoTx also cause muscle membrane depolarization. However, the time course and degree of depolarization may be different (Table 1).

TETRODOTOXIN-RESISTANT MUSCLE ACTION POTENTIALS

In normally innervated skeletal muscle, tetrodotoxin (TTX)
at concentrations between 10^{-5} and 10^{-6} M completely abolishes
directly elicited muscle action potentials, due to blockade of
sodium channels. After denervation, however, the muscle becomes partially resistant to the blocking action of TTX (8).
BoTx in a dose sufficient to cause complete paralysis is less
effective than surgical denervation in inducing the appearance
of TTX-resistant action potentials (7) (Fig. 2).

TABLE 1. *Resting Membrane Potential (E_m) from Extensor*
Digitorum Longus Muscles Recorded 8 Days after
Either Denervation or Injection of BoTx[a]

Control (mV)	Botulinum Toxin (mV)	Denervation (mV)
-75 ± 0.7[b]	-61 ± 0.8	-58 ± 0.7[c]
(58, 6)	(84, 9)	(66, 7)
≈ -80	-69 ± 0.5	-66 ± 0.6[d]
	(77, 6)	(28, 3)

[a] *Local nonlethal injection of 5-10 mouse LD_{50} of type A
toxin.*
[b] *Numbers in parentheses indicate total number of fibers
sampled and the number of muscles in each group, respectively.*
[c] *Sellin and Thesleff, rat muscle (unpublished).*
[d] *Mathers and Thesleff, mouse muscle (7).*

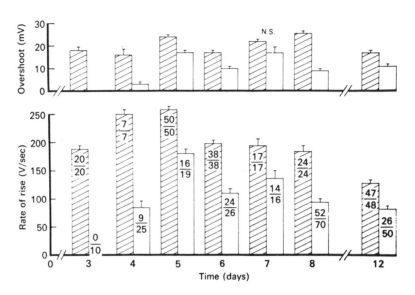

FIGURE 2. Maximum rates of rise and overshoot of action potentials in the presence of TTX (10^{-6} M) after the period of denervation (striped columns) or BoTx poisoning (open columns) as indicated on the ordinate. The columns give means $\pm$ S.E. of mean and the differences between denervated and BoTx poisoned muscles are significant at P < 0.005 with the exception of the value indicated by N.S. (Student's t test). The figures show the number of fibers responding with an action potential over the number of fibers examined (7, reprinted by permission).

EXTRAJUNCTIONAL ACETYLCHOLINE RECEPTORS

At the neuromuscular junction, acetylcholine (Ach) released from the presynaptic nerve terminal crosses the synaptic cleft by diffusion where the Ach molecules bind to specialized receptor proteins. The interaction of Ach with its postsynaptic receptors increases ionic permeability through channels at the end-plate region, resulting in depolarization of the muscle membrane and subsequent contraction of the muscle fibers. In normally innervated skeletal muscle, only the end-plate region, where receptors are present in high density (3×10^4 receptors/μm^2 of membrane), is sensitive to the depolarizing effect of Ach. Within 10-15 μm from the end-plate region, the density of receptors falls to less than 1/1000th that of the synaptic region (9).

After surgical denervation or during development (i.e., before innervation), receptors are distributed over the entire surface of the muscle membrane, where their density may be as high as 10^3 receptors/μm^2. The density of these "extrajunctional" receptors is several hundred times greater than that seen in innervated muscle, but remains less than the density of receptors at the synaptic region (9).

The new receptors appearing in the extrajunctional membrane are initially present as clusters randomly distributed over the membrane surface. While the junctional and extrajunctional receptors are basically similar (i.e., application of Ach still increases membrane permeability of sodium and potassium ions and the action of Ach is blocked by curare), they do differ in certain chemical and pharmacological properties, which suggests that they are different proteins (9, 10).

Thesleff (11) showed that after a local nonlethal injection of BoTx, the muscle became sensitive to applied Ach to a similar degree and with approximately the same time course as denervated muscle (Fig. 3). In a subsequent study (12), other investigators demonstrated that the number of extrajunctional Ach receptors induced by BoTx poisoning was somewhat less than that induced by denervation. Since the toxic effect occurs without any apparent ultrastructural change in the nerve terminal, it is unlikely that the "denervation-like" effects are the result of nerve degeneration (11).

END-PLATE ION CHANNELS

Loring and Salpeter (13) reported that, following denervation, the apparent halftime of receptor turnover at the end-plate is only 2-3 days, compared to 10 days in the innervated end-plate, and about 1 day in the extrajunctional membrane of denervated muscles. One interpretation was that the end-plate after denervation contains a dual population of receptors: the original receptors with a slow turnover time and new ones with a turnover rate similar to that of extrajunctional receptors (14). Several investigators have reported that the receptors which are inserted extrajunctionally, following denervation, or at the end-plate, during embryonic development,

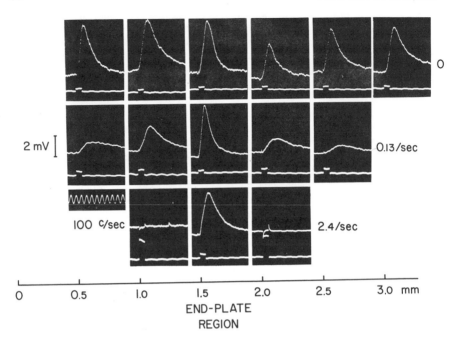

FIGURE 3. In a tenuissimus muscle, intoxicated 3 weeks
earlier with a small amount of BoTx, muscle fibers were observed in which the Ach-sensitive surface varied in size. The
sensitivity of the membrane to Ach was tested by iontophoretic
micro-application of the drug. The membrane potential of the
fiber is recorded in the upper tracing of each record and the
current passing through the pipette in the lower tracing. The
fiber used for the upper records was uniformly sensitive to
applied Ach over a distance of at least 1.5 mm at each of the
end-plates. The size of the Ach-sensitive surface in two
other fibers was smaller (middle and lower records). The frequencies at which m.e.p.p. occurred are shown by the figures
to the right of the records (Thesleff, 11, reprinted by permission).

have a single channel[2] lifetime which is prolonged compared to
the receptors at the innervated adult end-plate (15-18).
Therefore, it was of interest to study the possible

[2] Acetylcholine receptors and these ion channels appear to
be two distinct entities, although they act in unison and are
always present together. For the sake of discussion, if not
clarity, they will be treated as a single unit.

alterations in the properties of end-plate ion channels due to chronic presynaptic blockade by BoTx.

Acetylcholine is synthesized in the motor nerve terminal, packaged, and released in vesicles as "quantal" units. The vesicles or quanta are released individually in a spontaneous and random fashion, or simultaneously in large numbers as a result of nerve stimulation. As mentioned in the previous section, Ach released from the nerve terminal binds with specific receptors on the postsynaptic end-plate regions and causes an increase in ionic permeability through channels in the membrane. It is possible to measure the electrical current due to this change in permeability by voltage clamp techniques, where a single spontaneously released quantum produces a miniature end-plate current (m.e.p.c.) and nerve-evoked multiple quantal release produces a larger postsynaptic response called an end-plate current (e.p.c.).

An analysis of m.e.p.c and e.p.c. by voltage clamp can be useful in elucidating the effects of BoTx poisoning on transmitter-receptor interactions at the end-plate, particularly those affecting the time course of these currents. Gage and McBurney (19) showed that the growth and decay phases of m.e.p.c. were governed by processes with different characteristics. They demonstrated that the growth phase was nonexponential, relatively insensitive to changes in clamp potential, and had a low Q_{10}[3]. In contrast, the decay phase was exponential, voltage-sensitive, and had a high Q_{10}. They suggested that the growth phase was determined by the rate of arrival of Ach at the postsynaptic receptors, while the factors controlling the decay phase were related either to the dissociation time of Ach from its receptor (20), or to a conformational change in a macromolecule with a dipole moment in the postsynaptic membrane (21). Thus, the growth phase results primarily from the transmitter release process or a presynaptic phenomenon, while the decay phase is related to the properties of the postsynaptic ion channel. Since, the presynaptic effects were discussed in a previous paper, this discussion will concentrate on the decay phase of the currents, which is primarily postsynaptic.

The decay phases of e.p.c and m.e.p.c. were shown to be affected by BoTx poisoning (22, Fig. 4). The time constant of the decay phase was not different from normal at 2 days after BoTx injection. However, at 7 days, the time constant of the decay phase was approximately twice that of normal muscle in both m.e.p.c. and e.p.c. Although BoTx poisoning prolonged

[3]Q_{10} is the alteration in magnitude of any measurable parameter as a function of a 10°C change in temperature.

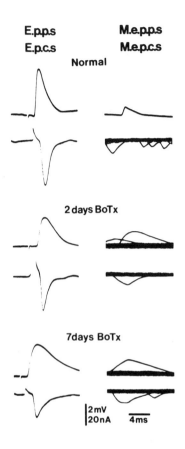

FIGURE 4. Examples of end-plate potentials (e.p.p., miniature end-plate potentials (m.e.p.p.), end-plate currents
(e.p.c.), and miniature end-plate currents (m.e.p.c.) recorded
from normal, and BoTx-poisoned muscles at 2 and 7 days. The
current recordings were made at a holding potential of -80 mV.
For the recording of e.p.c., transmitter release was depressed
in normal muscles by the addition of 12 Mg^{++} to the suffusate
(Sellin and Thesleff, 22, reprinted by permission).

the growth phase of m.e.p.c., the decay phase could still be
characterized by a simple exponential function (Fig. 5).
    The effect of membrane potential on the time constant (τ)
of the decay phase of m.e.p.c. for normal and BoTx-treated
muscles is shown in Figure 5. The relationship between the

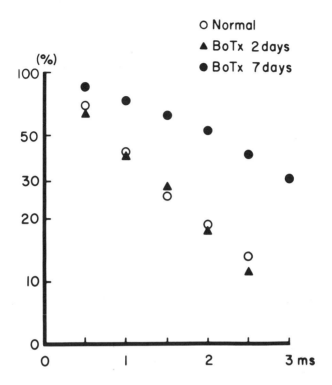

FIGURE 5. The time course of the decay phase of miniature end-plate currents recorded from normal and BoTx-treated
muscles are plotted semilogarithmically as a function of time
after peak current is attained. The normal (o), 2 days
after BoTx injection (Δ), and 7 days after BoTx injection
(●) were recorded from end-plates voltage-clamped at 80 mV
(Sellin and Thesleff, 22, reprinted by permission).

membrane potential and the time constant of the decay phase
has been described (22) as:

$$\tau(V) = \tau(0) \exp^{V/H},$$

where (V) is the time constant at clamped potential V, $\tau(0)$
is the time constant at zero potential, and H is the constant
indicating the voltage sensitivity. That is, H is the change
in membrane potential required to produce an e-fold change in
the time constant. This equation predicts an exponential

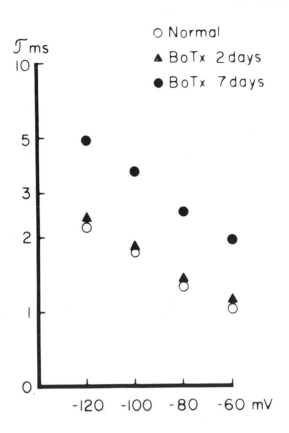

FIGURE 6. The mean time constant (τ) for the decay phase
of miniature end-plate currents recorded from normal (o),
2- (Δ), and 7- (●) day BoTx-treated muscles are plotted
semilogarithmically as a function of holding potential (Sellin
and Thesleff, 22, reprinted by permission).

decrease in τ as V goes in the depolarizing direction. The
results of the present experiment fulfilled this criterion
(Fig. 6).
    At 2 days after toxin injection, the time constant of the
decay phase of m.e.p.c. was unchanged from normal at all voltages examined. However, 7 days after toxin injection, the
time constant of the decay phase was increased compared to
normal muscle at all voltages (Fig. 6). This increase in the
time constant was accompanied by a decrease in the calculated
voltage sensitivity constant H, which was 75, 78, and 64 mV
for normal, 2-day, and 7-day BoTx-treated muscles, respectively.

The marked prolongation of the decay phase of m.e.p.c. and e.p.c seen 7 days after BoTx treatment suggests the appearance of receptors at the end-plate which have an increased channel open time, i.e., similar to those observed in the extrajunctional membrane of denervated muscle (19).

The possibility that the prolongation of the decay phase resulted from a repetitive binding of Ach to its receptor because of diminished cholinesterase activity cannot be excluded, but appears less likely, since BoTx-poisoned nerve terminals under appropriate conditions release transmitter quanta without a shift in the amplitude distribution towards higher values (23-25). Furthermore, there was an increase in the voltage sensitivity of the decay phase of m.e.p.c. indicative of altered receptor-channel properties which is not seen with cholinesterase inhibition alone (21).

CONCLUSIONS

These data indicate that BoTx may produce long-term alterations in the postsynaptic muscle membrane. These changes are not produced by direct action of the toxin, but by its ability to interfere with a trophic influence of neuronal origin, whether it be muscle activity, acetylcholine, or some yet unknown biochemical substance. It is clear, however, that the postsynaptic alterations due to BoTx poisoning are similar in mode, but not degree, to those changes observed after surgical denervation.

ACKNOWLEDGMENTS

The views of the author do not purport to reflect the positions of the Department of the Army or the Department of Defense.

REFERENCES

1. Drachman, D. B., *Ann. N.Y. Acad. Sci. 228,* 160 (1974).
2. Guyton, A. C., and MacDonald, M. A., *Arch. Neurol. Psychiatr. 57,* 578 (1947).

3. Jirmanová, I., Sobotková, M., Thesleff, S., and Zelena, J., *Physiol. Bohemoslov. 13*, 467 (1964).
4. Duchen, L. W., *J. Neurol. Neurosurg. Psychiatr. 33*, 40 (1970).
5. Albuquerque, E. X., and Thesleff, S., *Acta Physiol. Scand. 73*, 471 (1968).
6. Albuquerque, E. X., Schuh, F. T., and Kauffman, F. C., *Pfluegers Arch. 328*, 36 (1971).
7. Mathers, D. A., and Thesleff, S., *J. Physiol. (London) 282*, 105 (1978).
8. Redfern, P., and Thesleff, S., *Acta Physiol. Scand. 82*, 70 (1971).
9. Thesleff, S., and Sellin, L. C., *Trends Neurosci. 3*, 122 (1980).
10. Dolly, J. O., *Int. Rev. Biochem. 26*, 257 (1979).
11. Thesleff, S., *J. Physiol. (London) 151*, 598 (1960).
12. Pestronk, A., Drachman, D. B., and Griffin, J. W., *Nature 264*, 787 (1976).
13. Loring, R. H., and Salpeter, M. M., *Proc. Natl. Acad. Sci. (U.S.A.) 77*, 2293 (1980).
14. Levitt, T. A., Loring, R. H., and Salpeter, M. M., *Science 210*, 550 (1980).
15. Dreyer, F., Müller, K. D., Peper, K., and Sterz, R., *Pfluegers Arch. 367*, 115 (1976).
16. Sakmann, B., *Fed. Proc. 37*, 2654 (1978).
17. Gage, P. W., and Hamill, P. P., *J. Physiol. (London) 298*, 525 (1980).
18. Fischbach, G. D., and Schuetze, S. M., *J. Physiol. (London) 303*, 125 (1980).
19. Gage, P. W., and McBurney, R. N., *J. Physiol. (London) 244*, 385 (1975).
20. Adams, P. R., and Sakmann, B., *J. Physiol. (London) 283*, 621 (1978).
21. Magleby, K. L., and Stevens, C. F., *J. Physiol. (London) 223*, 151 (1972).
22. Sellin, L. C., and Thesleff, S., *J. Physiol. (London)* in press (1981).
23. Spitzer, N., *Nature New Biol. 237*, 26 (1972).
24. Boroff, D. A., del Castillo, J., Evoy, W. H., and Steinhardt, R. A., *J. Physiol. (London) 240*, 227 (1974).
25. Cull-Candy, S. G., Lundh, H., and Thesleff, S., *J. Physiol. (London) 260*, 177 (1976).

RELATIONSHIP OF BACTERIOPHAGES
TO THE TOXIGENICITY OF *CLOSTRIDIUM BOTULINUM*
AND CLOSELY RELATED ORGANISMS

M. W. Eklund
F. T. Poysky

Northwest and Alaska Fisheries Center
Seattle, Washington

INTRODUCTION

The most important characteristic in the identification
and differentiation of the pathogenic clostridia is the production of toxins. Based upon the production of antigenically
specific neurotoxins, the species *Clostridium botulinum* is
divided into types A through G. Even though the different
toxin types represent a heterogenous group of strains, they
have been placed into one species because of the similar pharmacological action of the toxins. When biochemical, physiological, and serological characteristics and deoxyribonucleic
acid homologies are used to characterize the different *C.
botulinum* strains, this species can be separated into four
groups. Group I cultures are proteolytic and produce toxin
types A, A_F, B, and F; group II cultures are nonproteolytic
and produce toxin types B, E, and F; group III cultures are
nonproteolytic and produce toxin types C_1, C_2, and D; and
group IV cultures are weakly proteolytic and produce toxin
type G.

The loss of the toxigenic characteristic has been observed
in pure cultures of *C. botulinum* during culture in laboratory
media. In addition, nontoxigenic clostridia resembling *C.
botulinum* have been isolated frequently from aquatic and ter-
restrial environments. The occurrence of nontoxigenic

[1]*This work was supported in part by the U.S. Army Research
Office.*

cultures coupled with the observations that all types of C. *botulinum* carry bacteriophages (2,3,14,24) suggested that the production of toxins by C. *botulinum* might be mediated by bacteriophages or plasmids analogous to the production of toxin by *Corynebacterium diphtheriae* (1,10,11).

This report provides evidence for the involvement of specific bacteriophages in the toxigenicity of C. *botulinum* types C and D and closely related organisms.

BACTERIOPHAGES AND THE TOXIGENICITY OF C. *BOTULINUM* TYPES C AND D

C. *botulinum* types C and D produce at least three different toxins designated as C_1, C_2, and D (5,7,17). Type C strains produce predominantly C_1 toxin and minor amounts of C_2 and D toxins. In contrast, type D strains produce predominantly D toxin and minor amounts of C_1 and C_2 toxins. The minor toxins are not produced by all strains of types C and D.

The relationship of bacteriophages to the toxigenicity of C. *botulinum* was first observed in type C and D strains (4,6, 15,16). Nontoxigenic derivatives were isolated from toxigenic strains following acridine orange or ultraviolet irradiation treatments. When these nontoxigenic derivatives were infected with bacteriophages from the toxigenic parent culture, toxigenic isolates were again recovered.

The roles that different bacteriophage play in the toxigenicity and in the interrelationship of C. *botulinum* types C and D and closely related organisms are discussed in further detail in the following sections of this paper.

Toxigenicity of Type C Strains

A bacterial culture is generally immune to the infection by bacteriophages that it carries or to antigenically related bacteriophages that are produced by other cultures. In order to determine the relationship of bacteriophages to the toxigenicity of a bacterial strain, one must therefore isolate bacteriophage-sensitive derivatives, preferably from known toxigenic strains.

Strain 468C was the first culture used in our laboratory to study the involvement of bacteriophages in the toxigenicity of type C cultures. This strain was grown in trypticase, yeast-extract glucose (TYG) medium containing acridine orange (AO) or cultures in logarithmic phase of growth were treated with ultraviolet (UV) irradiation to cure them of their prophages. Surviving colonies that developed on TYG agar following anaerobic incubation were tested for sensitivity to the parent phages. After a 60-second treatment with ultra-violet light, 15 of 106 cultures tested were cured of pro-phages and concomitantly ceased to produce C_1 and D toxins. In comparison, 2 of 68 colonies tested from the acridine orange treatment were cured of their prophages and toxigenic characteristic.

The inability of these phage-sensitive cultures to produce C_1 and D toxins was confirmed during subsequent passages in laboratory medium and indicated that the loss of the toxigenic characteristic was permanent. Later, it was learned (5) that the production of C_2 toxin was not governed by bacteriophages and that phage-sensitive cultures continued to produce C_2 toxin. This toxin, however, was detectable only after acti-vation with trypsin. For simplicity, the term "nontoxigenic" will be used hereafter in reference to cultures that failed to produce C_1 and D toxins.

To determine whether more than one bacteriophage was pro-duced by 468C, each phage-sensitive "nontoxigenic" derivative was tested for its sensitivity to the lysates of other cured derivatives using the agar-layer procedure (4,6). Derivative AO28 was the only isolate that was sensitive to the lysates of other cured cultures. This culture had therefore been cured of two of its prophages. Colony-centered plaques (phage $1C^{tox+}$) and turbid plaques (phage $2C^{tox-}$) were produced on bacterial lawns of strain AO28 by phages isolated from cell-free lysates of the parent strain 468C. These phages were purified by five successive single-plaque isolations on strain AO28.

Table 1. Relation of Phages of Type C Strain 468C to Toxigenicity and Sensitivity of Strain AO28

Bacterial strain and phage	Toxigenicity[a]	Sensitivity to phage	
		1C	2C
AO28	−	+	+
AO28 (1C)	+	−	+
AO28 (2C)	−	+	−
AO28 (1C, 2C)	+	−	−

[a]Production of predominant C_1 and minor D toxin

The relationship of each of these phages to the toxigenicity of strain AO28 was studied using procedures previously described (4). Table 1 summarizes the results of these experiments. When strain AO28 was infected with phage 1C, it concomitantly produced dominant C_1 and minor D toxins and displayed immunity to infection by the homologous phage. Phage 2C, however, did not induce strain AO28 to produce C_1 and D toxins, but the infected cultures, and all other cultures irrespective of phage involvement, did continue to produce C_2 toxin.

To determine whether the continued participation of phage 1C was necessary to maintain toxigenicity, strain AO28 (1C) was cultured in TYG medium containing antiserum against phage 1C and plated on TYG agar. Isolates that were resistant to phage 1C continued to carry phage 1C and to produce C_1 and D toxins. On the other hand, isolates cured of phage 1C simultaneously ceased to produce C_1 and D toxins. These "nontoxigenic" isolates, however, resumed the production of C_1 and D toxins after they were reinfected with phage 1C. This curing and reinfection cycle was repeated with strain AO28 and other "nontoxigenic" isolates from type C strain 468C and in every case the production of the C_1 and D toxins depended upon the continued participation of phage 1C. These results therefore emphasize the necessity of specific phages in the production of C_1 and D toxins by *C. botulinum* type C.

Strains of type C isolated from the different areas of the world were also examined to determine whether their phages also governed toxigenicity. In these experiments, spores from different strains were heated to 70°C for 15 minutes to inactivate free phage and plated on TYG agar. Vegetative cells were grown in TYG broth containing acridine orange or treated with ultraviolet irradiation and survivors plated on TYG agar. After anaerobic incubation, isolates were tested for phage-sensitivity and toxin production. All three methods yielded phage-sensitive derivatives which had simultaneously lost their ability to produce C_1 and D toxins. Strain 164 lost its phage and toxigenic characteristic during passage in EM medium (Table 2). Each of the "nontoxigenic" derivatives except the isolates from strain 6816 could be converted back to the toxigenic state (again produced C_1 and D toxins) when they were reinfected with specific TOX^+ bacteriophages from the toxigenic parent cultures. These converted cultures continued to produce TOX^+ phages and C_1 and D toxins during subculture in TYG or egg meat medium (EM). They also responded like type C strain 468C in being immune to the infection by the TOX^+ phages of the parent strain as long as they remained toxigenic and carried the corresponding TOX^+ phage.

With the exception of strain 162 or its phage-sensitive derivatives, all strains of type C produced the C_2 toxin

Table 2. *Relation of bacteriophages to the toxigenicity of different strains of C. botulinum type C*

Strain number	Method of obtaining cured cultures	Number of cultures		Producing C_2 toxin	Converted to toxigenicity by phage
		Tested	"Nontoxic"		
6816	Acridine orange	80	3	+	−
165	Spores	80	2	+	+
153	Spores	58	8	+	+
162	Acridine orange	64	2	−	+
162	Spores	40	1	−	+
3296	Spores	79	9	+	+
571	Spores	73	7	+	+
C_3	Acridine orange	92	9	+	+
C_8	Acridine orange	78	20	+	+
203	Acridine orange	89	5	+	+
2337	Acridine orange	102	40	+	+
6513	Acridine orange	160	86	+	+
SKM	Acridine orange	105	5	+	+
468C	Acridine orange	68	2	+	+
468C	Ultraviolet	106	15	+	+
460	Acridine orange	63	25	+	+
164	Passage in media	−−	−−	+	+

before and after they were cured of their TOX$^+$ prophages (Table 2). These results confirmed the earlier findings that the production of C_2 toxin was not governed by any of the bacteriophages used in these studies.

When the "nontoxigenic" isolates were tested for their sensitivity to the purified phages of the different type C cultures, five of the isolates were sensitive to numerous TOX$^+$ phages produced by toxigenic type C strains (Table 3). The remaining ten derivatives were sensitive only to the phages of the toxigenic parent culture. Each of the TOX$^+$ phages converted the "nontoxigenic" strains to the toxigenic state. Similar results have been reported with other type C strains (12,13,20-23). These results indicate that specific TOX$^+$ phages play a common role in the toxigenicity of different strains of type C.

Toxigenicity of Type D strains

The same procedures used to determine the involvement of bacteriophages in the toxigenicity of type C strains were also employed to study the toxigenicity of type D strains 1873 and South African. Strain 1873 produced the dominant D toxins and minor toxins C_1 and C_2. The South African strain, however, produced only the dominant D toxin.

*Table 3. Host Range of Bacteriophages Isolated
from C. botulinum Type C Strains*

		Number of type C strains	
"Nontoxigenic" host	*Tested*	*Produced phage that infected "nontoxigenic" host*	*Converted "nontoxigenics" to toxigenic state*
AO50	21	13	13
AO28	21	12	12
HS46	21	10	10
HS31	21	8	8
HS34	21	12	12

When the South African strain of type D was studied, a greater number of "nontoxigenic" isolates were obtained from sporulated cultures than from vegetative cells cultures in TYG medium containing acridine orange. All of the "nontoxigenic" isolates from both sources were sensitive to phage $1D^{tox+}$ from the toxigenic parent culture. This phage converted each isolate to produce the dominant type D toxin. Toxigenic isolates continued to carry and to be immune to phage 1D.

Further studies were made with "nontoxigenic" isolate AO20. This isolate maintained its "nontoxigenic" state and sensitivity to phage 1D during numerous passages in EM medium over a 5-year period. It also maintained the toxigenic characteristic as long as it was infected with phage 1D. Strain AO20 (1D) was permitted to sporulate and the spores were washed, centrifuged, and plated on TYG agar. Following anaerobic incubation, colonies were again tested for their toxigenicity and phage-sensitivity. Of the 39 isolates selected, 19 were "nontoxigenic" and sensitive to phage 1D. After infection with phage 1D, each of the 19 isolates were converted to the toxigenic state and continued to produce type D toxin as long as they carried phage 1D. Occasionally, a toxigenic culture would become "nontoxigenic" during passage in EM medium. These "nontoxigenic" cultures were invariably sensitive to phage 1D and could be converted to the toxigenic state merely by phage infection.

These studies were also extended to type D strain 1873 to determine whether phages were involved in the toxigenicity of other type D strains that produce not only dominant D toxin but also minor C_1 and C_2 toxins. This toxigenic culture carried two phages designated as phage $2D^{tox+}$ and $3D^{tox-}$. Of 214 isolates examined from strain 1873 following acridine orange treatment, 23 were "nontoxigenic" and sensitive to phage $2D^{tox+}$. One of these isolates, AOA113, was also sensitive to phage $3D^{tox-}$. Phage 2D converted each of the "nontoxigenic" isolates to the toxigenic state and dominant D and minor C_1 toxins were again produced. Phage 3D, however, did not participate in the production of any of these toxins. All of the "nontoxigenic" and toxigenic isolates from strain 1873 continued to produce C_2 toxin which required trypsin activation to demonstrate toxicity.

Strain 1873 resembled the South African strain in that subcultures would occasionally lose their ability to produce D and C_1 toxins. These "nontoxigenic" cultures were always sensitive to phage 2D and could be converted to the toxigenic state by phage 2D.

Production of C₂ Toxin by Type C and D Cultures

Of the 21 different type C cultures isolated from six
different countries, all except one produced C_2 toxin. This
strain was isolated in England. The C_2 toxin from 15 of the
strains cultured in EM medium required trypsin activation
before toxin could be detected.

Type C cultures that had lost their toxigenic properties
during transfer in laboratory media were received from other
research laboratories labeled as "nontoxigenic" strains.
Even though these strains did not produce C_1 and D toxins, 8
of the 15 strains did produce C_2 toxin which was detectable
only after trypsin activation.

Recent studies indicate that the production of the C_2
toxin is correlated with the sporulation of type C cultures
(18). The larger the sporulation, the higher the titer of C_2
toxin. When the spore populations were less than 10^4/ml of
culture, C_2 toxin was not detectable in the culture supernatant fluids.

The optimum pH for trypsin activation of toxins from nonproteolytic strains of *C. botulinum* types B, E, and F is 6.0.
When C_2 toxin was studied, the highest titers were obtained
following trypsin activation at pH 6.5 (5).

Strain 1873 was the only type D culture that produced C_2
toxin. This toxin required trypsin treatment to demonstrate
toxicity and was neutralized by antiserum prepared against
the toxin of type C strain 468C. The C_2 toxins from type C
and D strains therefore appear to be antigenically closely
related (5).

INTERCONVERSION OF *C. BOTULINUM* TYPE C AND D STRAINS BY
BACTERIOPHAGES

Strain 1873 was identified as *C. botulinum* type D because
it produced the dominant D toxin. When strain 1873 was cured
of phage $2D^{tox+}$, it could no longer be classified as type D
because of its inability to produce D toxin. These "nontoxigenic" phage-sensitive derivatives, however, continued to
produce C_2 toxin and became indistinguishable from "nontoxigenic" type C cultures.

The similarities in the characteristics of these cured
derivatives of type C and D strains suggested that type C and
D strains might arise from a common culture infected with different phages. To test this hypothesis, strain AOA113 was
tested for its sensitivity to the phages of different type C
strains. Phage $4C^{tox+}$ from type C strain 153 infected AOA113

and converted it to the toxigenic state in which C_1 toxin was dominant. When the cured derivatives of type C were tested for their sensitivity to phage $2D^{tox+}$ from 1873, only derivative HS15 from type C strain 153 was sensitive. Phage 2D converted HS15 to the toxigenic state and D toxin was dominant. As a result, derivatives HS15 and AOA113 became common hosts for both type D phage 2D and type C phage 4C. These cultures could therefore be converted to type D or to a type C merely by exchanging the TOX^+ phage (Table 5). Cultures infected with phage 4C were immune to infection by phage 2D and vice versa. Each culture irrespective of phage involvement produced C_2 toxin that required trypsin treatment to demonstrate toxicity.

Cultures AOA113(4C), AOA113(2D), HS15(4C), and HS15(2D) were permitted to sporulate and "nontoxigenic" derivatives were again isolated. These derivatives each became sensitive to phages 4C and 2D and when infected they again produced the dominant C_1 or D toxins, respectively.

These curing and reinfecting experiments were repeated three times and in each instance the production of toxin and the toxin type depended upon the continued presence of specific TOX^+ phages.

Interconversion of types C and D by bacteriophages was also observed in another group of strains that did not produce C_2 toxin. Strain HS37 (derived from type C strain 162) was not only sensitive to phage $3C^{tox+}$ of the parent strain but also to phage $1D^{tox+}$ from the South African strain of type D. Table 6 summarizes the results of the relationship of phage 1D and 3C to the type of toxin produced by strain

Table 5. *Relation of Bacteriophages 2D and 4C to the Toxigenicity of Bacterial Strains AOA113 and HS15*

| "Nontoxigenic" cured cultures | Phage | Number of cultures | | Toxin neutralized by antiserum |
		Toxigenic and phage producers	Tested	
AOA113	2D	20	20	Type D
AOA113	4C	37	37	Type C
HS15	2D	20	20	Type D
HS15	4C	20	20	Type C

Table 6. Relation of Bacteriophages 1D and 3C
to the Toxigenicity of Strain HS37

| Infecting phage | Number of cultures | | Toxin neutralized by antiserum |
	Tested	Converted to toxigenic state	
1D	40	30	Type D
3C	40	40	Type C

HS37. Infection of HS37 with phage 3C resulted in the production of dominant C_1 toxin whereas infection with phage 1D resulted in the production of the dominant D toxin. Of 40 TYG cultures arising from plaque material from phage 1D, only 30 were toxigenic. The ten "nontoxigenic" isolates were retested and found to be phage-sensitive and capable of producing D toxin when they were infected with phage 1D.

Strain HS37(1D) produced only 10 MLD of D toxin per ml. When the culture supernatant fluid was treated with trypsin, the toxicity increased to 2000 MLD/ml. In contrast, the South African type D strain which also carried phage 1D produced 10,000 MLD/ml of type D toxin and the titer was increased only 10-fold by trypsin treatment. This difference in the toxicity suggests a difference in the enzymes produced by the two cultures.

Strain HS37 (1D) often lost its phage and reverted to the "nontoxigenic" state after three or four transfers in TYG or EM medium. The production of the D toxin could be restored by merely reinfecting the "nontoxigenic" isolates with phage 1D. The maintenance of phage 1D and toxigenicity by strain HS37 could be continued for longer periods of time when the EM medium contained 2% sodium chloride.

INTERSPECIES CONVERSION OF *CLOSTRIDIUM BOTULINUM* TYPE C TO *CLOSTRIDIUM NOVYI* TYPE A BY BACTERIOPHAGES

C. botulinum and C. novyi are pathogenic anaerobes that are characterized by their ability to produce powerful toxins.

The *C. botulinum* group produce neuroparalytic toxins that are
responsible for botulism in man and animals. *C. novyi* also
produce lethal toxins and are often found in gas gangrene
infections of man and in other diseases of animals.
    The species *C. novyi* includes a heterogenous group of
organisms that is divided into types A, B, C, and D on the
basis of different toxins produced. The production of lethal
alpha toxin is the characteristic that unites types A and B.
When types A and B strains were cured of their TOX$^+$ phages,
they discontinued the production of the alpha toxin. As a
result, "nontoxigenic" type A cultures no longer resembled the
other *C. novyi* types, but instead became closely related to
"nontoxigenic" *C. botulinum* type C and D strains (8,9). In
comparison, when the *C. novyi* type B strains lost their TOX$^+$
phages and ceased to produce alpha toxin, they closely resembled *C. novyi* type D *(C. haemolyticum)* in that they continued
to produce the same lethal beta toxin and other minor antigens. The main characteristic in the identification and differentiation of *C. botulinum* types C and D and *C. novyi* type
A therefore is the toxins produced.
    To determine the relationship of these two clostridial
species, the phage-sensitive "nontoxigenic" derivatives of
types C and D were tested for their sensitivity to the phages
of 8 different strains of *C. novyi* type A. Strain HS37 (from
type C strain 162) was found to be sensitive to the phages of
C. novyi type A strain 5771. Cell-free lysates of strain 5771
contained two different phages. When phage NA1^{tox+} infected
strain HS37, the culture concomitantly produced the lethal
alpha toxin of *C. novyi*. Phage NA2^{tox-} also infected strain
HS37, but showed no relationship to any of the toxins produced.
    In earlier sections of this paper, strain HS37 was
reported to be sensitive to type D phage 1D and type C phage
3C. The relationship of the phages NA1, 1D, and 3C to the
toxigenicity of strain HS37 therefore was studied. When type
C strain 162 was cured of phage 3C, it became "nontoxigenic"
and a common host to phages NA1, 1D, and 3C (Table 7). Infection of strain HS37 with phage NA1 converted it to *C. novyi*
type A and dominant alpha toxin was produced. If this culture
was cured of phage NA1 and infected with phage 3C, then it was
converted to *C. botulinum* type C, and the C_1 toxin was dominant. Phage-sensitive derivatives isolated from type C culture HS37 (3C) could then be infected with phage 1D and the
culture was identified as type D because of the dominant D
toxin. A phage-sensitive strain of clostridia therefore could
be converted to *C. botulinum* type C or type D or to *C. novyi*
type A by merely exchanging the bacteriophages. These

Table 7. Effect of Different Phage on Toxigenicity
of Strain HS37

| Phage | Number of cultures | | | Neutralized by antiserum of: |
	Tested	Toxic	Produce phage	
$3C^{tox+}$	40	40	40	C. botulinum type C
$1D^{tox+}$	40	40	40	C. botulinum type D
$NA1^{tox+}$	40	40	40	C. novyi type A
$NA2^{tox-}$	40	0	40	-------------------

studies show that the toxigenicity of *C. botulinum* types C and
D and *C. novyi* types A and B depends upon the continued participation of specific TOX$^+$ phages.

STABILITY OF PHAGE HOST RELATIONSHIP

The high frequency of isolating "nontoxigenic" phage-
sensitive derivatives from toxigenic strains of *C. botulinum*
types C and D and *C. novyi* types A and B following acridine
orange and untraviolet irradiation treatments indicated that
the phage-host relationship was unstable. Further evidence of
this instability was obtained when isolates from toxigenic
sporulated cultures were tested for their phage immunity and
toxigenicity (Table 8). Even though the degree of instability
varied markedly from strain to strain, all of the toxigenic
strains yielded isolates that had lost their phages and immunity. These results suggested that a pseudolysogenic relationship existed between the phage and host.
    In order to confirm these findings, toxigenic strains were
transferred twice a day in TYG medium containing antiserum
against the specific phages. Examples of the results are summarized in Table 9. A very high percentage of the isolates
tested were phage-sensitive, and this percentage increased as
the number of passages in phage antiserum increased. These
results imply that the bacterial cells lose their phages
during culture but are protected from reinfection by phage

Table 8. Loss of Phage and Toxigenicity through Spore State
of C. botulinum Type C and C. novyi Type A

Strain	Number of colonies	
	Tested	"Nontoxigenic" and phage-sensitive
3296^a	79	9
571	73	7
165	80	2
460	23	12
J C	97	9
162	40	4
SKM	30	6
C_3	40	4
C_8	20	20
203	89	5
X-200	40	39
2337	40	40
6513	86	16
468C	37	10
201	2	2
SA^b	39	19
5771^c	50	25

[a]C. botulinum type C strain
[b]C. botulinum type D
[c]C. novyi type A

antiserum. In the absence of antiserum, toxigenic cultures
also lose their phages, but they can be reinfected by free
phages which are present in an actively growing culture.
These different results therefore support the fact that a
pseudolysogenic relationship exists between phages and their
host in C. botulinum types C and D and C. novyi type A and B
strains.

Results from these studies demonstrate the important role
that specific phages play in the production of C. botulinum
C_1 and D toxins and the alpha toxin of C. novyi types A and B.
Because of the pseudolysogenic relationship between the host
and phage, these cultures occasionally lose their phages in
nature and become "nontoxigenic." Depending on the presence

Table 9. *Effect of Cultivation of Toxigenic Cultures*
in TOX+ phage antiserum on phage-sensitivity and toxigenicity

Strain	Number of transfers in antiserum	Number of cultures	
		Tested	Phage-sensitive and "nontoxigenic"
SKM[a]	3	40	6
	7	40	15
468C[a]	7	39	27
S.A.[b]	7	37	29
8024[c]	6	194	19

[a]*C. botulinum type C*
[b]*C. botulinum type D*
[c]*C. novyi type B*

of other phages, these "nontoxigenic" strains could be induced to produce *C. botulinum* toxins C_1 or D or the alpha toxin of *C. novyi*. Because of this role, these bacteriophages are very important to the identification of the pathogenic clostridia and also to the corresponding disease that they cause.

REFERENCES

1. Barksdale, W. L., and Pappenheimer, A. M., *J. Bacteriol.* 67, 220 (1954).
2. Dolman, C. E., and Chang, E., *Can. J. Microbiol.* 18, 67 (1972).
3. Eklund, M. W., Poysky, F. T., and Boatman, E. S., *J. Virol.* 3, 270 (1969).
4. Eklund, M. W., Poysky, F. T., Reed, S. M., and Smith, C. A., *Science* 172, 480 (1971).
5. Eklund, M. W., and Poysky, F. T., *Appl. Microbiol.* 24, 108 (1972).
6. Eklund, M. W., Poysky, F. T., and Reed, S. M., *Nature (London) New Biol.* 235, 16 (1972).
7. Eklund, M. W., and Poysky, F. T., *Appl. Microbiol.* 27, 251 (1974).

8. Eklund, M. W., Poysky, F. T., Meyers, J. A., and Pelroy, G. A., *Science 186*, 456 (1974).
9. Eklund, M. W., Poysky, F. T., Peterson, M. E., and Meyers, J. A., *Infect. Immun. 14*, 793 (1976).
10. Freeman, V. J., *J. Bacteriol. 61*, 675 (1951).
11. Groman, N. B., *J. Bacteriol. 69*, 9 (1955).
12. Hariharan, H., and Mitchell, W. R., *Appl. Environ. Microbiol. 32*, 145 (1976).
13. Iida, H, and Inoue, K., *Japan. J. Microbiol. 12*, 353 (1968).
14. Inoue, K., and Iida, H., *J. Virol. 2*, 537 (1968).
15. Inoue, K., and Iida, H., *Japan. J. Microbiol. 14*, 87 (1970).
16. Inoue, K., and Iida, H., *Japan. J. Med. Sci. Biol. 24*, 53 (1971).
17. Jansen, B. C., and Ondersteport, J., *Vet. Res. 38*, 93 (1971).
18. Nakamura, S. Serikawa, T., Yamakawa, K., Nishida, S., Kozaki, S., and Sakaguchi, G., *Microbiol. immunol. 22*, 591 (1978).
19. Oguma, K., *J. Gen. Microbiol. 92*, 67 (1976).
20. Oguma, K., Iida, H., and Inoue, K., *Jpan. J. Microbiol. 17*, 425 (1973).
21. Oguma, K., Iida, H., and Inoue, K., *Japan. J. Med. Sci. Biol. 28*, 63 (1975).
22. Oguma, K., Iida, H., and Shiozaki, M., *Infect. Immun. 14*, 597 (1976).
23. Oguma, K., Iida, H., Shiozaki, M., and Inoue, K., *Infect. Immun. 13*, 855 (1976).
24. Vinet, G., Berthiaume, L., and Fredette, V., *Rev. Can. Biol. 27*, 73 (1968).

TOXIN PRODUCTION AND PHAGE IN
CLOSTRIDIUM BOTULINUM TYPES C AND D

Hiroo Iida
Keiji Oguma

Department of Bacteriology
Hokkaido University School of Medicine
Sapporo, Japan

Katsuhiro Inoue

Hokkaido Institute of Public Health
Sapporo, Japan

I. BACTERIOPHAGES OF *C. BOTULINUM*

Vinĕt et al (1) first presented electron micrographs of
bacteriophages obtained from *C. botulinum* type C, strain *468*.
It is large-sized phage, with length of 460 nm. We attempted
to demonstrate phages of each type and used each one toxigenic strain of types A, B, C, D, E and F. Induced lysates
were obtained by ultraviolet irradiation or mitomycin C
treatment. After lysis, the supernatants were centrifuged
at 60,000 g for 60 min. The pellets thus obtained were
resuspended in 0.1 M ammonium acetate solution, pH 6.8, and
were examined by an electron microscope using the negative
staining method with 2 % phosphotungustic acid, adjusted to
pH 6.8 with KOH.

The results of the induction experiments were reported
previously (2). The phages were classified into three
groups. The first group was type A phage which showed
mainly empty hexagonal heads. The second group consisted of
types C and D phages. They were large-sized phages of hexagonal heads, 120 nm in diameter and long flexible tails
which consisted of a tail tube, 350 to 450 nm long and 15 nm

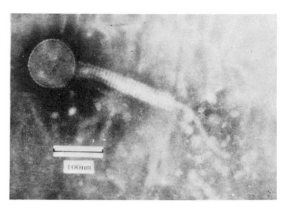

Fig. 1. Bacteriophages of C. botulinum type C.

in diameter, surrounded by a sheath, 30 to 35 nm in diameter
(Fig. 1). They were very similar to the type C phage reported by Vinét et al. The third group consisted of nonproteolytic types B, E and F phages. In most of our experiments on this group, only tails of phages were observed,
suggesting the abnormal and excessive production of tail
components. As the complete phages were observed only in
the second group, we started our experiments on the relationship between toxigenicity and lysogenicity with type c and D
strains.

Later Eklund et al (3) and Dolman and Chang (4) extended
our observaions and reported various phages in each type of
C. botulinum.

II.   PHAGE CONVERSION TO TOXIGENICITY IN *C. BOTULINUM*
      TYPE C

C. botulinum type C, strain *Stockholm,* was incubated at
37 C overnight in TYG medium which consisted of trypticase
(BBL) 3 %, yeast extract (Difco) 2 %, glucose 0.5 % and Na-
thioglycollate 0.1 %, pH 7.4. After incubation for 4 to 6
hr, mitomycin C (5 ug/ml, Kyowa Hakko Kogyo Co.) was added
and the tube was incubated for an additional 4 to 6 hr at 30
C   until lysis was complete. The lysate was clarified by
centrifugation and filtered through a membrane filter of
pore size 450 nm.

As toxigenic strains of *C. botulinum* were thought to be
lysogenized and produce phage by induction, we attempted
to obtain non-lysogenic and non-toxigenic indicator strains

TABLE I. Isolation of non-toxigenic strains

Conc. acridine orange, μg/ml	No. colonies tested	No. non-toxi genic strains	Percentage
30	56	2	3.75
20	100	3	3.33
12.5[a]	32	3	9.38
Total	188	8	4.26
None	120	0	0

[a]Colonies were picked from the third passage in TYG medium containing 12.5 μg/ml of acridine orange.

TABLE II. Conversion to toxigenicity by the filtrate of the induced lysate

Reaction time	No. colonies tested	No. colonies converted	Percent converted
0	50	0	0
30 min	50	0	0
1 hr	50	0	0
5 hr	50	48	96
24 hr	50	44	88

from these toxigenic strains (5). Ten non-toxigenic strains were isolated by incubating the toxigenic strain, *Stockholm*, in cooked meat medium containing acridine orange (Wako Pure Chem. Indust. Co.) in amounts of 12.5 to 30 μg/ml. The cultures were streaked on blood agar plates and incubated anaerobically at 37 C for 48 hr. As shown in Table I, eight out of 188 colonies grown on blood agar plates were found to be non-toxigenic. These non-toxigenic strains were non-lysogenic because these growing cells were lysed by the filtrate of the induced lysate though the parent strains did not show lysis. These non-toxigenic strains were stable and showed no toxin production even after 30 serial passages in cooked meat medium.

One of these non-toxigenic strains, *AO-2*, was incubated at 37 C for 4 to 6 hr in TYG medium and the induced lysate from the parent strain, *Stockholm*, was added to it. After incubation at 37 C for 2 hr, the cells showed a marked lysis. An aliquot of 0.1 ml of the culture was sampled at 30 min, 60 min, 5 hr and 24 hr of incubation, streaked on blood agar plates and incubated anaerobically at 37 C for 3 to 4 days and the isolated colonies were tested for toxicity by

TABLE III. Effects of various treatments

Treatment	No. colonies tested	No. colonies converted	Percent converted
Control	20	20	100
Trypsin[a]	20	18	90
DNase[b]	20	20	100
Filtration[c]	20	0	0
Heat[d]	20	0	0

[a] Trypsin: Sigma Chem. Co. 100 μg/ml, pH 8.2, 37 C, 2 hr.
[b] DNase: Worthington Biochem. Co. 20 μg/ml, 37 C, 2 hr.
[c] Gelman filter GA-10, pore size 50 nm.
[d] 60 C for 30 min.

injecting 0.5 ml of the culture supernatants intraperitoneally into mice. The results are shown in Table II.

As indicated in the table, 96 % of the colonies from surviving cells on the plates were found to be toxigenic after 5 hr. Later it was found that at least 75 % of the colonies were converted to a toxigenic state after 30 min contact with the filtrate of the lytic lysate obtained by repeating lysis of *AO-2* cells ten times. The converted culture showed no different biochemical characteristics from strain *AO-2* except toxigenicity.

The converting ability of the filtrate of the induced lysate was not destroyed by trypsin or DNase as shown in Table III. The filtrate of the lysate obtained through a membrane filter, pore size 50 nm, did not show any converting ability. Heat-treatment at 60 C for 30 min destroyed the converting ability of the lysate, but not at 55 C for 30 min. All of these results strongly suggested the possibility that the conversion is carried out by phage contained in the lysate from the parent strain. The high percentage of conversion suggested that the phenomenon is not transduction but phage-conversion.

III. PHAGE-CONVERSION TO TOXIGENICITY IN *C.BOTULINUM* TYPE D

Similar experiments were carried out with *C. botulinum* type D, strain *1873,* in parallel with type C, strain *Stockholm* (6). In this experiment, of 188 colonies from type C, 8 were non-toxigenic and 190 colonies from type D, 8 were also found to be non-toxigenic. These non-toxigenic

strains were found to be non-lysogenic by the lytic test
with induced lysates from the parent toxigenic strains.
A lysogenic but non-toxigenic strain, N-71, was isolated
from type C by the treatment with N-methyl-N-nitrosoguani-
dine. A non-lysogenic and non-toxigenic strain 151, obtained
from toxigenic D-1873 was employed for the conversion experiment. Similar experiments as described above were carried
out by adding the lysate from C-Stockholm and D-1873 to
young cultures of AO-2 and 151. In this case, 96 and 88 %
of the surviving cells were lysogenized and became toxigenic
in strains AO-2 and 151, respectively.

     Of particular interest was the results obtained with
strain 139 which derived from type D, strain 1873, by the
treatment with acridine orange. This non-toxigenic strain
was not converted to toxigenicity by the induced lysate
from its parent strain, but converted by the induced lysate
from type C, strain Stockholm, and the toxin produced by
the converted culture was found to be of type C by toxin-
antitoxin neutralization test.

     The characteristics of the converting agent in type D
were similar to those of type C, thus suggesting that the
converting agent is also a phage.

IV. AN ADDITIONAL EVIDENCE FOR PHAGE CONVERSION

     The high conversion rate as seen above experiments
showed that the phenomenon is phage-conversion. To obtain
more pieces of evidence, we attempted several experiments
using various phages and indicator strains (7).

     Each induced lysate from toxigenic parent strains was
filtered through a membrane filter, pore size 450 nm,
added to young cells of each non-toxigenic indicator
strains and incubated at 37 C for 3 hr. Then 0.2 ml of
each mixture was transferred to a tube containing 10 ml of
cooked meat medium and incubated at 37 C for 2 days. The
supernatant of each culture was diluted to 1:10 and 0.4 ml
amounts were injected intraperitoneally into mice.
Neutralization test was carried out by mixing 10 MLD of
each toxic culture and antitoxic sera of type C and type D
distributed by CDC, Atlanta, Georgia. The results obtained
with various induced lysates and non-toxigenic indicator
strains are summarized in Table IV.

     As can be seen from the table, lysates from type C,
strain Stockholm and 468, were found to convert non-
toxigenic strains AO-2 and 468-U 31, from type C and also

TABLE IV. Conversion to toxigenicity by induced lysates
          from toxigenic strains

Lysate from strain	Non-toxigenic strains						
	Type c					Type D	
	AO-2	468-U-31	201-NT	203-U-38	6813-NT	139	151
Type c							
Stockholm	C	C	–	–	–	C	–
468	C	C	–	–	–	C	–
203	–	–	–	–	–	–	C
6812	–	–	–	–	–	–	–
Type D							
1873	–	–	–	–	–	–	D

TABLE V. Conversion to toxigenicity by induced lysates
          from converted strains

Lysate from strain	Non-toxigenic strains						
	Type C					Type D	
	AO-2	468-U-16	468-U-31	203-U-28	203-U-38	N-71	139	151
AO-2(c-st)	C	C	C	–	–	–	C	–
468(c-st)	C	C	C	–	–	–	C	–
139(c-st)	C	C	C	–	–	–	C	–
151(c-203)	C	C	C	–	–	–	–	C
151(d-1873)	–	–	–	–	–	–	–	D

a non-toxigenic strain, *139*, from type D. On the contrary,
the lysates from type C, strain *203*, converted a non-
toxigenic strain *151*, from type D. The induced lysate from
toxigenic type D, strain *1873*, converted only *151*.

Then experiments on conversion by phages induced from
these converted strains were carried out. The results are
summarized in Table V. This table clearly showed that the
type of toxin produced by non-toxigenic strains which were
infected by phages induced from converted strains was
determined not by the propagating host bacterium but by the
phage. This is an additional evidence for phage-conversion.

From the data presented above there seemed to be at
least two groups of type C phages: (1) Phages carried by
strains *Stockholm* and *468*. (2) Phage carried by strain
203.

TABLE VI. *Conversion to toxigenicity with various
non-toxigenic strains and phages*

Non-toxigenic strain	Phage					
	c-468	c-st	c-203	d-1873	d-sA	d-4947
C-AO-2	C	C				
C-468-U-31	C	C				
C-203-U-28						
C-203-AO-1						
C-203						
C-N-71						
D-134			C	D		
D-151			C	D		
D-139	C	C				
D-SA					D	D

V.   ANTIGENICITY OF CONVERTING PHAGES

Later we succeeded in obtaining phages purified from
plaques by the procedure reported by Eklund et al (8).
Some non-toxigenic strains were converted to a toxigenic
state by specific phages, whereas the other strains were
not infected by these phages. So we investigated the
antigenicity of converting phages to clarify the basis for
the specific infection spectrum shown by these phages (9).
Various non-toxigenic strains were mixed with purified
phages and the conversion test was carried out. As shown
in Table VI, the converting phages were divided into three
groups on the basis of their infection spectrum. As
expected, the cells isolated from plaques had been converted
to a toxigenic state.
Then neutralization test was carried out ·using phages
and anti-phage sera, both diluted to 1:10. After incubating
at 37 C for 2 hr, conversion test was carried out. From
the results shown in Table VII, the converting phages were
also classified into three groups on the basis of the antigenicity. The quantitative neutralization test was carried
out using each phage diluted in serial 10-fold dilutions.
A partial cross-neutralization was observed between phages
belonging to group 1 and group 2.
As pointed out above, the conversion occurred only with
some combinations of phages and non-toxigenic strains. To
clarify the reason of this phenomenon, adsorption experiments were carried out using phage c-st (10). The phage

TABLE VII. Neutralization test of phages by
          antiphage sera

Phage	Group	Antiphage serum		
		c-468	d-1873	d-sA
c-468	1	s[a]	d[a]	d
c-st		s	d	d
d-1873	2	d	s	d
c-203		d	s	d
d-sA	3	d	d	s
d-4947		d	d	s

[a] s: *survived*, d: *died.*

was mixed at 4 C with cells of type C and D cultures and
non-toxigenic strains derived from them and the adsorption
tests were carried out.

Though strains *AO-2* and *139* were both converted to
type C toxigenicity by the phage, the conversion rate was
significantly higher for strain *AO-2*. This seems to be
related to the more effective phage adsorption to *AO-2* as
compared with *139*. Several reasons should be involved
in only certain phage-cell parings being productive of
conversion. Included are cases where the cells lack
receptors for phage attachment. In some of these strains,
it is possible that they carry a defective phage that
confers immunity against the phage; in others, host-
controlled restriction may be important in preventing
conversion. The phage adsorbed to some non-toxigenic
cultures without converting them to a toxigenic state.

VI. A NON-CONVERTING PHAGE OBTAINED FROM A NON-
     TOXIGENIC STRAIN OF TYPE C

As described above, a non-toxigenic strain, *N-71*,
obtained from a toxigenic parent strain, *C-Stockholm*,
with nitrosoguanidine treatment was found to be lysogenic
by the lysis test. Although the filtrate of a passaged
lysate of this non-toxigenic but lysogenic strain lysed
cells of non-toxigenic strain *AO-2* equally well as the
converting phage, *c-st*, it did not convert *AO-2* to a
toxigenic state. So we compared this non-converting

phage with converting one (11).

A toxigenic strain, type C *Stockholm,* was treated by nitrosoguanidine and three non-toxigenic strains were obtained. They were proved to be lysogenic by lysis test and one of them, strain *N-71,* was used in the experiment.

An electron micrograph of a complete phage which was similar in its morphology to that of *c-st* phage was obtained from the induced lysate of strain *N-71.* The anti-*c-n-71* phage rabbit serum was diluted in two-fold dilutions and mixed with equal volumes of either *c-st* or *c-n-71* phages. Conversion and lysis tests were carried out after the mixture was incubated at 37 C for 1 hr. By these experiments it was found out that anti-*c-n-71* phage serum neutralized both lytic and converting activities of the *c-st* phage.

Lysis curves and lysis spectra of *c-st* and *c-n-71* phages were also compared. The results clearly showed that the lysis curves and the lysis spectra of *c-st* and *c-n-71* phages against ten indicator strains were almost identical. As expected, the non-toxigenic strains which were lysed by these phages were converted to a toxigenic state only by the *c-st* phage.

VII. THE STABILITY OF TOXIGENICITY IN CONVERTED STRAINS

During these experiments, we often found that converted strains became non-toxigenic after several transfers in cooked meat medium. This suggested that the gene controlling toxin production of *C. botulinum* types C and D was not always integrated into the bacterial chromosome.

An experiment was carried out on the loss of toxigenicity in converted strains through serial transfers with or without anti-phage serum (12). During serial transfer, loss of toxigenicity was observed at varying rates with different combinations of phages and indicator strains (Table VIII). In only one strain, *151(d-1873),* toxigenicity was stable after ten transfers. With the other 4 strains, most colonies isolated at the 10th transfer were non-toxigenic. Loss of toxigenicity occurred more rapidly in the presence of anti-phage serum.

Most of the converted strains lost their toxigenicity even during transfer without antiserum, and the non-toxigenic strains that appeared were resistant to lysis and conversion by the original phage. In some combinations of phage and host bacterium, however, toxigencity was stable and the non-toxigenic strains that arose remained sensitive to lysis and conversion. When converted strains were transferred in

TABLE VIII. Appearance of non-toxigenic colonies
            during serial transfer

Antiphage serum	Conversion rate	Proportion of colonies originally toxigenic	Proportion of tox. colonies after transfer for following number of times				
			1	2	4	8	10
Without							
C-Stockholm		20/20	–	18/20	17/20	2/20	5/20
AO-2(c-st)	15/20[a]	18/20	–	20/20	10/20	8/20	2/20
139(c-st)	4/20[a]	19/20	–	5/5	1/20	2/20	0/10
151(d-1873)	10/10[b]	20/20	–	19/20	15/20	19/20	20/20
151(c-203)	10/10[b]	3/10	17/20	9/20	4/20	–	2/20
With							
C-Stockholm		20/20	–	7/10	3/10	0/10	0/10
AO-2(c-st)	15/20	18/20	–	10/10	6/10	0/10	0/10
151(d-1873)	10/10	20/20	–	18/20	15/20	8/20	6/20
151(c-203)	10/10	3/10	1/20	0/20	0/20	–	0/20

[a] *Conversion rate with filtrate of induced lysate*

[b] *Conversion rate with filtrate of passaged lysate*

medium containing anti-phage serum, toxigenicity was lost
more rapidly and the non-toxigenic strains that appeared
remained sensitive to lysis and conversion by the original
phage.

Filtrates of the supernatant of culture fluids of
strains transferred without anti-phage serum converted non-
toxigenic strains to a toxigenic state at varying rates.
However, a non-converting phage was also demonstrated in one
of these filtrates. The phage was almost identical to the
original converting phage in its morphology, host range and
antigenicity. Indicator strains infected by this phage
acquired resistance to lysis by the parent phage.

These results suggest that re-infection and conversion
to toxigenicity occurred in combinations showing stable
toxigenicity after ten transfers. However, in those combinations that lost toxigenicity, re-infection with non-
converting mutant of the original phage may have occurred
with the result that non-toxigenic variants became resistant
to the converting phage. This appears to be one of the
causes of the loss of toxigenicity which is common in some
type C and D strains.

VIII.   PHAGE CONVERSION AND NOMENCLATURE OF *C. BOTULINUM*

    The results above described show that the type of toxin
produced by *C. botulinum* is determined by the phage
infected. Eklund et al (13) reported that when *C. botulinum*
type C is cured of its prophage, it simultaneously ceases
to produce toxin. This non-toxigenic cultures can be
converted to *C. novyi* type A by its specific phage. This
interspecies conversion raises a problem in the nomenclature
of toxigenic *Clostridia*. The present classification based
on the immunological property of toxin is of course
important from the medical viewpoint. From the biological
point of view, however, species of genus *Clostridium* should
be classified on the basis of their biochemical properties,
DNA-homology, sensitivity to phages and so on. There are
some strains of *C. sporogenes* which show high DNA-homology
with proteolytic strains of *C. botulinum (14)* and if phages
from the latter organisms could convert the former ones
into a toxigenic state, we should not call them *C. sporogenes* but *C. botulinum* type A or type B. In this case,
C. sporogenes is thought to be non-toxigenic strain of
C. botulinum.

REFERENCES
    1. Vinét, G., Berthioume, L. and Frédette, V., *Rev.
        Canad. Biol. 27*, 73 (1968).
    2. Inoue, K. and Iida, H., *J. Virol. 2*, 537 (1968).
    3. Eklund, M.W., Poysky, F.I. and Boatman, E.S., *J. Virol.
        3*, 270 (1969).
    4. Dolman, C.E. and Chang, E., *Canad. J. Microbiol. 18*,
        67 (1972).
    5. Inoue, K. and Iida, H., *Japan. J. Microbiol. 18*,
        87 (1970).
    6. Inoue, K. and Iida, H., *Japan. J. Med. Sci. Biol.
        24*, 53 (1971)
    7. Oguma, K., Iida, H. and Inoue, K., *Japan. J. Micro-
        biol. 17*, 425 (1973).
    8. Eklund, M.W., Poysky, F.T., Reed, S.M. and Smith, C.A.,
        Science 172, 480 (1971).
    9. Oguma, K., Iida, H., Shiozaki, M. and Inoue, K.,
        Infect. Immun. 13, 855 (1976).
   10. Oguma, K. and Sugiyama, H., *Proc. Soc. Exper. Biol.
        Med. 159*, 61 (1978).
   11. Oguma, K., Iida, H. and Inoue, K., *Japan. J. Microbiol.
        19*, 167 (1975).
   12. Oguma, K., *J. Gener. Microbiol. 92*, 67 (1976).

13. Eklund, M.W., Poysky, F.T., Megers, J.A. and Pelroy,
     G.A., *Science 186*, 456 (1974).
14. Lee, W.H. and Rieman, H., *J. Gener. Microbiol. 64*,
     85 (1970).

FERMENTATION KINETICS OF BOTULINUM TOXIN PRODUCTION
(TYPES A, B AND E)

Lynn S. Siegel

U. S. Army Medical Research Institute of Infectious Diseases
Fort Detrick, Frederick, Maryland

INTRODUCTION

The botulinum toxoid currently in use for human immunization is derived from formalin-inactivated types A, B, C, D and
E toxins. It was produced in 1958 by Parke-Davis, under contract to the United States Army. For type A, the preparation
contains only about 10% neurotoxoid (1). Similar low percent-
ages of purity are to be expected for the other types. This
toxoid elicits sustained, measurable antibody titers only after a series of four injections over a period of one year (2).
Mild side-reactions are common, including itching, tenderness,
redness and swelling at the site of injection (3). A new product is required: one that includes types F and G, and that
is prepared from highly purified neurotoxins. This is the
goal of this research effort. To produce such a product,
suitable for human immunization against types A-G, methods
must be developed to: (a) produce each toxin in large quantities, (b) purify the neurotoxin from the culture fluid, and
(c) convert each neurotoxin into a neurotoxoid and combine
them into a polyvalent product.

To produce botulinum toxin in large quantities, previous
workers have used cultures grown statically in carboys. The
problems inherent in the use of carboys as growth vessels for
the production of clostridial vaccines are many, and have been
emphasized by Hepple (4). In contrast, we are employing a
fermentor for botulinum toxin production. The numerous advantages of using a fermentor system for the cultivation of anaerobic bacteria have been noted by Sargeant (5). A fermentor
allows for the precise, continuous measurement and control of

Copyright © 1981 by Academic Press, Inc.
All rights of reproduction in any form reserved.
ISBN 0-12-447180-3

temperature, pH, redox potential and the rate of agitation and sparging. Cultures in stirred fermentors are homogeneous and representative samples can easily be obtained without risk of aeration. In addition, the use of a fermentor facilitates the correlation of the appearance of the desired product with specific phases of growth. Thus, the aims of our fermentor studies are to determine the optimal conditions for toxin production (with respect to the initial concentration of growth medium components, pH, gas flow, agitation and temperature) and the relationship between bacterial growth and toxin production.

Studies have been conducted using a 70-liter fermentor containing 50 liters of medium. The medium consists of casein hydrolysate, yeast extract, plus an appropriate concentration of glucose. A complex medium is used, since such media have been reported to support approximately 10-fold more toxin production than do chemically defined media (6). This medium was chosen because of its suitability for toxin production and its economic feasibility for large-scale use.

CLOSTRIDIUM BOTULINUM TYPE A

We first examined the growth of C. botulinum type A, Hall strain, and the appearance of toxin in the culture fluid over a time course of 72 hours (Fig. 1). As measured by optical density, growth was exponential for about 6 hours (mean generation time, 76 min). The oxidation-reduction potential (Eh), recorded at the pH of the culture, declined from the time of inoculation to reach a minimum at 5 hours and then rose during the course of the experiment. The pH, which was not regulated, decreased to 5.4 by 24 hours and did not increase from that value for the remainder of the 72 hours.

The amount of toxin in the culture fluid increased during the first 24 hours to a maximum of 6.3 x 10^5 mouse intraperitoneal LD_{50}/ml. Toxin accumulation was not augmented by continued incubation. When the growth and the toxin curves are examined together, it is evident that the toxin titers rose during the logarithmic and stationary phases of growth, and that the maximum concentration of toxin was attained before the cells had lysed to an appreciable extent. Although previous investigators have maintained that autolysis is the mechanism by which toxin is liberated from C. botulinum type A (7, 8), cell lysis is apparently not required to obtain maximum toxin concentrations in the culture fluid when this organism is grown under the fermentation conditions described.

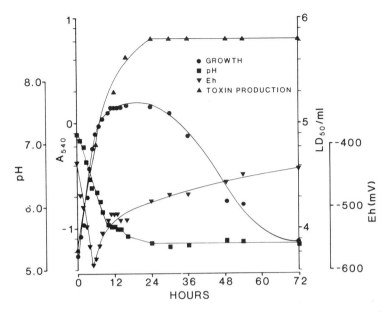

FIGURE 1.   Growth, toxin production and cultural condi-
tions of C. botulinum type A, Hall strain.   The medium consis-
ted of 2.0% casein hydrolysate and 1.0% yeast extract adjusted
to pH 7.3, plus 0.5% glucose.   Fermentation was at 35°C with
an agitation rate of 50 rpm and a nitrogen overlay (5 liters/
min).

In many fermentations by anaerobes, product yields have
been increased by changing the temperature, pH or some other
growth condition (5).   The goal in such efforts is to decrease
the rate of cell growth and thus to extend the production time.
Therefore, the effects of the rate of agitation, together with
the rate of nitrogen sparging of the culture versus a nitrogen
overlay, on growth and toxin production were determined (9).
Maximum growth was obtained in 16 hours in all studies, with
lysis essentially complete at 72 hours.   Using a nitrogen
overlay (5 liters/min) with an agitation rate of 50 rpm, the
maximum toxin concentration (6.3 x 10^5 LD_{50}/ml) was attained
within 24 hours.   Continued fermentation for up to 126 hours
did not augment toxin accumulation.   With nitrogen sparging at
5 liters/min and agitation at 50 rpm or at 10 liters/min and
agitation at 100 rpm, toxin appearance was delayed, and titers
subsequently decreased on continued incubation.   Data obtained
with CO_2 sparging (1 liter/min) were similar to those with
nitrogen sparging at 5 liters/min.
    Fermentations were conducted with varying concentrations of
glucose: 1.5, 1.0, 0.5 and 0.25%, as well as no added carbohydrate (9).   Growth was dependent on glucose concentration up

to 1.0%, but significant lysis occurred only in the presence of 0.5%. With 1.0 and 1.5% glucose, the maximum toxin concentration was attained in 24 hours; with 0.5% glucose, it was attained in 30 hours. Cultures supplemented with 0.25% glucose and those to which no carbohydrate was added produced much less toxin.

The addition of carbohydrate during growth has been reported to increase product yield (4). Therefore, after 8 hours of growth in a medium initially supplemented with 1.0% glucose, an addition of glucose was made to the culture to yield a further 1.0% glucose. However, this procedure did not increase toxin concentrations beyond those obtained with 1.0% glucose only (9).

The effect of temperature in the range from 30 to 45°C on growth and toxin production was examined (9). Growth occurred at all temperatures tested, but 40°C was optimal. However, of the temperatures tested, the optimum for toxin production was 35°C, with maximum titers produced in 24 hours. Toxin production was markedly reduced when an incubation temperature of 45°C was used.

Product yield has been reported to be increased by controlling the pH of the culture (4, 5). For type A, the pH (which was 7.1 after inoculation) was uncontrolled until pH 6.0 was reached, which occurred after approximately 8 hours of growth. The pH was then maintained at 6.0 for the duration of the experiment. The growth rate was unaffected by pH control, and the concentration of toxin was not increased by this procedure (9).

Thus, using a fermentor system, optimal production of C. botulinum type A toxin occurs at 35°C, with an agitation rate of 50 rpm and a nitrogen overlay of 5 liters/min, with an initial glucose concentration of 1.0%, in the absence of pH control. Under these conditions, maximum yields of toxin (6.3 x 10^5 LD_{50}/ml) are attained within 24 hours. In contrast, using static cultures requires 4 to 5 days incubation to obtain comparable toxin concentrations (10-13).

C. BOTULINUM TYPE B

Analogous studies have been performed with the bean strain of type B (14). The time course of growth and toxin production is shown in Figure 2. Growth was exponential for about 5 hours (mean generation time, 64 min), with maximum growth obtained in 12 hours. Lysis then occurred, followed by a resumption of growth, and a long stationary phase. The Eh decreased from the time of inoculation until 5 hours, remained

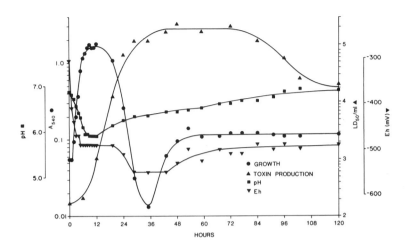

FIGURE 2. Growth, toxin production and cultural condi-
tions of C. botulinum type B, bean strain. The medium con-
sisted of 2.0% casein hydrolysate and 1.5% yeast extract ad-
justed to pH 7.0, plus 0.5% glucose. Fermentation was at 35°C
with an agitation rate of 50 rpm and a nitrogen overlay (5
liters/min).

constant until 19 hours, then declined to a minimum at 29
hours, and remained at this value until 43 hours. It then
increased over the remainder of the time period studied. The
pH decreased to 5.9 at 9 hours, but after 12 hours, increased
gradually for the duration of the run.

The toxin concentration in the culture fluid rose during
the first 48 hours to a maximum of 2.5 x 10^5 LD_{50}/ml. Toxin
titers were not increased by continued incubation, but declined with time after 72 hours. When the growth and toxin
curves are examined together, it is clear that the maximum
toxin concentration was attained only after lysis of the cells
had occurred.

The effects of a nitrogen overlay versus sparging with nitrogen or with CO_2 were determined. In all studies, maximum
growth was obtained in 12 hours. With the nitrogen overlay (5
liters/min), the maximum toxin concentration (4 x 10^5 LD_{50}/ml)
was obtained in 48 hours. Less toxin was produced when the
culture was sparged with nitrogen (5 liters/min) or with CO_2
(1 liter/min).

The effects of glucose concentration on growth and toxin
production were determined. Significant lysis of the culture
occurred with 0.25, 0.5 and 1.0% glucose, but increasing the
glucose concentration delayed the time at which lysis of the
culture began. In cultures supplemented with 0.5 and 1.0%
glucose, maximum toxin titers were attained in 48 hours. Less

toxin was produced with 0.25 and 1.5% glucose, and only low
toxin concentrations were obtained in the absence of added
carbohydrate.

The effects of temperature on growth and toxin production
were examined in the range from 25 to 40°C. A temperature of
40°C was optimal for growth, but growth occurred at all temperatures tested. However, the optimum for toxin production
was 35°C, with maximum concentrations produced in 48 hours.
Incubation at 25 or 40°C reduced toxin production.

Thus, the conditions required by the bean strain of type B
for maximum toxin production in the fermentor system (14) are
identical to those determined for the Hall strain of type A
(9). However, the highest toxin yields were obtained in 24
hours for type A (Hall), but 48 hours of incubation were required to attain the maximum toxin concentration for type B.
In contrast, incubation times of from 2 to 3 days, up to 10
days, are reportedly necessary to obtain comparable yields of
type B toxin in static cultures (15-18).

C. BOTULINUM TYPE E

The growth and toxin production of C. botulinum type E,
strain E43, were examined over a time course of 96 hours in
the fermentor system (Fig. 3). The mean generation time
during exponential growth was 62 min. Lysis of the culture
did not occur. The Eh decreased from the time of inoculation
to reach a minimum at 9 hours, remained at that value until 12
hours, then increased gradually over the remainder of the time
period. The pH of the culture fluid decreased to 4.8 at 24
hours and remained at that value for the duration of the run.
At the times indicated, samples of the whole culture were
treated with trypsin (100 µg/ml at 35°C for 60 min), diluted
serially and injected into mice to determine toxin concentration. The maximum amount of trypsin-activated toxin (2.0 x
10^5 LD_{50}/ml) was produced after 12 hours of fermentation.
Continued fermentation did not increase toxin concentration.

For type E, strain E43, fermentation at 30°C with an agitation rate of 50 rpm and a nitrogen overlay at 5 liters/min
yields a toxin concentration of 2.0 x 10^5 LD_{50}/ml (trypsin-
activated) in 12 hours.

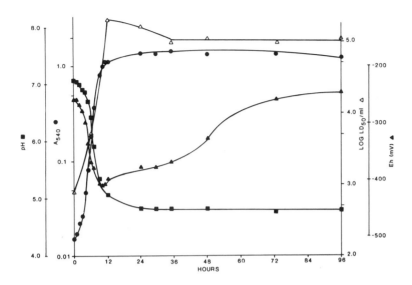

FIGURE 3. Growth, toxin production and cultural conditions of C. botulinum type E, strain E43. The medium consisted of 2.0% casein hydrolysate and 0.5% yeast extract adjusted to pH 7.2, plus 1.0% glucose. Fermentation was at 30°C with an agitation rate of 50 rpm and a nitrogen overlay (5 liters/min).

CONCLUSIONS

Thus, for types A, B and E C. botulinum, the concentrations of toxin produced using the fermentor are at least as high as those obtained with carboys. However, with the fermentor, toxin can be produced in a shorter period of time. In addition, the toxin concentrations obtained are reproducible from one batch to the next, using the same conditions.

ACKNOWLEDGMENTS

In conducting the research described in this report, the investigator adhered to the "Guide for the Care and Use of Laboratory Animals," as promulgated by the Committee on Care and Use of Laboratory Animals of the Institute of Laboratory

Animal Resources, National Research Council. The facilities are fully accredited by the American Association for Accreditation of Laboratory Animal Care.

The views of the author do not purport to reflect the positions of the Department of the Army or the Department of Defense.

REFERENCES

1. Boroff, D. A., Meloche, H. P., and DasGupta, B. R., *Infect. Immun. 2,* 679 (1970).
2. Metzger, J. F., and Lewis, G. E., Jr., *Rev. Infect. Dis. 1,* 689 (1979).
3. Fiock, M. A., Cardella, M. A., and Gearinger, N. F., *J. Immunol. 90,* 697 (1963).
4. Hepple, J. R., *J. Appl. Bacteriol. 28,* 52 (1965).
5. Sargeant, K., *Chem. Industr. 3,* 85 (1968).
6. Boroff, D. A., and DasGupta, B. R., *in* "Microbial Toxins" vol. IIA (S. Kadis, T. C. Montie, and S. J. Ajl, ed.), p. 1. Academic Press, New York (1971).
7. Bonventre, P. F., and Kempe, L. L., *Appl. Microbiol. 7,* 374 (1959).
8. Bonventre, P. F., and Kempe, L. L., *J. Bacteriol. 79,* 18 (1960).
9. Siegel, L. S., and Metzger, J. F., *Appl. Environ. Microbiol. 38,* 606 (1979).
10. Abrams, A., Kegeles, G., and Hottle, G. A., *J. Biol. Chem. 164,* 63 (1946).
11. Duff, J. T., Wright, G. G., Klerer, J., Moore, D. E., and Bibler, R. H., *J. Bacteriol. 73,* 42 (1957).
12. Sugii, S., and Sakaguchi, G., *Infect. Immun. 12,* 1262 (1975).
13. Sugiyama, H., Moberg, L. J., and Messer, S. L., *Appl. Environ. Microbiol. 33,* 963 (1977).
14. Siegel, L. S., and Metzger, J. F., *Appl. Environ. Microbiol. 40,* 1023 (1980).
15. Lamanna, C., and Glassman, H. N., *J. Bacteriol. 54,* 575 (1947).
16. Duff, J. T., Klerer, J., Bibler, R. H., Moore, D. E., Gottfried, C., and Wright, G. G., *J. Bacteriol. 73,* 597 (1957).
17. Beers, W. H., and Reich, E., *J. Biol. Chem. 244,* 4473 (1969).
18. DasGupta, B. R., and Sugiyama, H., *Infect. Immun. 14,* 680 (1976).

BOTULINUM A AND TETANUS TOXIN - SIMILAR ACTIONS
ON TRANSMITTER SYSTEMS IN VITRO

Ernst Habermann

Rudolf Buchheim Institute of Pharmacology
Justus Liebig University
Gießen, FRG

I. INTRODUCTION

Tetanus and botulinum toxins share many properties. They
are produced by clostridia. The original gene product is a
peptide chain of about 150,000 daltons in either case which
may then be nicked, yielding a molecule consisting of two
chains of about 100,000 and 50,000 daltons, respectively. The
large chains of both botulinum (A and B) and tetanus toxin
contain a disulfide loop in a similar position. Moreover
their LD_{50} in mice is in the same range (for review see (18)
on botulinum toxin, and (20) on tetanus toxin). It is still
a matter of controversy how both toxins interact with neuronal
matter. Without doubt tetanus toxin is fixed by polysialo
gangliosides, whereas the binding of botulinum A toxin to
these lipids has been claimed and denied (19). However, contrary to many assumptions it is not clear whether the effects
of tetanus toxin are mediated through the ganglioside binding
sites. Like tetanus toxin, clostridium botulinum A toxin is
fixed to grey but not to white matter. It binds to synaptosomes in a neuraminidase sensitive manner (8). Tetanus and
botulinum A toxin certainly bind to different sites, as shown
by cross-competition experiments (7).

Whereas tetanus and botulinum toxins share important
chemical properties as well as their ability to interact with
central nervous system matter, differences are considerable
in other aspects. Tetanus is characterized by spasticity, and
botulism by paralysis. Nevertheless peripheral paralysis may
also occur in tetanus (for review see 10). The reason why

botulinum toxins do not produce central effects *in vivo* may
stem from their pharmacokinetics. Tetanus toxin is known for
its considerable axonal and even transsynaptic transport.
Thus it reaches not only the pericarya of the motoneurons but
also the synaptic boutons contacting them (for review see 20).
In contrast, the ascent of botulinum A ^{125}I-neurotoxin is very
weak (7,21). The small amounts reaching the central nervous
system may be insufficient to elicit symptoms.

Some pitfalls are inherent in every work with botulinum
toxin. Neglecting them might be responsible for differences
in the literature. Firstly, some authors disregard that
"crystalline" botulinum A toxin is a relatively firm complex
between neurotoxin and haemagglutinins. Thus neurotoxin might
be linked not directly to brain and spinal cord matter but
through the haemagglutinins. Moreover haemagglutinin itself
might be the causative agent when crystalline botulinum A
toxin is applied in higher concentrations to isolated systems.
Such experiments should be repeated with purified neurotoxin.
Secondly, botulinum toxins have to be subclassified into A -
H according to the producing strains, whereas only one kind of
tetanus toxin exists. Novel findings with one botulinum toxin
should not be extrapolated to the others.

Our work to be presented here started with the central
hypothesis that tetanus and botulinum A toxin act in a basically similar manner. To circumvent the pharmacokinetic
problems already discussed we compared tetanus and botulinum
A toxin on various isolated systems. I shall first compile
our recent results and then deduce some generalizations.

II. RESULTS

A. *Isolated Phrenic Nerve-Hemidiaphragm of the Mouse*
    (See Table I)

The action of botulinum A toxin on the rat preparation
has been extensively studied (for review see 15). Tetanus
toxin has been applied mainly by injection into muscles *in
situ*. Nevertheless, similarities to botulinum toxin had
already become apparent (for review see 20). We (10) preferred the *in vitro* poisoning because it allowed a larger
variation of conditions and a better comparison with the
data obtained by previous authors with botulinum toxin on
isolated nerve-muscle preparations.

In general, there is a striking parallelism between the
two toxins. Both depress the transmitter release, which
manifests itself by a drop of the number of m.e.p.p's. Both

TABLE I. *Tetanus and Botulinum A Toxin — A Comparison on Isolated Systems, Contractile Organs*

Neuromuscular junction poisoned in vitro, presynaptic paralysis	Tetanus toxin	Botulinum A toxin
Detection limit	0.05-0.1 µg/ml, mouse (10)	1 ng/ml mouse (10)
Due to neurotoxin	Yes (10)	Yes (10)
Latency period	Pronounced (10)	Pronounced (4)
Subdivided into two stages	Yes (10,14)	Yes (4,16,17)
Q10 of paralysis calculated –		
From time dependence	2.7 (10)	High (4)
For the paralytic step	> 20 (14)	4.2 (17)
Partial reversibility by 4-amino-pyridine	Yes (10)	Yes (16)
Dependence on synaptic activity	Yes (10,14)	Yes (12)
Pretreatment with neuraminidase	Ineffective (10)	Ineffective (unpubl.)

Plexus myentericus-muscle strip from guinea pig, presynaptic paralysis	Tetanus toxin	Botulinum A toxin
Detection limit	0.1-1 µg/ml (1)	0.01-0.1 µg/ml (1)
Latency period	Pronounced (1)	Pronounced (1)
Partial reversibility by 4-amino pyridine	Yes (1)	Yes (1)
Dependence on synaptic activity	Yes (1)	Yes (1)
Acetylcholine content	Not decreased (1)	Not decreased (1)
Acetylcholine release due to veratridine	Depressed (1)	Depressed (1)

become active not before a considerable lag period has passed. Within this time, poisoning becomes resistant first to washing, then to an excess of antibodies. The paralysis due to both botulinum A toxin (4) and tetanus toxin (10) strongly depend on temperature. Q_{10} for tetanus toxin is 2.7 over a wide range, and the activation energy has been calculated to be 17.8 kcal/mol from the Arrhenius plot. These data already indicate that it is not binding but a subsequent, chemical process which limits the rate of paralysis. The work has been extended (14) and led to a three-step model of tetanus toxin action, close to that constructed for botulinum A toxin (16,17). The first two steps are insensitive to temperature and differ by their sensitivities against washing (first step) and antitoxin (second step). The third step much depends on temperature and leads to paralysis. As with botulinum A toxin (12), the action of tetanus toxin depends on the activity of the neuromuscular junction. Time to paralysis is shortened by raising the stimulation frequency and delayed by rest, or when the preparation is stimulated in the presence of Mg^{2+}, or in the absence of Ca^{2+}. However, paralysis by tetanus toxin can not be postponed infinitely by the measures mentioned. As with botulinum toxin, a partial paralysis by tetanus toxin is temporarily overcome by 4-aminopyridine (10^{-5}M) or guanidine (10^{-3}M).

We conclude that tetanus and botulinum A toxin are qualitatively indistinguishable as to their effects on the neuromuscular junction, whereas the quantitative differences are considerable. When calculated for the neurotoxin, botulinum A toxin is about 1,000 times more potent than tetanus toxin (10).

B. *Postganglionic Cholinergic Nerve Endings in the Myenteric Plexus (See Table I)*

The data obtained with both toxins on the isolated myenteric plexus-muscle strip from the guinea pig resemble those from the phrenic nerve-hemidiaphragm of the mouse. Again, onset and course of paralysis are slow. Washing and antitoxin are effective during the latency period only, and the efficacy of the toxins depends on the activity of the preparation. Substances like 4-aminopyridine, sea anemone toxin II and scorpion toxin which prolong the membrane depolarization restore temporarily the contraction of partially paralyzed muscle strips. Again, the difference between tetanus and botulinum A toxin is only quantitative, in that the former toxin is about eight times less potent than the latter (1).

C. Particulate Preparations from Brain and Spinal Cord

Studies on isolated organs may be considered as indirect since contraction serves as an indicator for transmitter release. Moreover, peripheral and central synapses might behave differently. Therefore we have studied both uptake and release of various transmitters directly using particles from brain and spinal cord, as influenced by tetanus and botulinum A toxin (2,3,11).

1. Uptake (Table II). Crude rat synaptosomes (P_2-fraction) were pretreated with tetanus or botulinum A toxin, then exposed to labeled choline (11), glycine, gamma amino-butyric acid (GABA), or noradrenaline (3). The uptake was terminated by dilution, followed by filtration and washing.

With any transmitter studied, tetanus toxin was more potent than botulinum A toxin. However, even the inhibition of choline uptake by maximal concentrations of tetanus toxin did not exceed 50%. At least 10 times lower amounts of tetanus toxin were required in order to achieve an inhibition comparable to that by botulinum A toxin of choline uptake into forebrain synaptosomes. The efficacy of both toxins depended on time. The effect of botulinum toxin was reproducible by using neurotoxin, and no longer obtained with preheated toxin. Pretreatment of the synaptosomes with neuraminidase did not influence the efficacy of tetanus toxin, and only moderately diminished that of botulinum A toxin.

Inhibition of glycine or GABA uptake due to tetanus toxin was by 25% only and that of noradrenaline was not affected at all. Accordingly, these uptake processes were not influenced by botulinum A toxin to a statistically significant degree.

2. Transmitter Release from Superfused Poisoned Particles (Table III). It might be argued that inhibition of uptake prevents the subsequent assessment of release. However, we have shown both on guinea pig ileum strips (1) as well as on particles preloaded with choline, glycine, GABA or noradrenaline that neither tetanus toxin nor botulinum A toxin in the concentrations used, promote the release of transmitter once taken up. Thus preloaded particles were incubated for 2 hours with tetanus toxin or botulinum A toxin, transferred to a superfusion apparatus and depolarized with 25 mM potassium. In agreement with the data obtained on isolated organs and with previous work on synaptosomes (22), botulinum A toxin and its neurotoxin inhibited the release of acetylcholine (2). However, tetanus toxin was about 10 times more potent. Thus the inhibition of release mirrors the inhibition of uptake, although the former process is not causal to the latter.

TABLE II. Inhibition of Transmitter Uptake into Forebrain Synaptosomes

Transmitter	Tetanus toxin	Botulinum A toxin
Choline		
Detection limit	0.1 µg/ml (11)	1 µg/ml (11)
Degree of inhibition	Up to 50% (11)	Up to 40% (11), or less (6)
Type	Noncompetitive (11)	Noncompetitive (11)
Latency period	Yes (11)	Yes (11)
Becomes measurable above 29°C only	Yes (11)	Yes (11)
Antitoxin becomes ineffective soon after poisoning	Yes (11)	Yes (11)
Pretreatment with neuraminidase	Ineffective (11)	Slightly effective (11)
Fixation of toxin precedes its effect considerably	Yes (11)	Not tested, but probable
Glycine		
Detection limit	~ 0.03 µg/ml (3)	Above 6 µg/ml (3)
Degree of inhibition	Up to 25% (3)	Not regular (3)
Time dependence	Prominent (3)	
GABA		
Detection limit	~ 0.01 µg/ml (3)	Above 6 µg/ml (3)
Degree of inhibition	Up to 25% (3)	Not regular (3)

TABLE III. Inhibition of K^+-Evoked Release from Superfused Particles

Transmitter	Tetanus toxin	Botulinum A toxin
Acetylcholine		
Detection limit	0.1 µg/ml[a] (2)	1 µg/ml[a] (2)
	0.01 µg/ml[b] (3)	
Due to neurotoxin	Yes[a] (2)	Yes[a] (2)
Pretreatment with neuraminidase	Ineffective[a] (2)	Slightly effective[a] (2)
Degree of inhibition	Up to 80%[a,b] (2,3)	Up to 80%[a] (2)
Glycine		
Detection limit	0.001 µg/ml[b] (3)	1 µg/ml[b] (3)
	0.01 µg/ml[a] (3)	
Caused by neurotoxin	Yes[b] (3)	Yes[b] (3)
Degree of inhibition	Up to 90%[b] (3)	Up to 50%[b] (3)
	Up to 50%[a] (3)	
GABA		
Detection limit	0.002 µg/ml[b] (3)	5 µg/ml[a] (3)
	0.01 µg/ml[a] (3)	
Caused by neurotoxin	Yes[b] (3)	Not tested
Degree of inhibition	Up to 75%[b] (3)	Up to 50%[a] (3)
	Up to 50%[a] (3)	
Noradrenaline		
Detection limit	0.05 µg/ml[b] (3)	2 µg/ml[c] (3)
	0.05 µg/ml[c] (3)	
Caused by neurotoxin	Yes[c] (3)	Yes[c] (3)
Degree of inhibition	Up to 75%[b] (3)	Up to 75%[c] (3)
	Up to 80%[c] (3)	

[a]from forebrain, [b]from spinal cord, [c]from c. striatum

135

Now the question arose whether either toxin influences
the acetylcholine release only. Otherwise it might be non-
specific like in the uptake studies. It turned out that both
toxins inhibit the release of glycine, GABA and noradrenaline
too. The effect of botulinum A toxin could be mimicked by its
neurotoxin, and was no longer demonstrable with heated or
antitoxin-treated toxin. The concentration-effect curves were
similar with both tetanus and botulinum toxin, particularly in
that the inhibition reached a maximum which depended on the
transmitter. Using botulinum A toxin, GABA release from forebrain and glycine release from spinal cord was inhibited by
about 50%, noradrenaline (c. striatum) and acetylcholine
(forebrain) release was inhibited by about 80%. Again the
difference was quantitative in that botulinum A toxin was
about 40 times less potent with respect to noradrenaline
release and about 1,000 times less potent in diminishing
glycine and GABA release (3).

*3. Transmitter Release from Particles Depolarized in
Bulk (Table IV)*. As compared with the superfusion experiments, release of transmitters from particles in bulk is not
only simpler and faster, but also allows comparative studies
of spontaneous and evoked release under the influence of the
toxins. Therefore we made use of this technique in our
recent work (Habermann, submitted).

Briefly particles were prepared from rat brain cortex by
triturating and washing in Krebs-Ringer solution buffered with
Hepes (KR-H, see 11), loaded with ^{3}H noradrenaline for 15 min
and washed with KR-H. They (0.2 ml) were then incubated with
0.1 ml KR-H containing 0.1% bovine serum albumin or toxins
under various conditions, depolarized with 24 mMK$^+$ (final
concentration) for 15 min and centrifuged at 6,000 xg. An
aliquot of the supernatant was counted for radioactivity.
Under our conditions, depolarization increased the release by
a factor of 2 to 2.5.

The evoked noradrenaline release was inhibited in a dose
dependent manner, 100 ng of tetanus toxin per ml being still
demonstrable. Similar to the superfusion experiments with
striatal particles, botulinum toxin was about 10 times less
potent than tetanus toxin. Its effect depended on its neurotoxin content. Heating abolished the effects of either toxin.
The efficacy of either toxin increased for at least 2 hours
with the duration of preincubation and strongly depended on
temperature. It was measurable at 37°C but not at 23°C or
30°C. As in the experiments concerning choline uptake, pretreatment with neuraminidase did not at all influence the
effects of tetanus toxin, and only partially diminished those
of botulinum A toxin. At the same time, neuraminidase had

TABLE IV. Inhibition of K^+-Evoked Release of Noradrenaline from Forebrain Particles in Batch (Habermann, submitted)

	Tetanus toxin	Botulinum A toxin
Detection limit	0.1 µg/ml	1 µg/ml
Caused by neurotoxin	Yes	Yes
Degree of Inhibition	Up to 75%	At least 40%
Basal release	Slightly inhibited	Slightly inhibited
Ca^{++}-independent release	Partially inhibited	Not measurably inhibited
Time dependence of inhibition	Pronounced	Pronounced
Temperature dependence Inhibition is present at 37°C but not at 30°C	Pronounced	Pronounced
Sensitivity to pretreatment with neuraminidase	No	Moderate

transformed quantitatively the polysialo gangliosides into the monosialo ganglioside GM1. It is concluded that only a part of the binding sites for tetanus and botulinum toxin are true receptors, since fixation of labeled tetanus toxin is much reduced under these conditions.

As expected, potassium evoked release is much depressed by omission of Ca^{2+} and addition of $10^{-4}M$ EGTA. This diminished release is further depressed by tetanus toxin. Thus at least this toxin does not act exclusively on Ca^{2+} movements or its consequences.

A survey of the work from this laboratory devoted to the comparison of tetanus and botulinum toxin is given in Tables I to IV.

III. DISCUSSION

A. Both Tetanus and Botulinum Toxin Act on Many Central
    Transmitter Systems

In fact, so far any central transmitter system studied was found to be influenced by either toxin. We started with the neuromuscular synapse, proceeded to the myenteric plexus, and arrived at the central cholinergic synapses. Then we switched to the central adrenergic system and inhibited noradrenaline release by either toxin. In contrast to the cholinergic system, we were so far not able to inhibit peripheral nor-adrenergic synapses in the cat nictitating membrane, in the rat m. anococcygeus and in the mouse vas deferens by either toxin (9). As a type of inhibitory synapses we included those handling amino acid transmitters glycine and GABA. Here, tetanus toxin was very much more potent than botulinum A toxin. Our data contradict the previously assumed specificity of tetanus toxin for inhibitory synapses, and of botulinum toxin for cholinergic synapses. Our findings basically agree with those of others (5) who injected tetanus toxin into the basal ganglia of the rat and inhibited, by that way, the release of not only GABA but also of dopamine. Into the same direction point observations that the release of more than one amino acid is depressed by tetanus toxin (13)

B. Both Uptake and Release Are Depressed

Gundersen and Howard (6) for the first time observed that choline uptake can be depressed by botulinum A toxin. We have confirmed this finding and reproduced it with tetanus toxin

which is about 10 times more potent. The uptake of glycine
and of GABA was also sensitive to tetanus toxin, however to a
smaller degree. So the question might be raised as to the
interdependence of uptake and release. Is the depression of
release due to a depression of uptake? This is not true of
noradrenaline whose uptake was not measurably inhibited at
all. It is very improbable with the aminoacid transmitters
whose uptake is only mildly influenced by tetanus toxin, and
not regularly by botulinum toxin. As with the cholinergic
system, no decision is possible. The reversed hypothesis,
i.e., whether the inhibition of the release leads to the
eventual inhibition of uptake, can at present not be challenged in an unambiguous system.

The multiple effects of both toxins still lack a common
denominator. If it exists, it must be involved in the release
process of any central transmitter studied. In addition, it
must participate in uptake processes, albeit to a smaller
degree. The changes triggered by the toxins are not of the
all or nothing type since so far neither uptake into nor
release of any transmitter from brain matter could be
inhibited completely.

In our hands, neither toxin inhibited the basal or depolarization evoked $^{45}Ca^{2+}$ uptake into particle preparations
(2). Neither toxin depressed the activity of the Na^+, K^+
ATPase from brain. There was also no evidence for an ADP
ribosylation process similar to that triggered by cholera-
toxin, and also no effect on sodium channels or cyclic
nucleotides, or on the polymerization of microtubuli, or on
the GABA-stimulated benzodiazepine binding (unpublished
experiments).

Per exclusionem we assume a direct membrane effect of
both toxins which leads to a partial loss of the ability to
handle transmitters into either direction. This membrane
effect strongly depends on time and temperature.

*C. How Can We Explain the Clinical Symptoms of Tetanus and
     Botulism?*

The effects of both toxins differ by their relative and
absolute potency on various synapses. For instance, on the
neuromuscular junction tetanus toxin was about 1,000 times
less potent than botulinum toxin, whereas with respect to
inhibition of glycine release it was about 500 times more
potent, yielding a discrimination index of 500,000. This
tremendous quantitative difference certainly contributes to
the expression of the contrasting symptoms in tetanus and
botulism. However, other differences should not be neglected.

For instance, the effects of botulinum toxin can be partially
overcome by pretreatment with neuraminidase, which has not
been observed with tetanus toxin. The fixation of the toxins
occurs at different binding sites, and cross competition is
negligible (7). Finally, the neuronal ascent of botulinum
toxin is weak (7,21) whereas tetanus toxin is a now classical
tracer of the axonal transport (see 20). Hence the differences between tetanus and botulism are based on both pharma-
codynamics and pharmacokinetics.

This work is supported by the Deutsche Forschungsgemein-
schaft, SFB 47, and by the Bundesinnenministerium. It has
been communicated shortly by H. Bigalke, I. Heller and E.
Habermann [*Naunyn-Schmiedeberg's Arch. Pharmacol. (1980) 313,
R 26*]. A short communication deals with the inhibition of
release of various transmitters by botulinum A toxin
[Bigalke, H. and E. Habermann, *IRCS Medical Science (1981) 9,
105*].

REFERENCES

1. Bigalke, H., and Habermann, E., *Naunyn-Schmiedeberg's
    Arch. Pharmacol. 312,* 255 (1980).
2. Bigalke, H., Ahnert, G., and Habermann, E., *Naunyn-
    Schmiedeberg's Arch. Pharmacol.* (in press, 1981).
3. Bigalke, H., Heller, I., Bizzini, B., and Habermann, E.,
    Naunyn-Schmiedeberg's Arch. Pharmacol. (in press, 1981).
4. Burgen, A.S.V., Dickens, F., and Zatman, L.J., *J.
    Physiol. (London) 109,* 10 (1949).
5. Collingridge, G.L., Collins, G.G.S., Davies, J., James,
    T.A., Neal, M.J., and Tongroach, P., *J. Neurochem. 34,*
    540 (1980).
6. Gundersen, G.B., and Howard, B.D., *J. Neurochem. 31,*
    1005 (1978).
7. Habermann, E., *Naunyn-Schmiedeberg's Arch. Pharmacol.
    281,* 47 (1974).
8. Habermann, E., and Heller, I., *Naunyn-Schmiedeberg's
    Arch. Pharmacol. 287,* 97 (1975).
9. Habermann, E., Bigalke, H., Dreyer, F., and Streitzig,
    P., *in* "Natural Toxins" (D. Eaker and T. Wadström (eds.),
    p. 593. Pergamon Press, Oxford (1980).
10. Habermann, E., Dreyer, F., and Bigalke, H., *Naunyn-
    Schmiedeberg's Arch. Pharmacol. 311,* 33 (1980).
11. Habermann, E., Bigalke, H., and Heller, I., *Naunyn-
    Schmiedeberg's Arch. Pharmacol.* (in press, 1981).

12. Hughes, R., and Whaler, B.C., *J. Physiol. (London) 160*, 221 (1962).
13. Osborne, R.H., and Bradford, R.F., *Nature New Biol. 244*, 157 (1973).
14. Schmitt, A., Dreyer, F., and John, C., *Naunyn-Schmiedeberg's Arch. Pharmacol.* (in press, 1981).
15. Simpson, L.L., *in* "The Specificity of Animal, Bacterial and Plant Toxins" (P. Cuatrecasas, ed.), p. 271. Chapman and Hall, London (1977).
16. Simpson, L.L., *J. Pharmacol. Exp. Ther. 206*, 661 (1978).
17. Simpson, L.L., *J. Pharmacol. Exp. Ther. 212*, 16 (1980).
18. Sugiyama, H., *Microbiol. Rev. 44*, 419 (1980).
19. Van Heyningen, W.E., and Mellanby, J., *Naunyn-Schmiedeberg's Arch. Pharmacol. 276*, 297 (1973).
20. Wellhöner, H., *Rev. Physiol. Biochem. Pharmacol.* (in press, 1981).
21. Wiegand, H., Erdmann, G., and Wellhöner, H.H., *Naunyn-Schmiedeberg's Arch. Pharmacol. 292*, 161 (1976).
22. Wonnacott, S., and Marchbanks, R.M., *Biochem. J. 156*, 701 (1976).

USE OF CRYSTALLINE TYPE A BOTULINUM TOXIN IN MEDICAL RESEARCH

Edward J. Schantz

Food Research Institute/
Department of Food Microbiology and Toxicology
University of Wisconsin-Madison
Madison, Wisconsin

Alan B. Scott

Smith-Kettlewell Institute of Visual Sciences
San Francisco, California

The various toxins produced by *Clostridium botulinum* are extremely potent neurotoxins. Type A toxin (one of the 6 recognized types) is easily produced in deep culture and the first to be obtained in a highly purified crystalline form. It is a high molecular weight simple protein (about 900,000) and dissociates under certain conditions of pH and ionic strength into a protein of about 150,000 molecular weight having the neurotoxin properties and another possessing hemagglutinating properties which appears very important in stabilizing the toxic portion of the molecule. The toxin has the specific physiological action of causing a presynaptic block by inhibiting in some manner the release of acetylcholine at the myoneural junction and producing a flaccid paralysis of the muscle which requires about three weeks or more for recovery.

The work of Scott (1) originally presented at the 84th Annual Meeting of the American Academy of Ophthalmology in San Francisco, California, 1979, and recently published in Ophthalmology (2) has taken advantage of this property of the toxin to treat strabismus in humans by injecting a small amount of toxin under carefully controlled conditions directly into the extraocular muscle pulling the eye out of

BIOMEDICAL ASPECTS OF BOTULISM

143

alignment. The amount of toxin used in the treatment depends
upon the condition of the patient. At the present time the
toxin used for this treatment is an ultrafiltered preparation
of 0.05 micrograms (μg) of crystalline toxin (116 mouse IP
LD_{50}) lyophilized with human serum albumin and saline in
small ampoules kept under vacuum. This preparation appears
to be appropriate and reliable in every respect for medical
use in the treatment of strabismus in humans. Although the
specific toxicity of the crystalline toxin of 3 x 10^7 mouse
IP LD_{50} per mg, or 1.5 x 10^3 LD_{50} for the 0.05 μg in an
ampoule, drops more than one log during filtration and lyophilization, this drop is relatively constant from one preparation to another and close to 116 mouse LD_{50} remains, in the
ampoule. For treatment 0.64 ml or more, depending upon the
dose to be given, of sterile saline is introduced aseptically
into the ampoule to dissolve the toxin and a water clear
solution is produced. A 0.1 ml of this solution, using an
electromyrographic needle, is injected into the muscle.
Experience gained by Scott indicates that about 1 mouse LD_{50}
is a starting dose and this is repeated or increased according
to the response of the patient. Upon recovery the muscle
tends to stay in the proper position and corrected cases, now
over 2 years old, have remained so. The maximum time of
paralysis occurs 4 or 5 days following the injection, and
then gradually diminishes, depending on the dose. The maximum
correction of strabismus has been 20 degrees. The maximum
follow-up following injection is 6 months. The results after
the treatment of 43 cases in humans have been remarkably good
and the simplicity of the treatment definitely makes it an
alternative to surgery for the correction of strabismus.
Details of the treatment are given in publications by Scott
(2). One concern regarding this preparation is the presence
of detoxified toxin in the presence of active toxin. One
injection however would deposit less than one ng of detoxified
toxin. This amount seems to be inconsequential and probably
insufficient to ilicit any antibody production. At least
detoxified toxin appears to have no observable effect when
injected IP or IV into mice and Dr. Scott has observed no
effects on humans.

Although the preparation described above is, for all
practical purposes, satisfactory for the treatment of strabismus, the ideal preparation for this treatment, or for any
other medical use of the toxin would be one in which the full
toxicity was maintained during preparation and on long time
storage.

Studies have been undertaken to accomplish the ideal
preparation. One of the purposes of this paper is to describe some of the important problems regarding the nature

and properties of the toxin that are involved in its preparation for medical use; that is the use of the toxin as a drug. Botulinum toxin, like other proteins that possess biological activity, such as some enzymes, possesses its extreme toxicity due to its conformational structure (3,4). It is therefore detoxified in solution by heat, various chemicals, dilution to low concentrations, surface stretching and surface drying. To make a preparation suitable for medical use it was necessary to find means to preserve the toxicity and considerations were given to: (a) purity; (b) factors involved in making a reliable and stable preparation; (c) some data on dose response in animals; and (d) sterility of the preparation.

In regard to purity, the crystalline toxin, upon ultracentrifugation at pH 5.6 or below, is a homogeneous substance of constant composition and activity. From the time Lamanna (5) found that the crystalline toxin could be dissociated into toxin and hemagglutinin by treating with red blood cells at pH 7.3 there has been a question about the advisability of using crystalline toxin in physiological research because of the possible effects of the hemagglutinin on the action of the neurotoxin. The separation of the neurotoxin from hemagglutinin by physical means by others (6,7) has pointed out the marked instability of the neurotoxin without the hemagglutinin (8). It is believed that the hemagglutinin is dissociated from the neurotoxin in the body when consumed orally and that the neurotoxin only reaches the site of action. When a solution of the crystalline toxin is injected directly into a muscle both the toxin and hemagglutinin are present. The work of Scott (2) has not indicated any undue side effects of the hemagglutinin when the crystalline toxin was injected into the extraocular muscle. An important point regarding the use of the purified neurotoxin besides its instability is the fact that it cannot be prepared with constant composition and activity.

The stability of the toxin in a preparation or medical use and its long time storage without loss of toxicity is a very important factor if the dose is to be reliable. Crystals of the toxin are stable for several years when suspended in 0.9 M ammonium sulfate solution and refrigerated. Dispensing a suspension of such extremely toxic crystals into units of 10 ng is not practical and cannot be done accurately. Our studies therefore have been directed toward the development of a suitable medium for solution of the toxin that would retain the specific toxicity over a reasonable length of time, perhaps for 2 years. The specific toxicity of the crystalline toxin in solution is 3×10^7 mouse IP $LD_{50} \pm 10\%$ per mg using the white mice available in

our laboratory. The specific toxicity varies with different
kinds of mice and the conditions under which the assay is
carried out. To get around this variation and consistently
produce a uniform preparation the crystalline toxin must be
measured by its extinction coefficient of 1.65 for one mg
per ml at 278nm in a one cm light path and must have a 260nm
to 278nm absorption ratio of 0.55 or less. Solutions of the
toxin at concentrations of 2 mg or more per ml in 0.05 M
acetate buffer at pH 4.2 are stable for long periods, but
dilution to much lower concentrations results in its detoxification within a short period of time. Addition of other
proteins such as gelatin or serum albumin greatly helps to
prevent detoxification in dilute solution and the addition
of gelatin is customarily made when diluting the toxin for
the mouse assay. The addition of protein to a solution of
the toxin at pH 4 to 4.5 was used for the establishment of a
reference standard for the bioassay of toxin in foods and
body fluids for the Food and Drug Administration (9). For
this preparation a solution of 3X crystalline toxin in
acetate buffer at pH 4.2 at a concentration of 2 to 4 mg per
ml, accurately determined by its absorbance at 278nm, was
diluted to a concentration of 100 ng per ml with a 0.05 M
sodium acetate buffer at pH 4.2 containing 3 mg of bovine
serum albumin and 2 mg of gelatin per ml. When 0.5 ml of
this solution was sealed in 1 ml glass ampoules and stored
at room temperature, the toxicity remained at the original
level of 2500 LD_{50} for two years but gradually fell off to
about 1000 LD_{50} or 50% within 5 years. Such a solution
should be satisfactory for medical use except for the fact
that the toxicity is destroyed upon freezing and no assurance
can be made against the possibility that it might be frozen
in shipping and handling. Some recent preliminary tests
show that citrate buffers at pH 4.8 with gelatin and serum
albumin make good stable solutions of the toxin at low
concentrations stored at 22°C or frozen at -20°C. After
three months storage the toxin at these temperatures and a
concentration of 65 ng per ml showed no detectable loss.
The toxin is also stable to freezing in succinate or oxalate
buffers (4).

Because a lyophilized preparation seemed more practical
for a wide variety of conditions we carried out lyophilization of crystalline toxin with gelatin and bovine serum
albumin in phosphate buffers at pH 6.2 and 6.8. These
buffers were used because freezing did not destroy the
toxin. However upon lyophilization there was a certain loss
in toxicity which amounted to as much as one log or 90
percent in cases, leaving only 10 percent of the toxin
remaining with 90 percent detoxified toxin. Use of the

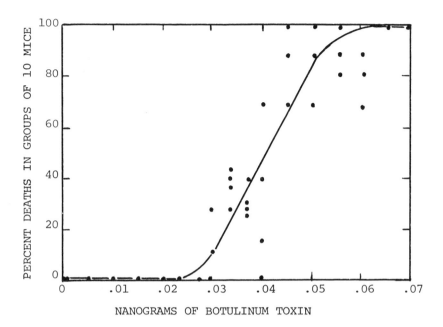

FIGURE 1. *Dose response of white mice to type A botulinum toxin. Each mouse challenged intraperitoneally with the dose contained in 0.5 ml of 0.05 M sodium phosphate buffer at pH 6.2 containing 0.2% gelatin. Deaths recorded in a 96 hour period.*

toxin in the phosphate-protein buffers would make a good preparation if kept frozen and used immediately after thawing. Standing at room temperature at pH 6.2 or 6.8 results in a gradual loss of toxicity. We are now investigating the use of a variety of different substances along with proteins such as some of the dextrans for stabilization of the toxin during lyophilization.

The toxicity or dose response of crystalline toxin for any medical use in humans must be determined in each particular case. However animal experimentation is indicative of the potency and nature of the toxin. The extrapolation from animal to man cannot be made directly on a weight basis, of course, but the IP dose response in mice, as illustrated in Figure 1, points out the nature of a dose response curve. These data are based on about 350 white mice weighing 18 to 22 grams to increases doses of the crystalline toxin from

0.001 to 0.065 ng contained in 0.5 ml of a 0.05 M sodium
phosphate buffer with bovine serum albumin and gelatin to
help stabilize the toxin at such dilute concentrations.
Each dot on the chart represents the percent dead mice in a
group of ten and the combined 35 dots represent the total of
three separate trials with 100 to 120 mice on each trial.
Some mice showed signs of botulism at about 0.01 ng up to
0.025 ng above which deaths began to appear. Those that did
not die recovered within two to three weeks. A dose of
0.065 and above killed all mice in these trials. At least
in our mice signs of botulism without death occurred in some
mice over a 2 to 3 fold dose and the same was true over the
period where death began to occur and where the dose killed
all mice.

Other animals have been used. A collection of animal
data of various investigators by Smith (10) indicates that 5
mouse LD_{50} will kill a 500 gram guinea pig by IP injection
but 700 LD_{50} were required by the oral route. Botulism and
death occurred in monkeys at 650 mouse LD_{50} per kg of body
weight by the oral route. Swine are very resistant to the
toxin and 20,000 mouse LD_{50} were required per kg by IV
injection to cause death and 1.6×10^6 LD_{50} by the oral
route. Dogs are also very resistant to the toxin. In our
laboratory 20,000 mouse LD_{50} of type A toxin per kg by oral
route caused no detectable signs of botulism, but 500 LD_{50}
caused signs of botulism by IV injection. These dogs had no
antibodies or other toxin neutralizing substances in their
blood. Most of the toxin passed through the intestinal
tract without absorption and was found in the feces.

One important concern is the amount of toxin to cause
botulism in a person. Information on this point can only be
obtained, and some has been collected, from accidental cases
of poisoning. Estimates from a variety of sources (11)
indicate that the dose would be between 0.1 and 1 microgram
or about 3,000 to 30,000 mouse LD_{50}, but data collected by
Smith (10) from various investigators over the past 60 years
indicated a dose as high as 250,000 by the oral route. Most
of these data are of little value for cases where the toxin
would be injected because they are based on the absorption
of the toxin through the alimentary tract and this amount
varies greatly from person to person and from one animal
species to another. Injection of the toxin and bypassing
the alimentary tract makes the response much more uniform.
The guinea pig appears to be the most sensitive animal to
the toxin by IP injection that we know. If we assume a
similar sensitivity for humans and 0.1 ng (2.5 mouse LD_{50})
was injected there would be a safety factor of more than
1000 and for one ng (25 mouse LD_{50}), the highest amount used

by Scott, there would be a safety factor of more than 1000, which is better than most drugs. Another safety factor to be considered is the sterility of the toxin preparation. Pasteurization by heating toxin solutions buffered at pH 4.2-4.8 in the presence of gelatin or other proteins at 62°C for 30 minutes can be accomplished without detectable loss of the toxicity but heating at 80°C for one minute would destroy practically all of the toxin. Attempts at sterilization of toxin solutions by ultrafiltration in our laboratory caused a 60 percent loss in the toxicity. Sterilization by the addition of bactericidal substances may be the best approach. The two most important functions of antimicrobial preservatives in pharmaceutical products are: (a) protecting the patient from microbial contamination; and (b) preventing loss of toxicity by microbial action. According to the United States Pharmacopeia XVIII multiple dose containers must contain a suitable substance to prevent the growth of microorganisms regardless of the method of sterilization employed. Because multiple dose containers have the advantage of saving medication we are investigating the effect of some of the parabens, organic mercury compounds (thimersal) and substances like chlorohexidine on the toxin during long time storage.

Another point that should be considered here is the name of the toxin, which of course being the most lethal substance known, is scaring indeed to a patient. It is suggested that crystalline type A botulinum toxin to be used in medical practice be called OCULINUM which is derived from the words ocular and botulinum. Other bacterial products, used in medicine, have been designated by names in this manner.

REFERENCES

1. Scott, A. B., *84 Annual Meeting Am. Acad. Ophthalmology*, San Francisco, California, November, 1979.
2. Scott, A. B., *Ophthalmology 87,* 1044 (1980).
3. Schantz, E. J., Stefanye, D., and Spero, L., *J. Biol. Chem. 235,* 3489 (1961).
4. Schantz, E. J., *in* "Botulism" (K. H. Lewis and K. Cassel Jr., eds.), p. 91. U.S. Public Health Service, Cincinnati, Ohio, (1964).
5. Lamanna, C., and Lowenthal, J. P., *J. Bacteriol. 61,* 751 (1951).
6. Wagman, J., and Bateman, J. B., *Arch. Biochem. Biophys. 45,* 375 (1953).

7. DasGupta, B. R., and Boroff, D. A., *J. Biol. Chem. 243,* 1065 (1968).
8. Ohishi, I., Sugii, S., and Sakaguchi, G., *Infect. Immun. 16,* 107 (1977).
9. Schantz, E. J., and Kautter, D. A., *Assoc. Official Anal. Chem. 61,* 96 (1978).
10. Smith, L., "Botulism", Publisher C. C. Thomas, Springfield, Illinois (1977).
11. Schantz, E. J., and Sugiyama, H., *Agri. and Food Chem. 22,* 26 (1974).

PRODUCTION OF BOTULINUM TOXIN
IN THE GUT[1]

Hiroshi Sugiyama

Food Research Institute and Department of Bacteriology
University of Wisconsin
Madison, Wisconsin

The multiplication and accompanying toxin production by
Clostridium botulinum in the gut is the basis of infant
botulism. Since the human illness is considered in a separate presentation of this Conference (1), my subject can be
put in perspective by merely emphasizing the restricted age
incidence of the disease. At the time the toxicoinfectious
origin of infant botulism was recognized, it was known that
the development of some gastrointestinal infections was
affected by the microorganisms in the gut (2) and that the
intestinal microbiota of infants differed from that in older
individuals (3). Thus, it was reasonable to propose that
the multiplication of *C. botulinum* in the infant gut was
related in some way to the microorganisms that normally
inhabit that organ.

Historically, the possibility of enteric botulinum
infection had been a part of the early studies that were
motivated by concerns about the pathogenicity of the ubiqui-
tous *C. botulinum* spores (4-7). However, the results of
feeding spores in toxin-free suspensions to adult laboratory
animals and the practical experience with foods indicated
that ingesting the numbers of spores which may be on foods
was not a health problem. Nevertheless, several suggestions
were made during the course of the years that *in vivo* formation of toxin could be part of the pathogenesis of at least

[1]*Research was supported by the College of Agricultural
and Life Sciences, University of Wisconsin-Madison and by
Public Health Service grant AI5336, U.S. Department of Agriculture grant 58-32U5-9-100 and the Sioux Honey Association.*

some cases of food poisoning botulism (8-10). This viewpoint
was supported by the finding of *C. botulinum* and toxin in
the stool of a food poisoning case on the 32nd day from the
onset of illness (11).

The best evidence for the production of botulinum toxin
in the gut was the natural outbreaks of type C botulism in
broiler chickens. These outbreaks have occurred in circum-
stances in which a direct source of the toxin is not found
but the spores are present in large numbers in the litter of
the areas in which the birds are being raised (12). That
the illness could be a strict toxicoinfection was shown
experimentally when all 14-day-old chickens fed 100 type A,
C or D spores developed botulism. The toxin production
occurs in the cecum since this is the most proximal part of
the gut where significant amounts of toxin are found and the
chickens are resistant when their ceca are tied off (13).

The mouse has an age-dependent susceptibility to enteric
botulinum infection, if this event is monitored as the
production of toxin in the gut instead of overt botulism
(14). When suckling mice are challenged intragastrically
with 10^5 *C. botulinum* spores (type A, strain 62A) in a
toxin-free suspension, those mice 7-13 days old at time of
challenge are infected; younger or older mice are not (Table
I). The infection rates indicate that 8- to 10-day-old pups
are the most susceptible.

The toxin is found in the lumen of the colon; some may
be in the cecum but this is difficult to prove because the
organ is very small in infant mice. The toxin is first
detected as early as 18 hr of the spore challenge but is
most likely to be found at 2 and 3 days postchallenge (Table
II). It is not present on the eighth day when mice have
reached the age when they would be resistant to a challenge
with spores (14). Thus, the mouse is susceptible to enteric
botulinum colonization during a narrow age span and the
colonization disappears naturally within a few days. The
colonized suckling mice remain asymptomatic despite their
intestinal tracts containing toxin amounts which are much
greater than the minimum needed to kill the mouse if the
toxin is in the abdominal cavity (up to 2,000 mouse, i.p.
LD_{50}).

In agreement with the observations of others, the adult
mouse is not colonized by challenge doses of 10^5 or 10^6
spores. As later retitrated, the 50% infective dose of the
routinely used spore suspension is less than 200 spores per
8- or 9-day-old mouse (15). Spores in an unheated suspension
are as infective as those in suspensions which are heated to
further insure that the inocula do not contain free toxin.

TABLE I. *Dependence of Enteric Botulinum Colonization on Age of Suckling Mice[a]*

Age (days)	Number colonized among 12 mice
4	0
5	0
6	0
7	9
8	11
9	10
10	10[b]
11	9[b]
12	1
13	1
14	0
15	0

[a]10^5 C. botulinum spores administered intragastrically.
[b]11 mice in test group.

TABLE II. *Botulinum Toxin in Intestines of Mice[a] at Different Times after Spore Challenge*

Day after challenge	No. with toxin among 20 tested
0.5	0
0.75	1
1	15
2	20
3	18[b]
4	16
5	11
6	6
7	7
8	0

[a]Nine-day-old mice injected intragastrically with 10^5 spores.
[b]19 instead of 20 mice.

The infant rat has an age-determined susceptibility to
enteric botulinum colonization very similar to suckling mice
(Table III; ref. 16). Again, the colonization does not
cause overt botulism and its short duration is shown by the
absence of toxin by the seventh postchallenge day. Nevertheless, the similar responses of two animal species give some
confidence that these animals can be used as models in which
to study some aspects of human infant botulism.

From birth to past the age when the rodents become
resistant to enteric botulinum colonization, the microorganisms constituting the intestinal microbiota are changing in
a sequence characteristic of the animal species (3). Therefore, the susceptible age could be that period when the gut
has transient microorganisms which give rise to conditions in
which the pathogen can grow. Or, the reverse situation is
possible: the susceptible age could be the period before
competitors of C. botulinum become established as part of
the intestinal microflora.

The second of the two possible explanations was indicated
to be correct when germfree adult mice were tested (17).
Since inocula of 10 spores infected all the test animals
(Table IV), C. botulinum does not need the help of other
bacteria in order to colonize the gut. From 2,000 to 110,000
mouse, i.p. LD_{50} of botulinum toxin could be assayed in the
gut of infected animals on the third or fourth postchallenge
days. In contrast to the colonized conventional infant mice
which are asymptomatic, adult mice monoassociated with C.
botulinum developed botulism. The toxin responsible for the
illness was probably that absorbed from the lower gut where
it is produced, but that ingested by the coprophagic animals
could contribute to the toxic response.

TABLE III. Infection Rates among Infant Rats
            of Different Ages Fed 10^5 C. botulinum
            Spores

Age (days)	% Infected among 20 rats
3	0
5	0
7	6
9	17
11	7
13	0

TABLE IV. Susceptibility of Germfree Adult Mice to
Challenge of 10 C. botulinum Spores

Test[a]	Infected/ Tested	LD_{50} in intestine[b]	Days to botulism[c]
1	3/3	3,000-33,000	-, 3, 3
2	4/4	1,700-22,000	3, 4, 4, 4
3	2/2	NT-112,000	4, 4

[a]Separate isolator for each experiment.
[b]Total in lower ileum, cecum and colon; NT, not tested
since animal found dead in morning.
[c]-, Not ill when sacrificed on third postchallenge day.

The data indicated a critical role of intestinal organisms in determining whether or not the gut is receptive to
colonization by C. botulinum. The conclusion was supported
by the resistance developed by the highly susceptible axenic
mice when they were allowed to acquire the intestinal microorganisms of normal mice (17). Germfree mice were transferred from their isolators into a room housing conventional
mice and at different residence times in the new environment
were challenged orogastrically with 10^5 C. botulinum spores.
All mice receiving spores at the time of their relocation
were enterically colonized by C. botulinum since botulinum
toxin was present in the gut 3 days postchallenge (Table V).
However, the challenge was ineffective when given to mice
which had 3 or more days of the conventionalizing exposure,
at which time microscopic examination of feces showed many
different bacteria had already colonized the gut.
Like their mouse counterparts, germfree adult rats were
infected by inocula of 10 spores and developed overt botulism
within 5 to 6 days (16). Total toxin amounts in the gut at
4 to 7 days postchallenge were greater than 130,000 mouse,
i.p. LD_{50} of which less than 1,500 is in the ileum and the
remainder distributed so that the cecum had 4 to 20 times
the amount in the colon. The ex-germfree rat resulting from
a 3 day conventionalizing exposure was resistant to challenges of 10^5 spores.
These observations were consistent with the interpretation that the susceptibility to enteric botulinum infection
depends on the absence from the gut of organisms which act

TABLE V. Development of Resistance to Enteric
Botulinum Infection during Conventionalization
of Axenic Mice

Days[a]	No. infected/no. tested	LD_{50} in gut[b]
0	7/7	300-9,900
3	0/6	Nil[c]
6	0/3	"
9	0/4	"c
12	0/3	"

[a]Days of conventionalizing treatment before spore
challenge.
[b]One with 300 LD_{50}; remaining six with >1,000 LD_{50}.
[c]See reference 17 for details.

as barriers to the multiplication of the pathogen. A predic-
tion of this interpretation is that the resistant conventional adult mouse would be susceptible if they are compromised
by altering its gut microflora. Such a conversion from
resistance to susceptiblity should result when adult mice
are fed antibiotics which inhibit a wide spectrum of bacteria.

Conventional adult mice were fed a mixture of 5 mg
erythromycin and 4 mg of kanamycin at 12-hr intervals for a
total of five doses. Drinking water during the treatment
period contained 100 μg and 80 μg of the respective antibiotics per ml. At different times after the last controlled
dose, the animals were challenged with 10^5 C. botulinum
spores (18).

When challenges were given 15 to 60 hr after discontinuing the antibiotic treatment, most mice were enterically
colonized by C. botulinum (Table VI). Progressively lower
colonization rates resulted with increases in times between
antibiotic treatment and challenge. The apparent resistance
during the first few hours following the last feeding of
antibiotics was most likely an artifact caused by antibiotic
concentrations persisting at levels inhibitory to the pathogen.

Gram stains of smears made of feces excreted at 1 to 60
hr postantibiotics showed that the drugs had greatly reduced
the variety as well as the total number of bacteria in the
gut. By 116 hr, the flora was indistinguishable from that
in normal mice. Since mice not treated with antibiotics are

TABLE VI. *Colonization Rates when 10^5 C. botulinum*
           Spores Are Fed to Mice at Different Times
           After Erythromycin-Kanamycin Treatment[a]

Hr. postantibiotics	No. colonized among 12 tested
1	0
7	2
15	11
23	12
36	12
60	10
83	6
116	1
168	0

[a] *5 doses of 5 mg erythromycin-4 mg kanamycin at 12 hr intervals.*

resistant to challenges of 10^6 spores and the 50% infective
dose for mice at 36 hr postantibiotics was slightly less
than 10^4 spores, the antibiotics had significantly reduced
the resistance of mice to colonization by *C. botulinum*. However, resistance was not completely abolished since all germfree adult mice are infected when fed 10 spores (Table IV).
   The *in vivo* produced toxin lasted in the gut for up to 5
days. As much as 15,000 mouse, i.p. LD$_{50}$ could be titrated
in some gut but the animals were asymptomatic, as is the
situation with suckling mice and rats. However, minor toxic
effects might be missed by the gross observations being used
to determine the health of animals. This possibility was
tested by a procedure based on a report that administering
aminoglycosides to infant botulism patients precipitates a
rapidly developing but transitory worsening of the clinical
condition (19). In studying this phenomenon in mice, a
gentamicin dose just below the toxic level for normal mice
elicited mild paralysis in some mice which had not developed
botulism after receiving a sublethal dose of botulinum toxin
(20). Injection of this amount of gentamicin into botulinum-
colonized but asymptomatic mice had no observable effect (D.
Burr and H. Sugiyama, unpublished observations). The results
indicated that *in vivo* formed toxin did not affect the host
to a degree which could be augmented into a detectable
response by a normally subtoxic dose of aminoglycoside.

TABLE VII.   Cumulative Death among 30 Germfree and
             30 CRASF Mice Following Orogastric
             Challenge with 50 C. botulinum Spores

Day	Germfree	CRASF
1	0	0
2	0	0
3	16	0
4	26	0
5	27	2
7	29^a	8
14		8
21		13^b

[a]Observation terminated on 10th day.
[b]One mouse died on day 45.

Attempts are being made to identify the kinds of bacteria
which make the gut unsuitable for multiplication of C.
botulinum. A screening approach is used since it is imprac-
tical to test individually the many species that are in the
cecum-colon of an animal. In the procedure, germfree adult
mice with a "defined" intestinal flora are challenged with
C. botulinum spores.

The first trial was with mice carrying the Charles River
Altered Schaedler Flora (CRASF) which consists of two Lactobacillus, one Bacteroides, four fusiform-shaped and one
spirochete species.[2] The flora had some protective effect
since challenges of 50 C. botulinum spores killed 29 of 30
control germfree mice within 7 days but only 8 of 30 CRASF
mice (Table VII). However, all CRASF mice were infected by
C. botulinum and became severely ill (21).

A different set of nine bacteria is used as the intestinal microflora of mice in a special colony maintained at
the Gnotobiote Laboratory of the University of Wisconsin
(UW-GLF). The UW-GLF was established in axenic adult mice
and the animals were challenged first with 50 C. botulinum
spores (Table VIII). When the animals did not become ill or

[2]These mice were obtained through the generosity of Dr.
Roger P. Orcutt, Director of Research and Development,
Charles River Breeding Laboratories, Inc.

TABLE VIII. Resistance of UW-GLF Mice[a] to Enteric
Botulinum Colonization

Exp.	Day	Spore dose	Response	Fecal toxin
1[b]	0	50	–	–
	5	–	Healthy	Nil
	6	50	"	NT[c]
	11	–	"	Nil
	13	2×10^4	"	NT
	18	–	"	Nil
	29	–	"	"
2[d]	0	1×10^5	–	–
	7	–	Healthy	Nil
	14	–	"	"
	21	–	"	"

[a]Obtained by feeding suspensions of feces from stock UW-GLF mice or placing UW-GLF mice in cage holding germfree mice.
[b]Second and third challenges given when tests for toxin showed animals had not been colonized by prior dose. Total of 30 mice.
[c]Not tested.
[d]20 animals.

excrete toxin during the next 5 days, each was given a second dose of 50 spores. The second challenge also had no effect, so 2×10^4 spores were fed. This dose was also ineffective (21,22). The resistance to the third dose was not the result of immunity having been stimulated by the two earlier contacts with a few spores. When 10^5 spores were used as the first challenge dose (second experiment), none of 20 mice were colonized by C. botulinum (K. Kim and H. Sugiyama, unpublished observations).

It seems reasonable to suggest that not all the organisms in the UW-GLF are active in making the gut resistant to enteric botulinum colonization; the barrier effect of the flora could be due to only one species or to a few acting together. To identify these organism(s), pure cultures must be used. Since the isolates used to start the UW-GLF mouse line were not available, pure cultures had to be isolated from stock UW-GLF mice. Nine different cultures were recovered. The Wisconsin State Laboratory of Hygiene has determined these to be three Clostridium species, three Bacillus, one

Lactobacillus, one *Bacteroides* and one organism which may be
an Enterobacteriaceae. Thus, the components of the UW-GLF
may be different from that originally reported (23), but the
difference is not important since the flora protects mice
against colonization by *C. botulinum*.

It seemed prudent to show first that mice associated
with all the isolated organisms are resistant to *C. botulinum*.
Ten germfree adult mice were fed a mixture having all the
organisms and again after one week. When continued excretion
of all organisms (>10^7 per g feces) indicated that the
complete flora was established in the gut, the animals were
challenged with 50 *C. botulinum* spores (Table IX). All mice
remained healthy and did not excrete botulinum toxin during
the following 7 days. A second challenge of 1 x 10^5 spores
was also ineffective (K. Kim and H. Sugiyama, unpublished
observations). These results give hopes that the protective
organism(s) of the UW-GLF can be identified by an elimination
process in which a series of gnotobiotic animals having a
gut flora of progressively fewer species are tested for
resistance to the pathogen.

There have been several suggestions that bile acids play
a role in the natural resistance to gastrointestinal infections and in determining the composition of the indigenous
intestinal microbiota. They are based on *in vitro* tests in
which the bile acids inhibit the growth of certain bacteria

TABLE IX.   *Resistance to Challenges of 1 x 10^5*
            C. botulinum Spores of Ex-germfree Mice
            Obtained by Feeding Pure Cultures of UW-GLF
            Organisms to Germfree Mice

Day	Spore dose	Response[a]	Fecal toxin[a]
0	50	–	–
3	–	Healthy	Nil
7	–	"	"
10	1 x 10^5	"	NT[b]
17	–	"	Nil
24	–	"	"
29	–	"	"

[a]*Ten animals in test group.*
[b]*Not tested.*

(3,24). When effective, the free bile acids are more inhibitory than the same bile acid that is conjugated with glycine or taurine. Similar tests have found that growth of pure cultures of *C. botulinum* is affected by certain bile acids, with lithocholic acid being most inhibitory and deoxycholic and chenodeoxycholic acids being the next most active (25).

These observations suggested that the feeding of bile acids might make susceptible mice less receptive to enteric botulinum colonization. Twenty conventional adult mice were treated with an erythromycin-kanamycin combination (Table VI). At 36 hr postantibiotics, each mouse was fed 10^5 spores. Additionally, ten of these mice were each fed 19 mg of deoxycholic acid within 1 hr of the spore challenge and again 24 and 36 hr later.

All mice were sacrificed 3 days postchallenge and their intestinal tracts were tested for type A botulinum toxin. In accord with expectations, all 10 controls not fed deoxycholic acid were enterically colonized by *C. botulinum* but only 5 of the test mice were colonized (P<0.05). Thus, deoxycholic acid has a significant *in vivo* anti-*C. botulinum* action in the conditions of the experiment (D. Burr and H. Sugiyama, unpublished observations).

The observations made on animal models support the thesis that the production of botulinum toxin in the gut depends primarily on the absence of intestinal microorganisms which would prevent *C. botulinum* from multiplying. Since these competitors of the pathogen are acquired during postnatal development, susceptibility to infection is normally restricted to infants who have not reached this critical phase. Those who have acquired the barrier organisms become susceptible when their gut flora is altered. *C. botulinum* is, therefore, an opportunistic pathogen.

The mechanisms by which the competitors prevent *in vivo* growth of *C. botulinum* could be direct ones such as production of a bacteriocin-antibiotic type of substance, competition for space or nutrients, and the like (2). However, indirect antagonistic actions are possible. The supporting information is admittedly inadequate, but it can at least be suggested that multiplication of *C. botulinum* in the gut could be affected by organisms which actively free bile acids from their glycine or taurine conjugates.

An intestinal flora of a few species can be an effective barrier against *C. botulinum* but it is likely that there is more than one barrier against a pathogen (26). Multiple barriers would be an obvious advantage since the host would have some protection if one should fail. The partial but incomplete reduction by erythromycin-kanamycin treatment of resistance of the conventional adult to enteric botulinum

colonization could be a case where one barrier is suppressed
but a different one remains to give partial protection.

REFERENCES

1. Arnon, S. S.,   (This Symposium).
2. Savage, D. C., *in* "Microbial Ecology of the Gut" (R. T.
    J. Clarke and T. Bauchop, eds.), p. 277. Academic
    Press, New York, (1977).
3. Savage, D. C., *Annu. Rev. Microbiol. 31,* 107 (1977).
4. Orr, P. F., *J. Infect. Dis. 30,* 118 (1922).
5. Coleman, G. E., and Meyer, K. F., *J. Infect. Dis. 31,*
    622 (1922).
6. Dack, G. M., and Hoskins, D., *J. Infect. Dis. 71,* 260
    (1942).
7. Keppie, J., *J. Hyg. (London) 49,* 36 (1951).
8. Burke, V., Elder, J. C., and Pischel, D., *Arch. Intern.
    Med. 27,* 265 (1921).
9. Shvedov, L. M., *Zh. Mikrobiol. Epidemiol. Immunobiol.
    30,* 72 (1959).
10. Minervin, S. M., *in* "Botulism 1966" (M. Ingram and T.
    A. Roberts, eds.), p. 336. Chapman and Hall, London,
    (1967).
11. Dowell, V. R., McCroskey, L. M., Hatheway, C. L.,
    Lombard, G. L., Hughes, J. M., and Merson, M. H., *JAMA
    238,* 1829 (1977).
12. Smart, J. L., and Roberts, T. A., *Vet. Rec. 100,* 378
    (1977).
13. Miyazaki, S., and Sakaguchi, G., *Jpn. J. Med. Sci.
    Biol. 31,* 1 (1978).
14. Sugiyama, H., and Mills, D. C., *Infect. Immun. 21,* 59
    (1978).
15. Sugiyama, H., *Rev. Infect. Dis. 1,* 683 (1979).
16. Moberg, L. J., and Sugiyama, H., *Infect. Immun. 29,* 819
    (1980).
17. Moberg, L. J., and Sugiyama, H., *Infect. Immun. 25,* 653
    (1979).
18. Burr, D. H., Jarvis, G., and Sugiyama, H., *Annu. Meet.
    Am. Soc. Microbiol. Abst. B15,* p. 19 (1980).
19. L'Hommedieu, C., Stough, R., Brown, L., Kettrick, R.,
    and Polin, R., *J. Pediatr. 95,* 1065 (1979).
20. Burr, D. H., Korthals, G. J., and Sugiyama, H., *Annu.
    Meet. Am. Soc. Microbiol. Abst., B33,* p. 20 (1981).
21. Wells, C. L., and Sugiyama, H., *Annu. Meet. Am. Soc.
    Microbiol. Abst. B16,* p. 19 (1980).

22. Sugiyama, H., *in* "Proc. of International Symposium on
     Bacterial Vaccines" (J. B. Robbins and J. C. Hill,
     eds.), Thieme-Stratton, New York (in press).
23. Helstrom, P. B., and Balish, E., *Infect. Immun. 23,* 764
     (1979).
24. Folch, M. H., Gershengoren, W., Elliott, S., and Spiro,
     H. M., *Gastroenterology 61,* 228 (1971).
25. Huhtanen, C. M., *Appl. Environ. Microbiol. 38,* 216
     (1979).
26. Ducluzeau, R., Ladire, M., Callut, C., Raibaud, P., and
     Abrams, G. D., *Infect. Immun. 17,* 415 (1977).

LABORATORY INVESTIGATION OF HUMAN
AND ANIMAL BOTULISM

Charles L. Hatheway
Loretta M. McCroskey

Centers for Disease Control
Atlanta, Georgia

I. CONFIRMATION OF BOTULISM

A. *General*

The most convincing proof that the illness of a patient
showing typical neurological signs and symptoms is botulism
is the demonstration of botulinal toxin in the patient's
serum. However, as we will point out here, confirming botulism with a positive serum toxicity and neutralization test
is possible only in a minority of cases. The investigation
must go further, not only to confirm the diagnosis but also
to establish the cause or the source of the botulism. If
the botulism is foodborne, the causative food must be identified, if possible, to prevent additional exposures. Mild
cases and virtually all infant botulism cases are likely to
give negative serum results. Adequate food samples for
laboratory examination often are not available. Analysis of
fecal specimens has contributed much to the success of laboratory investigations (1) and serves as the only means for
confirming infant botulism. A variety of specimens, which
includes serum, stool, food, autopsy, vomitus, tissue or
exudate from wounds, gastric fluid, and environmental
samples, can be chosen for examination as deemed appropriate
for each incident. Methods for examining specimens are
published in detail elsewhere (2,3). Laboratory confirmation is similar for foodborne, wound or infant botulism in
humans as well as for botulism of animals. For wound

botulism one would not ordinarily expect to find evidence in
the feces, but one must be aware that even though a patient
exhibiting signs of botulism has a wound, he may still have
a case of foodborne botulism.

Detecting and identifying botulinal toxin in the serum
or feces of a patient exhibiting appropriate signs and symptoms is usually considered sufficient evidence for confirming
the diagnosis. Demonstrating botulinal toxin in a food epidemiologically implicated in an outbreak of illness clinically consistent with botulism is also very good confirmatory evidence. Experience has shown that *Clostridium
botulinum* is very rarely isolated from the feces of humans
without botulism; it is often isolated from the feces of
patients with foodborne botulism and is always isolated from
the feces of infant botulism cases (1,4,5). Culturing of
food specimens which contain no detectable amounts of toxin
is not very helpful. *C. botulinum* is widely distributed
in soils and can often be found in produce and other foods.
Unless the spores germinate, multiply and produce toxin, no
botulism will occur. Easton and Meyer have reported that
fecal specimens from persons who had eaten produce known to
contain *C. botulinum* yielded none of the organisms upon
culturing (4). Thus, it appears that in order to recover
C. botulinum from the feces, larger numbers have to be
present because the organism had multiplied either in the
food before ingestion or in the gut after ingestion.

B. *Laboratory Methods*

1. *Detecting and Identifying Botulinal Toxin.*
Although there are criticisms of using the mouse toxicity
and neutralization test for demonstrating botulinal toxins,
it is the method of choice in the Centers for Disease
Control (CDC) Anaerobe Laboratory for a number of reasons.
It is extremely sensitive; it will detect as little as 10
picograms (10^{-8}mg) of toxic protein in the injected
sample. Identifying the toxin by neutralization with antitoxin is quite specific. Even if there are other antigen-
antibody (nonspecific) reactions taking place in the test
mixture, the only one that will be apparent is the specific
neutralization, which allows the mouse to live. Often the
objection is that the test is too time consuming. Although
it is generally described as a 4-day test, the results when
moderate amounts of toxin are present in the specimen (or

specimen extract) are evident much sooner, usually within 12
hours or overnight. Some *in vitro* tests may require a
similar length of time for results. The biggest problems
with the mouse tests are that they cannot be readily performed in laboratories that do not have mice available on a
regular basis, and that many specimens, especially stools,
can contain materials other than botulinal toxin which are
toxic and can cause death in mice. The latter problem is
sometimes referred to as nonspecific toxicity. This problem
can sometimes be overcome by diluting the test material to a
point at which the nonbotulinal factor is no longer toxic,
but at which the botulinal toxin is still sufficient for
reliable identification. On some occasions, low molecular
weight substances such as salt in extracts of salted fish or
medicinal residues in fecal extracts have interfered with
mouse tests, but such problems can be solved by dialysis.
On at least three occasions, stools from botulism patients
were found to contain pyridostigmine or neostignine because
the patient was treated earlier with the drug after a diagnosis of myasthenia gravis had been made (6; CDC, unpublished).

     2. *Cultural Approaches to Laboratory Confirmation.*
Although results from culturing specimens for *C. botulinum*
provided confirmatory evidence more often than the direct
toxicity tests on specimens, more time is required to obtain
those results. The procedure used in the CDC Anaerobe laboratory has been to inoculate liquid media (chopped meat
glucose) with some of the specimen and then to test for
toxicity after 3 to 5 days' incubation. Direct streaking of
solid media (egg yolk agar) with suspensions of stool specimens are often unsatisfactory because of the very high
number of other anaerobic and facultative organisms and the
relatively low numbers of *C. botulinum* present. Enrichment cultures inoculated after spore selection (heat or
alcohol treatments) are usually more satisfactory. Toxic
enrichment cultures usually contain *C. botulinum* in high
enough numbers for easy isolation when streaked on agar
plates, although sometimes a spore selection technique on
the enrichment culture before streaking is helpful or even
necessary. Recently, a selective egg yolk agar medium
containing antibiotics (cycloserine, sulfamethoxazole and
trimethoprim) has been developed (7), and a current laboratory evaluation shows that it is very useful in confirming
botulism, especially in infants. Direct streaking of

positive fecal suspensions on this selective agar,
Clostridium botulinum isolation (CBI) medium, results in
the appearance of lipase positive colonies, recognizable
after 24 hours, which can be picked. The isolates still
must then be tested for toxigenicity before positive
identification can be made. In cases of infant botulism,
the lipase positive colony-formers, typical of *C. botulinum*,
are often the predominant organism on the CBI plate
streaked with the stool specimen. In some cases, the plate
looks almost as though it had been streaked with a pure
culture. By picking from the directly streaked plates, the
time and effort of toxicity testing the enrichment cultures
can be saved.

Using fluorescent antibody (FA) techniques for pre-
sumptively identifying *C. botulinum* in fecal specimens,
enrichment cultures, and individual colonies isolated from
agar media can be very helpful in giving an early indication
of whether on not confirmation will be made on the basis of
culture results. The success with this method depends on
the reliability of the reagents. Some reagents do not
distinguish between *C. botulinum* and *C. sporogenes*. In
addition, *C. botulinum* strains appear to have considerable
serological variability, and some reagents do not react with
strains of the same toxin type and physiologic group as the
homologous strain. FA reagents have been prepared and
evaluated recently in the CDC Anaerobe Laboratory (8). The
type A and B antisera produced at least a 2+ staining
intensity with 100% of a wide selection of strains of the
homologous toxin types (89 type A and 46 type B). The cross
reactions between these two types were 30% for the type A
reagent and 22% for the type B reagent. Very little cross
reaction occurred between these two reagents with 23 strains
of *C. sporogenes* or with any other bacterial species.
Since one case of type F infant botulism has been confirmed
(9), a polyvalent ABF FA reagent has been prepared for
screening infant botulism specimens. Twenty-nine (85%) of
34 infant stool specimens which were culture positive, were
FA positive by examination of direct smears (10). Some of
the specimens had been stored in the refrigerator or freezer
for several months. Those which were negative by FA tests
on the direct smears, showed positively staining bacteria in
the enrichment cultures after incubating for 24 to 72
hours. Two of 31 culture negative specimens gave FA
positive results, one on the direct smear and the other in
an enrichment culture. Testing direct smears of specimens
with monovalent or polyvalent reagents may provide early

presumptive evidence for a diagnosis of botulism. Screening
of cultures using FA reagents may save much effort and
expense by eliminating unnecessary toxicity testing of many
negative cultures.

II. CONFIRMING HUMAN BOTULISM

A. *Foodborne Botulism*

   In reviewing laboratory data from examination of serum
and stool specimens in 135 foodborne botulism investigations
over a 3-year period, Dowell et al. (1) reported the following (Table 1): (a) 31 of the incidents were confirmed as
botulism outbreaks, involving 72 cases; (b) 33.3% of the
patients tested were confirmed by demonstrating botulinal
toxin in their serum; (c) 33.9% were confirmed by showing
the presence of toxin in their stools; (d) 60% had stools
which were culture positive for *C. botulinum*; and (e)
overall, about 64% of the cases were confirmed by laboratory
evidence from either serum or stool.
   The success rate in confirming foodborne botulism
outbreaks varies from incident to incident. Table 1 shows
three examples of large outbreaks in which the confirmation
rate varies from 0 to 76.5%. In the outbreak in Oklahoma in
1976 (11), toxin was not detected in the serum or stools of
any of the seven patients nor was *C. botulinum* isolated
from any of the stools. Since no toxin was detected in the
suspect food (cherry peppers), the diagnosis of botulism was
made solely on the basis of clinical and epidemiological
evidence. The largest documented outbreak of botulism in
the United States, which occurred in Michigan in 1977,
involved 59 clinical cases (12). Botulinal toxin was not
detected in the serum of any of the patients. Stools from
only eight of the patients were positive for either type B
botulinal toxin, *C. botulinum* type B, or both. Thus, only
13.6% of the cases in this outbreak were confirmed by evidence in clinical specimens. None of the home-processed
jalopena peppers from the jar served in the restaurant to
the victims were available, but type B botulinal toxin was
identified in 2 unopened jars of the same lot. The second
largest outbreak, which occurred one year later in New
Mexico (13,14), was most convincingly confirmed by laboratory evidence from clinical specimens from 26 of the 34
victims (76.5%). Type A botulinal toxin was detected in

Table 1. Confirmation of Foodborne Botulism Cases with Laboratory Evidence in Patients' Serum and Stool Specimens.

Incident	Year	Causative Food	No. Cases	Serum (toxin)	Stool		Overall Confirmation
					Toxin	C. botulinum	
31 outbreaks United States	1972-1975	Various	72	20/60 (33.3)[b]	19/56 (33.9)	36/60 (60.0)	46/72 (63.9)
Oklahoma	1976	Cherry peppers[a]	7	0/7 (0)	0/7 (0)	0/7 (0)	0/7 (0)
Michigan	1977	Jalapeno peppers	59	0/59 (0)	4/59 (6.8)	5/59 (8.5)	8/59 (13.6)
New Mexico	1978	Salad items	34	16/30 (53.3)	7/22 (31.8)	19/24 (79.2)	26/34 (76.5)

[a]No botulinal toxin detected in any of the peppers available for examination.

[b]Figures in parentheses are percent positive.

the serum of 16 of 30 patients tested and in the stools of 7 of 22 patients. *C. botulinum* was isolated from 19 of 24 stool cultures. Type A botulinal toxin was detected in one of the epidemiologically implicated foods (potato salad) but not in the second (bean salad).

The data from investigations such as these point out that a number of cases of actual botulism will not be confirmed by laboratory evidence. In a large outbreak, this is inconsequential if at least one of the cases is confirmed, because the confirmation of one case adequately confirms the diagnoses of the others. In cases involving only a single case in which no food has been identified, negative results on the clinical specimens may leave the diagnosis doubtful. The data also point out the importance of examining stool specimens.

Success in confirming individual foodborne botulism cases appears to be at least partly related to the amount of toxin ingested and to the time of collection of clinical specimens, in relation to the time of ingesting of peccant food. The severity of illness is also likely due to the amount of ingested toxin, and this in turn has an influence on the time of specimen collection. The more severe cases have a more rapid onset of signs and symptoms and have more pronounced signs and symptoms which are more clearly recognizable. These factors facilitate an early diagnosis.

B. *Wound Botulism*

Laboratory confirmation of wound botulism is usually attempted by testing the patient's serum for botulinal toxin and culturing the wound for *C. botulinum*. Since 1943, 23 cases have been diagnosed and reported to the Center for Disease Control (Table 2). Sixteen of the cases were

TABLE 2. *Laboratory Confirmation of Wound Botulism in the U.S., 1943-1980*

23 cases: 13 type A, 3 type B, 7 unknown		
Serum positive[a]	7/20	35%
Culture positive[b]	14/22	63.6%
Both specimens positive	5/19	26.3%
Total cases confirmed	16/23	69.6%

[a]*Botulinal toxin identified in serum.*
[b]*C. botulinum isolated from wound*

confirmed in the laboratory. The rate for confirming wound botulism on the basis of positive sera, 35%, is about the same as has been reported for foodborne botulism (1). Culturing of the wounds in addition to testing the sera doubled the confirmation rate.

C. Infant Botulism

In addition to those infant cases investigated by various state and local health departments, specimens from 163 cases of suspected infant botulism have been examined in the CDC Anaerobe Laboratory (Table 3). Forty-four of these were confirmed with laboratory evidence. This confirmation consists of detecting botulinal toxin in the feces or isolation of C. botulinum, or both. All cases for which C. botulinum was isolated from the stool were considered confirmed. In testing the stools for botulinal toxin, one case was found negative. The specimen was obtained 2 weeks after the onset of illness. The tests on stools from four cases were inconclusive because of nonspecific toxicity of the extract. Some of the specimens in which botulinal toxin was detected also were nonspecifically toxic, but we were

TABLE 3. *Confirmation of Infant Botulism in the CDC Anaerobe Laboratory, 1975 - 1981[a]*

Investigations		163
Culturally Confirmed Cases		44
type A	15	
type B	28	
type F	1[b]	
Feces from Confirmed Cases Tested for Toxin		42
no. positive	37	
no. negative	1	
no. inconclusive[c]	4	
Serum from Confirmed Cases Tested for Toxin		28
no. positive	1	
no. negative	27	

[a]*Through February 28, 1981.*
[b]*Investigated simultaneously with New Mexico Health Dept.*
[c]*Toxin test inconclusive because of nonspecific toxicity of fecal extract.*

able to test them at a dilution at which the nonspecific factor was inactive in mice but at which we were able to demonstrate and identify the botulinal toxin by specific neutralization. In tests on 28 of the cases for botulinal toxin in the serum, the test was positive for only one.

Specimens from 49 cases of *Sudden Infant Death Syndrome* from 12 states were also examined for *C. botulinum* and botulinal toxin. In each case, at least one stool or intestinal specimen was examined. For some cases, sera, visceral, and multiple intestinal specimens were seen. Neither toxin nor the organism was found in any of the specimens.

III. INVESTIGATIONS OF SUSPECTED ANIMAL BOTULISM

A. *Botulism in Dogs*

Occasionally, specimens pertaining to suspected animal botulism are sent to the CDC Anaerobe Laboratory. In the past 5 years, specimens from 12 incidents involving dogs have been examined. Evidence has been found in five of the incidents to support a diagnosis of type C botulism (Table 4). One incident involved a group of foxhounds which was believed to have found and eaten some discarded chicken carcasses in a wooded area (15). Type C botulinal toxin was identified in the feces of one of the affected dogs and in a fecal culture of another dog. *C. botulinum* type C was not isolated from the toxic enrichment culture nor from fecal cultures from three other affected dogs. On the other hand, *C. botulinum* type A was isolated from an autopsy liver specimen from the dog which had type C toxin in the fecal specimen obtained while he was living.

A case of type C botulism resulted in Ohio after a coonhound had eaten some dead chickens (Table 4). The chickens had become ill and died sometime after they were observed eating maggots on discarded groundhog carcasses (16). When the veterinarian was examining the paralyzed dog, he noted feathers in the vomitus and then concluded that the illness was possibly foodborne. The diagnosis of botulism was confirmed by identifying type C botulinal toxin in the serum and vomitus from the dog. No toxin was identified in the dog's feces.

Three other cases, each involving a single dog were confirmed as type C botulism by demonstrating type C toxin

TABLE 4.   *Confirmation of Botulism in Dogs*

	specimens	toxin	culture (C.botulinum)
Georgia, Oct. 76			
19 dogs (ate dead chickens)			
dog #1	stool	type C	negative
	liver	negative	type A
dog #2	serum	inconclusive	
	stool	inconclusive	negative
dog #3	serum	negative	
	stool	negative	negative
dog #4	serum	negative	
dog #5	serum	negative	
	stool	inconclusive	type C[a]
dog #6	serum	negative	
Georgia, Aug. 77			
1 dog (ate dead animal)			
	serum	negative	
	stool	type C	---
Ohio, Aug. 77			
1 dog (ate dead chicken)			
	serum	type C	
	stool	inconclusive	---
	vomitus	type C	---
Georgia, Nov. 78			
1 dog (source unknown)			
	serum	negative	
	stool	type C	type C[a]
Georgia, Sept. 80			
1 dog (source unknown)			
	serum	negative	
	stool	type C	type C[a]

[a]*Type C toxin detected in culture; no toxigenic organism isolated.*

in the feces (Table 4). The sera from these cases were
negative in mouse toxicity tests. One of the cases was
related to the dog's eating a dead animal, and in the other
2 cases, the source was not known. In none of these 5
incidents were we successful in isolating toxigenic C.
botulinum type C, even from enrichment cultures which
contained type C toxin. Nontoxigenic organisms resembling
C. botulinum type C were isolated from some of the
cultures.

B. *Shaker Foal Syndrome*

In 1967, Rooney and Prickett described a condition in
Kentucky foals known as *shaker foal syndrome* (17). The
condition affects foals usually between 3 and 8 weeks of age
and is characterized by sudden onset of severe muscular
weakness and prostration. An affected foal which is down
may be able to stand for a few minutes if helped to its feet
but will soon develop generalized muscular trembling (thus,
the term "shaker") and then fall to the ground. Death
occurs in most cases within 72 hours and is attributable to
respiratory failure. Rooney and Prickett considered a
botulism etiology and observed the same clinical presentation in foals given botulinal toxin experimentally.
However, they could not conclude that this was the natural
cause of the shaker foal syndrome because they could not
identify botulinal toxin in the dead foals or in suspect
feed materials. They commented that the most disturbing
problem in postulating that the condition was caused by a
toxin was that it was seen only in this distinctly restricted age group. This aspect, in addition to the observation
that an associated constipation occurs, leads one to
speculate on the similarities to infant botulism.

In 1978, Dr. James Klyza, a veterinarian in Lexington,
Kentucky observed that cultures from fecal specimens from
shakers had FA positive bacilli when tested with the
commercially available reagents specific for C. botulinum,
whereas cultures from normal foals generally did not.
Examination of the specimens from the foals in the CDC
Anaerobe Laboratory confirmed Dr. Klyza's findings. C.
botulinum type B was identified in enrichment cultures of
specimens from 11 of 12 shakers and isolated from 9 of those
cultures. The presence of the organism was established by
demonstrating type B botulinal toxin in culture supernatants
by using mouse toxicity and neutralization tests. C.
botulinum type B was detected in the fecal culture of 1 of

14 normal foals but was not isolated. No botulinal toxin
was detected in either the serum or in the fecal specimens
of any of the foals. The one shaker which was culture
negative had an infected wound on the lower jaw; this may
represent a case of wound botulism, rather than a
gastrointestinal toxico infection.

C. botulinum was found in fecal specimens of some
adult horses from the same farms. Cultures from 3 of 17
mares were positive for type B toxin, and C. botulinum
type B was isolated from cultures from 2 of those cultures.
All 3 culture positive mares were dams of shaker foals.
Four other dams of shakers and 9 dams of normal foals were
culture-negative.

The question arises as to why botulinal toxin was not
detected in any of the fecal specimens. Extracts of 7 of 10
specimens from shakers which were tested for toxin were
nonspecifically toxic. The extracts killed mice, but the
toxicity was not neutralized by botulinal antitoxins; the
signs of illness in the mice before death did not indicate
botulism. The nonspecific toxicity may mask the presence of
botulinal toxin. In addition, the activity of the botulinal
toxin may have been destroyed before it could be tested in
the feces. The lack of detectable toxin in the serum of
shaker foals is similar to the findings in infant botulism
(3,5). Furthermore, Swerczek has shown that horses are very
sensitive to type B toxin (18). If they are relatively as
sensitive as or more sensitive than the mice which are used
to detect the toxin, the toxin level in affected horses is
not likely to be detectable by injecting 0.5 ml of serum per
mouse. That the toxin type of C. botulinum encountered in
the specimens from these Kentucky foals and mares was type B
in all cases is consistent with the findings in the soil
survey reported by Smith (19). Soil samples taken in
Kentucky very often yielded C. botulinum, and in each case
the toxin type was B.

IV.   CHARACTERISTICS OF CLOSTRIDIUM BOTULINUM STRAINS
ISOLATED FROM BOTULISM INCIDENTS

Almost all cases of human botulism in the United States
have been caused by C. botulinum strains which produce
type A, B, or E toxin. Three incidents of type F botulism
have been documented in this country: a foodborne outbreak
due to venison jerky in California in 1966 (20), a case of

infant botulism in New Mexico in 1979 (9), and a case in
February 1981 of undetermined classification in an adult
male in Florida. One incident of suspected human botulism
in the U.S. was suggested as possibly type C because an
organism resembling *C. botulinum* type C was isolated from
the stomach contents of a patient who had died of an illness
with symptoms suggestive of botulism (21). No toxin was
detected, and the suspect food was not available for
examination. Excluding the latter incident, all confirmed
human botulism in the U.S. has been caused by strains
belonging to physiological groups I and II (22) (sometimes
referred to as proteolytic and nonproteolytic *C. botulinum*, respectively). Group I consists of strains which
produce either type A, B, or F toxin; group II strains
produce either type B, E, or F toxin. Although the group I
organisms have strong proteolytic activity, they generally
cause botulism by their growth in low protein foods such as
vegetables, whereas the group II organisms with low proteolytic activity usually, if not exclusively, cause botulism
by way of high protein foods such as fish. All infant botulism cases confirmed in the United States to date have been
caused by group I strains. The strains isolated from infant
botulism cases do not differ in any physiological aspect
from the group I strains which cause human foodborne botulism (23), although 2 strains isolated from infants have
been found to produce toxin with unusual serological
properties. The only outbreak of botulism in the United
States in the past 6 years in which a nonproteolytic strain
of type B was implicated was caused by salted fish
(Akiachak, Alaska, Dec. 1976). The type B botulism in
Europe so often caused by ham (usually home processed) is
believed to be due to group II strains (personal communication, Prof. L. Leistner, Kulmback W. Germany). A nonproteolytic strain of type F was implicated in the botulism
outbreak in California caused by venison jerky (20).
    Types C and D comprise group III. These organisms are
generally considered to cause botulism only in birds and
animals (21). Type C has been implicated in canine botulism
in the CDC Anaerobe Laboratory, but attempts to isolate the
organism were not successful. The failure was either
because the media or cultural procedures were inadequate or
because the organisms present in the specimens no longer
produced toxin after isolation.
    Usually, the serological characteristics of the toxin
produced by the organism causing an outbreak of human

TABLE 5.   Neutralization of Type B and Strain 657
Botulinal Toxins with Antitoxins

	Antitoxin	
Toxin Source	type B(1 IU)	Anti 657(0.1ml)
Strain 657	10 LD[a]	1,000 LD
Beans Strain	10,000 LD	10,000 LD

[a]No. of lethal doses of toxin neutralized by 1 IU or
0.1 ml of the indicated antitoxin

botulism conform with those of the classical types A, B, E,
or F.   However, two cases of infant botulism were caused by
strains with serologically anomalous toxins.   The one strain
(strain 657) which caused botulism in a Texas infant, produces a toxin which requires an exceedingly large amount of
type B antitoxin (24).   One international unit of type B
toxin neutralizes only about 10 mouse lethal doses of strain
657 toxin, while it will neutralize about 10,000 lethal
doses of conventional type B toxin from the "Beans" strain
(Table 5).   One tenth ml of an antiserum prepared against
the 657 strain toxin will neutralize 10-fold more conventional type B toxin than homologous toxin.   This strain is
a group I organism.   The deviant serological properties of
the toxin may be similar to those of the toxin of the QC
strain reported by Shimizu and Kondo (25).   The QC is a
nonproteolytic (group II) type B strain.   Recently, the New
Mexico State Health Department confirmed a case of infant
botulism in which the toxin in the specimen extracts and in
the cultures of the isolated organism requires a combination
of type B and type F antitoxins for neutralization (New
Mexico State Health Dept./CDC Anaerobe Laboratory, unpublished data).   The toxin in pure cultures appears to be
roughly 90% type B and 10% type F.   This is analogous to the
toxin of strain 84 of Gimenez and Ciccarelli, which is a
mixture of type A and F toxins (26).

V.   CONCLUSION

The CDC Anaerobe Laboratory has been examining specimens
pertaining to cases and outbreaks of suspect botulism since
1962.   The experience gained over this period has provided

valuable insights into laboratory confirmation of botulism as well as into some aspects of the disease and the nature and varied characteristics of the causative organisms. The laboratory approaches to the investigation of human botulism are applicable to the investigation of botulism in animals.

REFERENCES

1. Dowell, V. R., Jr., McCroskey, L. M., Hatheway, C. L., Lombard, G. L., Hughes, J. M., and Merson, M. H. *J. Am. Med. Assn. 238*, 1829 (1977).
2. Center for Disease Control., *in* "Botulism in the United States, 1899-1977." Handbook for Epidemiologists, Clinicians and Laboratory Workers. (Issued May 1979).
3. Hatheway, C. L., *Rev. Infect. Dis. 1*, 647 (1979).
4. Easton, E. J., and Meyer, K. F., *J. Infect. Dis. 35*, 207 (1924).
5. Arnon, S. S., *Annu. Rev. Med. 31*, 541 (1980).
6. Horwitz, M. A., Hatheway, C. L., and Dowell, V. R., Jr., *Am. J. Clin. Pathol. 66*, 737 (1976).
7. Dezfulian, M., McCroskey, L. M., Hatheway, C. L., and Dowell, V. R., Jr., *J. Clin. Microbiol. 13*, 526 (1981).
8. Glasby, C., and Hatheway, C. L., *in* "Abstracts, 81st Annu. Meeting, American Society for Microbiology, Dallas, Marh 1-6 (1981).
9. Center for Disease Control, *Morbid. Mortal. Wkly Rept. 29*, 85 (1980).
10. Glasby, C., "Doctor of Public Health Dissertation." University of North Carolina, Chapel Hill (1981).
11. Center for Disease Control, *Morbid. Mortal. Wkly. Rept. 25*, 134, 148 (1976).
12. Center for Disease Control, *Morbid. Mortal. Wkly. Rept. 26*, 117, 135 (1977).
13. Center for Disease Control, *Morbid. Mortal. Wkly. Rept. 27*, 138, 145 (1978).
14. Mann, J., Hatheway, C. L., and Gardiner, T., Manuscript in preparation (1981).
15. Barsanti, J. A., Walser, M., Hatheway, C. L., Bowen, J. M., and Crowell, W., *J. Am. Vet. Med. Assn. 172*, 809 (1978).
16. Richmond, R. N., Hatheway, C. L., and Kaufmann, A. F., *J. Am. Vet. Med. Assn. 173*, 202 (1978).
17. Rooney, J. R., and Prickett, M. E., *Mod. Vet. Pract. 48*, 44 (1967).
18. Swerczek, T. W., *Am. J. Vet. Res. 41*, 348 (1980).
19. Smith, L. DS., *Health Lab. Sci. 15*, 74 (1980).

20. Midura, T. F., Nygaard, G. S., Wood, R. M., and Bodily,
     H. L., *Appl. Microbiol.* *24*, 165 (1972).
21. Meyer, K. F., Eddie, B., York, G. K., Collier, C. D., and
     Townsend, C. T., *Proc. VI Internat. Congr. Microbiol. 2*,
     276 (1953).
22. Smith, L. DS., "Botulism: The Organism, Its Toxin, The
     Disease." C. C. Thomas, Springfield, Ill. (1977).
23. Dezfulian, M., and Dowell, V. R., Jr., *J. Clin. Micro-
     biol. 11*, 604 (1980).
24. Hatheway, C. L., McCroskey, L. M., Lombard, G. L., and
     Dowell, V. R., Jr., *J. Clin. Microbiol.*, in press (1981).
25. Shimizu, T., and Kondo, H., *Japan J. Med. Sci. Biol. 26*,
     269 (1973).
26. Gimenez, D. F., and Ciccarelli, A. S., *Zbl. Bakt. I. Abt.
     Orig. 215*, 212 (1970).

ISOLATION AND IDENTIFICATION OF BOTULINUM TOXINS
USING THE ELISA

Servé Notermans

Laboratory for Zoonoses and Food Microbiology
National Institute of Public Health
Bilthoven, The Netherlands

Shunji Kozaki

Department of Veterinary Science
College of Agriculture
University of Osaka Prefecture
Sakai-shi, Osaka, Japan

INTRODUCTION

Determination of botulinum toxin is an essential part of
botulism research. The presence of *Clostridium botulinum* in
samples is determined by culturing these samples in an enrichment medium. The presence of toxin in the culture fluid indicates the presence of *C.botulinum* in the original sample.
Growth of *C.botulinum* in food is mostly determined by toxin
production. A method frequently used for detecting and typing
of toxins produced by *C.botulinum* is the mouse-bio-assay. For
quantitation and typing of the toxin relatively high numbers
of mice are needed. The test, however, is found to be unsuitable for examination of samples containing other toxic substances that may cause non-specific deaths.
    A sensitive serological test system for detecting the
presence of toxin, and its immunological type, is time saving
and may supplant the use of mice. One of the most promising
serological tests is the enzyme linked immunosorbent assay
(ELISA). The ELISA is similar in design to the radio-immuno-
assay; however, instead of a radio-active label an enzyme
label is used.

The enzyme label may be conjugated either to the toxin or
to the antibody for use in the competitive and the sandwich
ELISA respectively. Since labeling of botulinum toxin with an
enzyme requires extreme care and as an active immunity of laboratory personnel is essential only the sandwich ELISA has so
far been described (6, 7, 8). The procedures of the ELISA for
botulinum toxins as well as details of production of the different reagents used were recently summarized by Notermans et
al. (9). The sandwich ELISA can be performed as a "sandwich"
or as a "double sandwich". The "sandwich" ELISA is carried out
using polystyrene or polyvinyl tubes which are coated with
antibotulinum Ig (e.g. from rabbits). After incubation with
the toxin, the amount of adsorbed toxin is measured using antibotulinum Ig conjugated to an enzyme. The amount of enzyme is
determined spectrophotometrically after the addition of a
suitable substrate. In the "double sandwich" ELISA an antibotulinum Ig originating from another species than rabbit (e.g.
horse) is bound to the adsorbed toxin. The amount of these adsorbed antibodies is measured with antihorse Ig enzyme conjugate. An advantage of the "double sandwich" technique is that
the same anti-Ig-enzyme conjugate can be used for the detection
of all botulinum toxins. Furthermore it was found by Kozaki et
al. (5) that compared with the "sandwich" the "double sandwich"
was somewhat more sensitive. A drawback is that antibotulinum
Ig has to be prepared in two animal species.
    Detection of the various types of botulinum toxins re-
quires type specific antisera. These can be prepared by immunization of animals with only purified derivative toxin (neurotoxin). They are produced from L- or M-toxin complexes by
DEAE-Sephadex chromatography as described by Sugii and Sakaguchi (11), Kozaki et al. (6) and Kitamura et al. (4).
    However, in spite of the use of type specific antisera
slight cross-reactions have been observed (5, 8). These cross-
reactions, however, were limited to culture filtrates of only
some of the *C.botulinum* strains. In the ELISA for toxin type B,
cross-reactions were observed with culture filtrates of *C.botu-
linum* type A. In the ELISA for toxin type E, cross-reactions
were found with culture filtrates of *C.botulinum* type A and
proteolytic *C.botulinum* type B. No cross-reactions were observed for any of the other Clostridia strains tested. The lowest
reliably detectable quantities of botulinum toxin is ca 100
mouse i.p. LD_{50} for toxin types A and E (7, 8), and ca 400
mouse i.p. LD_{50} for toxin type B (5).
    This paper presents the results of investigations to pre-
vent cross-reactions and attempts to increase the sensitivity
of the ELISA. Examples are also given of application of the
ELISA for detection and identification of *C.botulinum* strains.

PREVENTION OF CROSS-REACTIONS

Non-specific reactions which occur in the ELISA can be caused by cross-reacting antibodies and/or by non-immunological binding of proteins. Cross-reacting antibodies may be formed if the toxic component used for immunization is not completely free from non-toxic components. In the double sandwich ELISA as described by Kozaki et al. (5) and Notermans et al. (7, 8) only the rabbit IgG used for coating was prepared using the derivative toxin, contrary to the horse serum which was of commercial origin. This latter serum may have caused the observed cross-reactions. Therefore a sheep has been immunized with the derivative toxin to produce antibodies to be used instead of the horse serum. From the results it became clear that non-specific binding was not prevented. This means that cross-reacting antibodies are still present or that non-immunological binding occurs.

In earlier experiments cross-reacting antibodies have been removed by adsorption of the IgG with culture filtrates containing different types of botulinum toxins immobilized with CNBr-activated Sepharose 4B (Pharmacia Fine Chemicals AB, Uppsala, Sweden). However, in the ELISA these cross-reactions did still occur. In this study cross-reacting antibodies were removed by adsorption of the antibotulinum IgG to the toxic component immobilized with CNBr-activated Sepharose 4B (11). After washing, the immunologically bound IgG was eluted with 0.2 M glycine-HCl buffer, pH 2.3, containing 0.5 NaCl and dialysed immediately against 0.15 M PBS pH 7.2. With this specifically purified rabbit and horse antibotulinum IgG all false-positive reactions could be prevented in the double sandwich ELISA (Table 1).

INCREASING THE SENSITIVITY

The results of Kozaki et al. (5) showed that the "double sandwich" ELISA is about 5-10 times more sensitive than the "sandwich" ELISA. Yolken and Stopa (14) claimed that the sensitivity of the ELISA can be improved by using a fluorogenic substrate (4-methylumbelliferyl phosphate) which yields a fluorescent product upon enzyme action. By using a fluorogenic substrate approximately 10^{-12} moles of alkaline phosphatase in one-tenth of 1 ml should be detectable whereas with nitrophenylphosphate only 10^{-10} moles of alkaline phosphatase are detectable.

TABLE I. Prevention of cross-reactions in the ELISA of botulinum toxine type
B in 1:4 diluted culture supernatants of some C.botulinum strains

Type of ELISA applied	C.botulinum type (and strains)			
	A(73A)	A(141A)	E(RIV1)	E(Beluga)
Double sandwich coat : rabbit IgG anti 7S toxin type B label: commercial horse serum	0.7[x]	0.7	0.0	0.3
Double sandwich coat : rabbit IgG anti 7S toxin type B label: sheep IgG anti 7S toxin type B	0.7	0.6	0.0	0.2
Double sandwich coat : specific rabbit IgG anti 7S toxin type B label: specific horse IgG anti 7S toxin type B	0.0	0.0	0.0	0.0
Sandwich coat : rabbit IgG anti 7S toxin type B	0.0	0.0	0.0	0.0

[x]extinction value

We tested the fluorogenic substrate for the detection of
botulinum toxins with the double sandwich ELISA using alkaline
phosphatase as enzyme. However, no improvement in sensitivity
was obtained in comparison with nitrophenylphosphate as colorogenic substrate. This result indicates that the limiting
factor of the immuno-assay may not be the measurement of the
enzymatic reaction but rather the formation of the initial antigen-antibody complex. This hypothesis was tested in the
ELISA by using increasing amounts of horse specifically purified IgG and of rabbit antihorse IgG enzyme conjugate. Peroxidase was used as enzyme and 5-amino salicylic acid (ASA) as
colorogenic substrate. The results are presented in Fig. 1.
It is clear that the concentrations of IgG and of IgG∞enzyme
complex influence the blanc-values. Since the use of higher
concentrations of these reagents magnify the extinctions values of the blanc as well as of the samples it is extremely unlikely that the use of higher energy substrates such as the

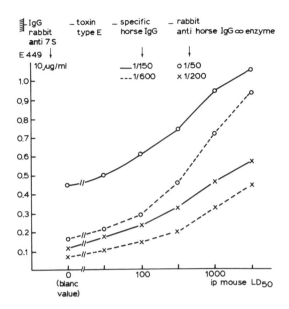

FIGURE 1. The "double sandwich" ELISA for determining of botulinum toxin type E, using increasing amounts of specific horse IgG and IgG∞enzyme conjugate.

fluorescent ones will lead to an increased degree of sensitivity. This is demonstrated in the sandwich ELISA for toxin type E using orthophenyldiamine (OPD) as colorogenic substrate. In the liquid phase 12 times less peroxidase can be detected with OPD than with ASA. However, it is also clear that again the blanc value increased with the amount of conjugates used (see Fig. 2).

PRACTICAL APPLICATION

Testing for Toxin Production by C.botulinum in Food Samples

Several factors can be considered for preventing growth and toxin production by C.botulinum in food, i.e. heating, lowering pH, lowering water activity or addition of inhibiting substances like sorbate and nitrite. Before a new additive is introduced into a food it is important to test whether it will prevent toxin production by C.botulinum. For this type of investigations, the ELISA can be used successfully. De Wit et al.

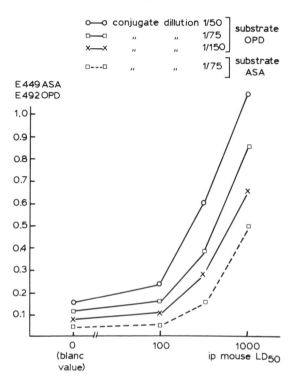

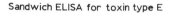

FIGURE 2. "Sandwich" ELISA for determining botulinum toxin type E using increasing IgG∞enzyme conjugate and OPD and ASA as substrate.

(1) tested the effect of garlic oil and onion oil on toxin production by *C.botulinum* in meat slurry. Toxin production by *C.botulinum* type A was successfully detected using the ELISA. This was also the case when testing the effect of glycerylmono-laurate on toxin production by *C.botulinum* in meat slurry (un-published data). In these experiments similar results were ob-tained with the mouse-bio-assay and with the ELISA. In another experiment toxin production by *C.botulinum* in vacuum packed cooked potatoes was readily detectable using the ELISA (10). From these examples it becomes clear that the ELISA gives re-liable results. This was mainly due to a high contamination level of the test samples with spores of *C.botulinum* and

optimal incubation conditions. If no toxin is detected using
the ELISA then for absolute safety small amounts of toxin can
be detected using the mouse-bio-assay.

Testing for the Presence of Toxin in Enrichment Cultures

The presence of *C.botulinum* in samples is determined by
culturing these samples in an enrichment medium. From earlier
results obtained with the ELISA (9) it is concluded that when
enough toxin is produced in the enrichment cultures (e.g. for
type E > 100 mouse i.p. LD_{50}/ml) the toxin can easily be detected with the ELISA. However, toxin production by *C.botulinum*
in enrichment cultures depends on the sample composition and
on the enrichment medium used. From the results of Smith (12)
it becomes clear that *C.perfringens* from soil represses the
growth and toxin production of *C.botulinum*. It also repressed
growth and toxin production of *C.botulinum* in mixed cultures
of soils in which *C.botulinum* naturally occurred if cooked
meat medium was used but not if trypticase medium was used.
Graham (3) found that *C.botulinum* could not always be detected
in mud samples due to the presence of *Bacillus* ssp, gram-positive non-sporing rods and gram-positive cocci which inhibited
growth of *C.botulinum* type C. As a result of this inhibition
only small amounts of toxin or even no toxin is produced in
the enrichment cultures. Therefore a search must be made to
develop media in which such inhibition is suppressed. DezFul-
lian and Dowell (2) showed that *C.botulinum* exhibited a high

TABLE 2. Recovery of Clostridium botulinum *from sewage sludge
using Fortified Egg Meat Medium (FEM) and FEM containing cycloserine, sulfamethoxazole and trimethoprim (FEM +) as enrichment media.*

Number of samples tested	Heat treatment	Incubation medium	Number with toxin production	B	C	E
26	$70^{o}C$/10 min.	FEM	8	6	1	1
		FEM +	3	3	0	0
26	not treated	FEM	13	11	1	1
		FEM +	10	9	1	0

degree of resistance to cycloserine, sulfamethoxazola and trimethoprim. They suggested that addition of these antibiotics
to the enrichment medium may prove to be useful in the isolation and identification of *C.botulinum* from mixed microbial
populations. This hypothesis was tested using Fortified Egg
Meat Medium (FEM) and FEM containing the three antibiotics.
Samples of sewage sludge were used. Results are presented in
Table 2, and it is clear that addition of the antibiotics to
the FEM does not result in a better recovery of *C.botulinum*
from the sludge samples. One explanation may be that the high
number of *C.perfringens* present in sludge may also be resistant
to the antibiotics present.

Besides developing better enrichment media which allow high
toxin production by *C.botulinum* the sensitivity of the ELISA
has to be improved. As long as the sensitivity of the ELISA
can not be increased, the mouse-bio-assay will be the method
of choice for detecting toxin in enrichment cultures.

DISCUSSION

The ELISA for botulinum toxins represents an important addition to the existing detection techniques for botulinum toxins. Although, as with all serological assays the immunological activity of the toxin is determined (not the biological
activity), serological assays do have some advantages over in
vivo quantitation. For example, if in samples other unknown
toxin substances are present, in vivo detection methods will
give irrelevant results. Furthermore botulinum toxins present
in a biologically non-active state (e.g., due to aging of samples) can be estimated if the molecule is still immunologically recognisable.

In vitro techniques for detection of botulinum toxin can
only be successful if highly specific antisera are used. To
avoid cross-reactions with culture filtrates of some other
C.botulinum strains it seems to be necessary to remove cross-
reacting antibodies by affinity chromatography in which IgG is
bound to immobilized toxin. However, it is our experience that
IgG obtained in this way has a decreased affinity to toxin molecules resulting in a lowering of the sensitivity of the ELISA.

In order to attain increased sensitivity the assay system
must be modified to provide for more favorable antigen-antibody
kinetics. One particularly promising way of accomplishing this
involves the use of monoclonal antibodies. If such antibodies
are carefully selected to insure a high activity it may be possible that extremely sensitive assay systems can be developed
since the sensitivity of such assays depends a great deal on

energy levels of the substrate utilized. There is no doubt that, if the sensitivity of the ELISA can be increased, this technique can compete with the mouse-bio-assay. Furthermore, the ELISA is a simple technique which can be automated and be performed by normally equipped laboratories. Although at this moment the ELISA is less sensitive than the mouse-bio-assay, a number of valuable practical applications exists.

REFERENCES

1. De Wit, J.C., Notermans, S., Gorin, N., and Kampelmacher, E.H. (1979). *J. Food Protection 41*, 222.
2. DezFulian, M., and Dowell,V.R. (1980). *J. Clin. Microbiol. 11*, 604.
3. Graham, J.M. (1978). *J. Appl. Bacteriol. 45*, 205.
4. Kitamura, M., Sakaguchi, S., and Sakaguchi, G. (1968). *Biochem. Biophys. Acta 168*, 207.
5. Kozaki, S., Dufrenne, J., Hagenaars, A.M. and Notermans, S. (1979). *Jap. J. Med. Sci. Biol. 32*, 99.
6. Kozaki, S., Sakaguchi, S., and Sakaguchi, G. (1974). *Infect. Immun. 10*, 750.
7. Notermans, S., Dufrenne, J., and Kozaki, S. (1979). *Appl. Environm. Microbiol. 37*, 1173.
8. Notermans, S., Dufrenne, J., and Van Schothorst, M. (1978). *Jap. J. Med. Sci. Biol. 31*, 81.
9. Notermans, S., Hagenaars, A.M., and Kozaki, S. (1981). Methods In Enzymology, Academic Press, ed. J. Langone (In Press).
10. Notermans, S., Dufrenne, J., and Keybets, M. (1981). *J. Food Protection 44* (In Press).
11. Sakaguchi, G., Sakaguchi, S., Kozaki, S., Sugii, S., and Ohishi, I. (1971). *Jap. J. Med. Sci. Biol. 27*, 161.
12. Smith, L.Ds. (1975). *Appl. Environm. Microbiol. 30*, 319.
13. Sugii, S., and Sakaguchi, G. (1975). *Infect. Immun. 12*, 126.
14. Yolken, R.H., and Stopa, P.J. (1979). *J. Clin. Microbiol. 10*, 317.

DIFFERENT TYPES OF CLOSTRIDIUM BOTULINUM
(A, D, and G) FOUND AT AUTOPSY IN HUMANS:
I. ISOLATION OF THE ORGANISMS AND IDENTIFICATION
OF THE TOXINS

Wolfgang Sonnabend

Institute of Medical Microbiology
St. Gallen, Switzerland

Ortrud Sonnabend

Department of Pathology
Kantonsspital St. Gallen
St. Gallen, Switzerland

In 1973, a program was initiated for collecting fluids and
tissues for microbiological studies during the routine postmortem examinations of patients being submitted for autopsy to
the Kantonsspital St. Gallen, in the northeastern part of Switzerland. Between 1973 and 1974, a standard method to obtain
sterile material at autopsy was elaborated and used by one of
us in 300 unselected necropsies. Certain base-line conditions
were defined in this first study to improve the reliability
and the value of the results. Since 1975, the postmortem microbiological study has been applied successfully as a part of
the autopsy routine (1).

I. MATERIALS AND METHODS

A total of 6'905 autopsies, consisting of 5'882 cases of
the Department of Pathology, and 1'023 cases of the Department
of Forensic Medicine, were done at the Kantonsspital St. Gal-

len between January 1, 1975, and December 31, 1980. Autopsies
were carried out at the earliest opportunity, usually within
24 hours, and rarely as late as 60 hours (range 1-60 hours)
after death. Before autopsy, the cadavers were kept refrigerated at 4°C.

A. *Routine Postmortem Microbiological Investigations*

From these 6'905 autopsies specimens of heart blood, lung,
liver, spleen, kidney, and brain of 882 selected cadavers were
tested by special enrichment techniques to isolate aerobic and
anaerobic bacteria as well as fungi. In many cases tissues and
intestinal contents were also tested for viruses, and necropsy
sera were investigated for the presence of antibodies. Tissue
specimens were obtained immediately at the beginning of the
autopsy by the following methods: A steel spatula was heated
to glowing in a gas flame and applied to the tissue surface
straight away, where 4 by 4 cm were seared to dryness. From
the center of the seared area a block of about 1 cubic centi-
meter was excised with a pair of sterile tweezers and scissors.
Separate instruments were used for each organ. After circular
craniotomy and cutting of the falx cerebri, the optic nerves,
basal arteries, and brain stem were cut with a sterile scal-
pel, the hemispheres of the cerebrum turned down and a block
of brain specimen was obtained from the left temporal area
with sterile instruments. 30 ml of heart blood were aspirated
with a sterile syringe after the surface of the right ventricle was seared. 5 ml were inoculated into a single-bottle culture medium, the rest was used for serological examinations.
Histological examinations were performed on tissues in all cases and the findings were correlated with the microbiological
results.

B. *Selection Procedure of Autopsies Studied*

The criteria of the selection was the exclusion of possibilities of an infection as a cause of death. Many patients
were studied where the infection was already proved by culture
or/and history, but where the clinicians wanted to know whether the treatment with antibiotics had eradicated the pathogen organisms. However, some of the patients studied postmortem died suddenly and unexpectedly at home, or died unexpectedly in the hospital without an obvious cause of death.

TABLE I. *Laboratory Procedures for Cases of Sudden and/or Unexpected Death*

Specimens taken at Autopsy	Specimens tested for
Heart blood	Aerobic and anaerobic
Tissues of lung, liver, spleen,	bacteria
kidney, and brain	Fungi
A segment of the small and	Viruses
large intestine	Specific antibodies
(Thymus, urine, cerebrospinal	Botulinal toxin
fluid, gastric content)[a]	Cytotoxin of C. difficile

[a] *Specimens taken in some cases.*

When pulmonary embolism was found at autopsy to be the cause of death the case was excluded from this study. If the cause of death remained unexplained after macroscopic and histological examinations, the possibility of poisoning was excluded by routine toxicological investigations.

C. *Detailed Investigations of Cases with Sudden and/or Unexpected Death*

In cases of sudden and/or unexpected death specimens were taken from heart blood, tissues of lung, liver, spleen, kidney, and brain, and in 70% a segment of the small and large intestine for routine cultures (Table I). In some cases, specimens of thymus, urine, cerebrospinal fluid, and gastric content were cultured. Specimens were placed in transport tubes and, immediately after collection, they were brought for prompt processing to the bacteriological laboratories which are situated next to the Department of Pathology. The specimens were investigated for aerobic and anaerobic bacteria, fungi, and viruses. Methods used for the recovery of anaerobic bacteria included examinations of the contents of the intestine for the presence of Clostridium botulinum (C. botulinum) organisms. Since 1977, bowel content was only tested for the presence of clostridia. Blood was tested by the standard mouse assay for botulinal toxin. Serological tests were performed to detect evidence of infection with common respiratory or gastrointestinal tract, or central nervous system pathogens. Since March 1980, specimens from the intestines have also been assayed for botulinal toxin, and for cytotoxin of C. difficile.

D. Laboratory Investigations

During the study period a systematic attempt was made to
recover anaerobes from all blood cultures, from tissue specimens, from body fluids, and from specimens of the small and
large intestine (Table II). Heart blood cultures were examined
with the Lederle Diagnostics one-bottle culture medium. The
bottles were incubated, without venting, at 35°C, and subcultures to solid media were made after seven and 14 days. Tissue
specimens were divided into two or more portions. For enrichment cultures, one tube each of thioglycolate and chopped
meat-glucose-starch medium were inoculated with the divided
materials, and incubated anaerobically at 35°C for seven and
14 days. The contents of the small and large intestine were
suspended in gelatin diluent, and an aliquot of these specimens were inoculated into two tubes of thioglycolate, and two
tubes of chopped meat-glucose-starch medium. After heat treatment, the heated and unheated enrichment cultures were incubated anaerobically at 30°C for five days.

Subcultures from all the enrichment cultures were done on
solid media, such as brucella blood agar, kanamycin-vancomy-
cin blood agar, and rifampin blood agar. Egg yolk agar to
check for lecithinase, lipase, and proteolytic enzyme production has been used since 1980. The plates were incubated anaerobically for four, seven, and 14 days at 35°C. Identification of anaerobes on the basic set of cultural and biochemical
characteristics was done following the procedures outlined by
Dowell and Hawkins (2), and gas chromatographic identification
was performed according to the Virginia Polytechnic Institute
system (3).

Most of the Clostridium cultures which were classified as
belonging to pathogenic species and all cultures designated
"unidentified" were tested in guinea pigs or mice for pathological changes. The presence or absence of toxin in clostridial
cultures was demonstrated in the mouse (ICR strain) following
the intraperitoneal inoculation of a culture supernatant from
a 3-5 day old chopped meat-glucose-starch culture. Animal protection tests with specific immune serum were performed to
identify the organisms. Examination of feces specimens for botulinal toxin was done according to the CDC laboratory procedures (4). Culture supernatant of C. difficile and that of
feces specimens were tested in tissue cultures assay for the
presence of cytotoxin, and, if detected, cytotoxicity was
neutralized by C. sordellii antitoxin (5)

TABLE II. Methods for Isolation of Anaerobic Bacteria from Autopsy Specimens

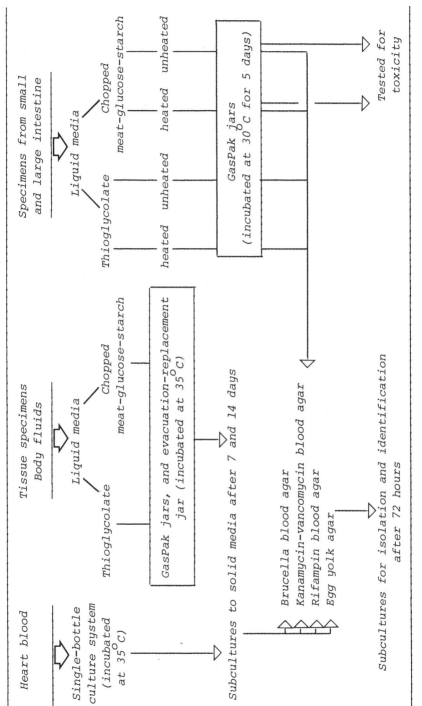

II. RESULTS AND DISCUSSION

A. *Classification of 116 Cases with Sudden and/or Unexpected Deaths after Autopsy and Microbiological Examination*

During the time interval of the study January 1975 through December 1980, 116 cases with no cause of death obvious before autopsy were tested microbiologically. Our findings enabled these 116 cases to be divided into the following three groups.

Group I: *Explained causes of deaths* - In 15 infants and 51 adults causes of deaths were found, e.g. myocardial infarction, respiratory infection, septicemia, meningitis, etc. In this group some causes of death could only be explained by carrying out microbiological investigations.

Group II: *Possible explanation of deaths* - No obvious macroscopic or histological changes were found that could explain cause of death, but certain microbiological results, sufficient to account for deaths in six infants and ten adults, were made.

Group III: *Unexplained deaths* - The thorough postmortem examinations failed to demonstrate an adequate cause of death in 26 infants and eight adults.

B. *Isolation and Identification of Botulinal Organisms and/or Toxins in Autopsy Specimens*

In one case of the first group, and in 11 cases of the second group, different types of botulinal organisms and/or toxins were found in specimens obtained at autopsy. Table III lists the different isolates of C. botulinum and botulinal toxins identified in necropsy sera recovered from these 12 cases.

1. Identification of Botulinal Toxin Type A in Autopsy Sera. In autopsy sera of three adults and a 27-week-old infant of group II, type A botulinal toxin could be demonstrated. No organisms of C. botulinum were found in specimens obtained at autopsy in these four cases (no. 1-4).

2. Demonstration of Mixed Botulinum Types A and G in Autopsy Specimens. In two autopsies of the group II (case no. 5 and 6) mixed botulinum types were identified. Type A botulinal toxin was demonstrated in the sera of these patients, and C. botulinum type G organisms were isolated from different specimens. In case no. 5, botulinum type G organisms were found in association with C. botulinum type A organisms.

TABLE III. Isolation and Identification of Botulinal
Organisms and/or Toxins in Autopsy Specimens

Case No.	Age (Years)	Toxin type of C. botulinum identified in serum	Type of C. botulinum organisms isolated from		
			Heart blood	Tissues	Intestinal contents
1	27 weeks	A	$-^a$	-	-
2	57	A	-	-	-
3	79	A	-	-	-
4	68	A	-	-	-
5^b	24	A	A + G	A + G	-
6^b	33	A	G	G	G
7	29	G	G	G	G
8	45	G	-	G	-
9	18 weeks	G	-	-	G
10	26	D	D	D	NA^c
11	44	D	-	D	D
12	55	D	D	D	-

a - means no isolation of C. botulinum organisms. b Cases
with mixed botulinum types. c Not available for testing.

3. Isolation and Identification of Botulinal Organisms and
Toxin of Type G in Autopsy Specimens. In group I, C. botulinum
type G organisms were isolated from the spleen in a 45-year-
old man, and in group II, from different specimens in an
adult and an 18-week-old infant. Type G toxin was demonstrated
in the sera of these three patients (case no. 7-9).

4. Isolation and Identification of Botulinal Organisms and
Toxin of Type D in Autopsy Specimens. In three autopsies of
group II, C. botulinum type D was isolated from different specimens, and type D botulinal toxin was identified in these
three necropsy sera (case no. 10-12). In only one of these
three isolates of type D was hemagglutinin production observed
in the supernatant fluids of LYG medium (6). Type D has been
incriminated in outbreaks of animal botulism, and only one
human outbreak due to type D has occured. This consisted of
six nonfatal cases of varying severity in Tschad (7).

C. Demonstration of Type G Organisms and Toxins in Humans

C. botulinum type G has been isolated only twice, from
soil samples in Argentina, the first time in 1969 from a corn-
field in the Mendoza Province by Gimenez and Ciccarelli (8);
nothing is known of its wider distribution, and the organism
has not been implicated until now in human or animal outbreaks.

*1. Problems Associated with the Isolation and Identifica-
tion of Type G from Mixed Cultures.* The first isolation of C.
botulinum type G from enrichment cultures inoculated with
autopsy specimens (case no. 5) has been extremely difficult.
This was the first autopsy case of our study involved with
botulinal organisms (9). In this case type G occured in combination with C. botulinum type A in mixed cultures associated
with other clostridial species. In contrast to all other known
types of C. botulinum (A-F), type G does not produce lipase,
so it may be difficult to isolate it, if only lipase-positive
colonies from egg-yolk agar are picked up for further identification. A rapid recognition of C. botulinum type G was also
complicated by the identification of botulinal toxin type A in
the serum of this patient. The procedures were somewhat time-
consuming.

*2. Cultural and Physiological Characteristics and Specifi-
city of the Toxin.* The mice inoculated with nontrypsin treated
and trypsin-treated culture supernatant died during the three-
day period of observation with symptoms typical for botulism.
Histologically, the mice presented a hemorrhagic edema of the
lungs. The botulinal-like toxin was not neutralized by antitoxin to any of the known botulinal toxins (types A-F).

The cultural and biochemical characteristics, and the analysis of short-chain acid products by gas—liquid chromatography of the isolated cultures, were identical to those of type
G described by Ciccarelli et al. (lo).

Type G antitoxin was not available commercially or from
the Center for Disease Control, Atlanta, to study the specificity of the toxin. The toxicity of these cultures of type G
sent to and tested by the Center for Disease Control was completely neutralized by C. botulinum antitoxin type G, but not
by antitoxin of types A, B, C_1, C_2, D, E, or F.

3. Toxic Dose of Type G in Serum Samples. After we had
prepared specific type G antitoxin by immunization of rabbits,
it was possible to demonstrate type G toxin in the sera of
three patients (case no. 7-9). A mouse-toxic substance that

TABLE IV. Toxic Dose of Type G Toxin in Serum Samples

Case/Age	Results obtained by laboratories	
	St. Gallen	CDC/Atlanta
7/29 years	7.0 MLD_{50}/ml	28.5 MLD_{50}/ml
8/45 years	2.0 MLD_{50}/ml	5.0 MLD_{50}/ml
9/18-week-old	6.0 MLD_{50}/ml	NA^a

^{a}Serum not available for testing.

killed mice with typical symptoms of botulism was identified as type G toxin by mouse neutralization test. The toxic dose of type G toxin ranged from 2.0 to 7.0 MLD_{50}/ml in the sera of these three patients (Table IV). In the titration of two of these three serum samples tested by the Center for Disease Control, it was found that the toxic dose was 5.0 MLD_{50}/ml and 28.5 MLD_{50}/ml, respectively (11). The results of toxin titration obtained by various laboratories can differ by as much as four- to fivefold (12).

4. Production of Type G toxin. Very low levels of toxin were produced in regular broth cultures in which type A strains can produce 10'000 to 1'000'000 MLD_{50}/ml. A subculture, isolate of case no. 7, contained 32 MLD_{50}/ml which increased to 36o MLD_{50}/ml after treatment with trypsin. The amount of dialysate toxin obtained by the cellophane tube techniques was 3 x 10^4 MLD_{50}/ml after seven days growth (9). It was stated that should such suitable conditions for toxin production occur naturally, or in food containing C. botulinum type G, this type of botulism could result (10).

5. Precipitation Tests with Type G Toxin of the Five Isolates. Crude, nonactivated type G toxin of each of the five isolates were studied by the Ouchterlony gel double diffusion technique against goat type G antitoxin. The toxic culture fluid of one strain that was identified in the small intestine of the 18-week-old infant (case no. 9), gave several distinct lines of precipitation, which appeared to be similar to the lines of precipitation formed by the strain isolated in Argentina. The other four strains, however, were different in gel precipitation tests (13).

D. *Evaluation of Bacteriological Data Obtained from Autopsy Specimens with Identification of C. Botulinum Organisms and/or Toxins*

In regard to the question of validity of our results, different conditions, which could influence postmortem bacteriological examinations, should be taken into consideration.

1. First of all *contamination* of the specimens during collection and processing may occur. This was excluded by an adequate technique, proved in 300 unselected autopsies in our first study. Furthermore, the comparison of results obtained from six different sites of a cadaver permits rapid recognition of contamination. It is rather unlikely that six different specimens, collected and processed one by one, are (if at all) contaminated by the same type of C. botulinum, and without other bacteria.

2. Most of the studies concerning postmortem bacteriology disagree with the idea of a quick *dissemination of bacteria in tissues after death.* Only one study supports a correlation between *time interval* of examination and number of isolated bacteria (14). In our experience, where cadavers are stored at 4°C before autopsy, bacteria can only be isolated, if (i) an *infection* had excisted anywhere *antemortem with bacteremia,* (ii) the patient had *aspirated,* (iii) there had been a hypovolemic hemorrhagic *shock* which, by increasing the permeability of the bowel, allows the spread of the intestinal bacteria, (iv) there had been a *severe bowel disease* associated with shock or mucosal lesions. Especially in patients who died from peritonitis or pancreatitis we found numerous fecal-type bacteria widespread in different organs. In cases with myocardial infarction, pulmonary embolism, etc., organs were sterile even after 6o hours after death.

3. Agonal aspiration of the patient could result in bacterial colonization of the lungs. Mixed cultures of aerobes and anaerobes were recovered from specimens of the lung in nine cases (no. 2, 4-9, 11, 12). Seven of these patients had aspirated to a slight or severe degree, and one had been reanimated (Table V). C. botulinum was isolated in only four of these mixed cultures of the lung (case no. 5-7, 11). In one patient with no signs of aspiration C. botulinum was found in pure culture (case no. 10). In our experience, bacteremia, following preterminal aspiration, rarely occurs and usually results in isolation of various organisms from different sites. Three

Table V. Bacteriological Findings in 12 Cases with Identification of Botulinal Toxins

Case No.	1	2	3	4	5	6	7	8	9	10	11	12
Age (years)	27 wks	57	79	68	24	33	29	45	18 wks	26	44	55
Time interval[a]	3	2	22	22	24	24	24	53	57	12	26	57
Toxin in serum	A	A	A	A	A	A	G	G	G	D	D	D
Heart blood	O[d]	O	O	E.coli / MF	A + G / MF	G	G	O	S.aureus D	D	MF	D
Liver, spleen, kidney, brain	O	O	O	E.coli	A + G / MF	G	O	G / MF	O	D	MF	D
Lung	O	MF[g]	O	E.coli / MF	A + G / MF	G	G / MF	O / MF	S.aureus D / MF	D	D / MF	MF
Aspiration[b]	none	RE[c]	none	++	none	(+)	+	++	(+)	none	++	+
Small intestine				NA[f]						NA		
C. botulinum	–[e]	–[h]	–		–	G	G	–	G		D	–
C. perfringens	–	+	–		+	–	–	+	–		–	+
Large intestine				NA						NA		
C. botulinum	–	–	–		–	G	G	–	–		–	–
C. perfringens	–	+	+		+	–	–	+	–		–	–
Intestinal lesions	none	focal	focal	subileus	none	none	none	none	none	none	none	none

[a] Hours. [b] Aspiration very slight (+), mild +, severe ++. [c] Reanimation. [d] Sterile. [e] Not isolated. [f] Not available for testing. [g] Mixed flora. [h] Isolated.

of our patients had sterile organs (case no. 1-3). In four cases (no. 6, 7, 11, 12) C. botulinum was found in pure culture
in all specimens except the lung. Mixed cultures in specimens
of other organs were only observed in three cases (no. 5, 8, 11).

4. *Lesions in the gastrointestinal tract* may result in an
invasion of the bloodstream by bacteria that normally populate
the bowel. Two patients (no. 2 and 3) had focal intestinal lesions, but sterile organs except the lung in one case (no. 2).
One patient had incomplete intestinal obstruction, causing an
increased permeability of the bowel. E. coli was isolated in
that case (no. 4) in pure culture from heart blood, kidney,
and brain, and in mixed cultures from the lung in association
with severe aspiration. A fecal-type flora, associated with
botulinal organisms, was found in specimens of different
organs (Table VI) in two patients (no.5 and 11). C. botulinum
type D was isolated from the content of the small intestine in
only one of these cases (no. 11).

5. *Shock prior to death* may be associated with an invasion
of the bloodstream by fecal-type flora of the gastrointestinal
tract. C. botulinum does not belong to the normal fecal flora
and was only isolated from stool specimens of persons who had
suffered from botulism or were involved, but not affected in
botulism outbreaks. We examined intestinal specimens of 181
cadavers to obtain information about the presence or absence
of C. botulinum organisms in humans. We found type G three
times and type D once (Table V), only in patients who died
suddenly and unexpectedly (no. 6, 7, 9, 11). However, *postmortem changes in the bacterial flora of the bowel* may occur
and, growth and toxin production of C. botulinum may be repressed in mixed cultures. The inhibition of type A, B, E, and
F strains by C. perfringens has been shown (15). In three
cases (no. 5, 8, 12) where C. botulinum was isolated from
tissue specimens, we found no botulinal organisms in the intestines, but C. perfringens in association with a predominantly
anaerobic intestinal flora. In four cases (no. 6, 7, 9, 11)
with isolation of botulinal organisms from tissues C. botulinum was found in the intestine with a fecal-type flora, but
C. perfringens was absent.

    In our study, C. botulinum organisms were present in pure
culture at multiple sites associated with botulinal toxin in
the serum. On the other hand, botulinal toxin type A was identified in necropsy sera of four patients, but no botulinal
organisms were isolated from tissue specimens or bowel content
in this group. C. botulinum organisms of type G and D were re-

Table VI.   Organisms and Site of Recovery in Cases With
            Mixed Botulinum Types A + G

	Case no. 5 24 yr / M	Case no. 6 33 yr / M
Time interval	24 hours	24 hours
Serum	Toxin type A	Toxin type A, HBsAg
Heart blood	C. botulinum A + G C. sordellii B. clostridiiformis P. vulgaris	C. botulinum G
Lung	C. botulinum A + G B. clostridiiformis	C. botulinum G P. productus Eubacterium sp Str. intermedius Str. faecalis
Aspiration	None	Very small amounts
Liver	C. botulinum A + G C. sordellii B. clostridiiformis B. fragilis	C. botulinum G
Spleen	C. sordellii B. clostridiiformis	C. botulinum G
Kidney	C. botulinum A + G C. sordellii B. clostridiiformis P. vulgaris	Sterile
Brain	Sterile	Sterile
Small and large intestine	C. perfringens C. sordellii B. clostridiiformis B. fragilis	C. botulinum G Fecal-type flora
Gastric content	Not available	Not available
Intestinal lesions	None	None

covered from the intestinal contents, but no botulinal toxin was detected in one tested sample. If botulinal organisms and toxins participate in causing these sudden and unexpected deaths, the exact mechanism by means of which they do so is unknown. The findings in these cases could represent: (i) single cases of fatal foodborne botulism, (ii) cases of possible infant-type botulism in adults, (iii) cases of sudden infant death syndrome due to a severe form of infant botulism, (iv) botulism, classification undetermined, or (v) post mortem changes. Data about clinical signs and symptoms prior to death as well as pathological and epidemiological findings will be shown in part II of this paper.

REFERENCES

1. Sonnabend, O., Sonnabend, W., Rauh, G., Bezzegh, T., Gloor, F., Amgwerd, R., Krech, U., *Schweiz. med. Wschr.* 1o7, 1209 (1977).
2. Dowell, V. R., Jr., and Hawkins, T. M., *in* "Laboratory Methods in Anaerobic Bacteriology. CDC Laboratory Manual", p. 96. Center for Disease Control, Atlanta, (1979).
3. Holdeman, L. V., Cato, E. P., and Moore, W. E. C., *in* "Anaerobe Laboratory Manual" (4th ed.), p. 132. Virginia Polytechnic Institute and State University Press, Blacksburg, (1977).
4. Center for Disease Control, *in* "Botulism in the United States, 1899 – 1977. Handbook for Epidemiologists, Clinicians, and Laboratory Workers", p. 41. Center for Disease Control, Atlanta, (1979).
5. Chang, T. W., Lauermann, M., and Bartlett, J. G., *J. Infect. Dis.* 14o, 765 (1979).
6. Oguma, K., Iida, H., and Mitsuko Shiozaki, *Infect. Immun.* 14, 597 (1976).
7. Demarchi, J., Mourges, E., Orio, J., and Prévot, A. R., *Bull acad. natl. méd.* 142, 58o (1958).
8. Gimenez, D. F., and Ciccarelli, A. S., *Zbl. Bakt., Abt. Orig. A.* 215, 221 (197o).
9. Sonnabend, O., Sonnabend, W., Heinzle, R., Sigrist, T., Dirnhofer, R., and Krech, U., *J. Infect. Dis.* 143 (1981), in press
10. Ciccarelli, A. S., Whaley, D. N., McCroskey, L. M., Gimenez, D. F., Dowell, V. R., Jr., and Hatheway, C. L., *Appl. Environ. Microbiol.* 34, 843 (1977).
11. Hatheway, C. L., *Personal communication* (1981).
12. Sugiyama, H., *Microbiol. Rev.* 44, 419 (198o).
13. Metzger, J. F., *Personal communication* (198o).
14. Carpenter, H. M., Wilkins, R. M., *Arch, Path.* 77, 73 (1964).
15. Smith, L. DS., *Appl. Microbiol.* 3o, 319 (1975).

PHYSIOLOGICAL CHARACTERIZATION OF *CLOSTRIDIUM BOTULINUM* AND DEVELOPMENT OF PRACTICAL ISOLATION AND IDENTIFICATION PROCEDURES

V. R. Dowell, Jr.
M. Dezfulian[1]

Centers for Disease Control
Atlanta, Georgia

I. INTRODUCTION

In a study reported recently (1), we compared the phenotypic characteristics of *Clostridium botulinum* isolates from foodborne and infant botulism cases in the United States. The isolates were compared on the basis of toxigenicity, cultural and biochemical characteristics, volatile and nonvolatile acid products, and susceptibility to antimicrobial agents. We found that, overall, the characteristics of the 78 strains, 42 from foodborne and 36 from infant botulism sources, were quite similar, and we were unable to differentiate isolates associated with foodborne botulism from those recovered from infant botulism cases on the basis of the tests performed. During the study, we found that all of the *C. botulinum* strains (35 type A, 43 proteolytic type B) produced one or more unidentified indole derivatives, detected with paradimethylaminocinnamaldehyde, and hydrocinnamic acid (3-phenylpropionic acid), detected by gas liquid chromatography. We also found that all of the strains exhibited a high degree of resistance to cycloserine, sulfamethoxazole and trimethoprim. Some of the strains exhibited two distinct types of colonies on CDC anaerobe blood agar which were designated opaque (Op) and translucent (Tr). The Op type appeared as raised, opaque white

[1]*present address: Johns Hopkins University, School of Medicine, Division of Infectious Diseases, Baltimore, Maryland.*

colonies, which could easily be distinguished from the flat, translucent, spreading gray Tr type colonies.

In this report, we review subsequent studies of the properties of Op and Tr variants of *C. botulinum* types A and B strains, a study of the production of phenyl-substituted fatty acids by *C. botulinum* (types A, B, C, D, E and F) and various other *Clostridium* species, and the development of a selective medium for isolation of *C. botulinum* from human feces. We also summarize some key differential characteristics of *C. botulinum* and related microorganisms and show how these can be used in a practical procedure for confirming the identity of *C. botulinum* isolates.

II. PROPERTIES OF OP AND TR VARIANTS

We studied the colony characteristics, morphologic features, growth kinetics, and physiological activities of several strains of *C. botulinum* types A and B (M. Dezfulian and V. R. Dowell, Jr., Abstract C58, Abstracts of Annual Meeting, American Society for Microbiology, 1981). Differences between the Op and Tr variants are summarized in Table 1. After purification, the Tr type cultures retained the same colony characteristics through repeated subcultures on anaerobe blood agar, but the Op type occasionally gave rise to Tr colonies. The Op variants regularly produced large numbers of spores in a suitable medium and the Tr variants rarely produced spores. The Tr variants of *C. botulinum* types A and B were similar to type G strains we examined (2) in respect to their inability to sporulate readily. The practical implication of this observation in regard to selective isolation of *C. botulinum* from mixed bacterial populations will be discussed in more detail in the section on development of a selective medium for *C. botulinum*.

The Op and Tr variants also showed distinct differences in their growth kinetics and in the production of certain volatile acids in Schaedler broth (BBL). The major differences in the growth kinetics of the Op and Tr variants were in the exponential phase of the growth curves. The Tr variants consistently grew faster in the exponential phase than their Op counterparts.

In general, the Op variants produce more butyric and isocaproic acids than Tr variants. No differences were noted in production of hydrocinnamic acid, the only nonvolatile acid produced by the Op and Tr variants in Schaedler broth.

In studies of a sporogenic strain and an asporogenic mutant of *C. botulinum* type E, Emeruwa and Hawirko (3) and Emeruva et al. (4) demonstrated a direct relationship between

TABLE 1. *Some differences between Op and Tr*
variants of Clostridium botulinum

Characteristic	Differences
1. Colonies on anaerobe blood agar	Op - raised, white, opaque Tr - flat, gray, translucent
2. Endospores	Op - usually abundant Tr - usually none or rare
3. Resistance to heat treatment (80 C for 10 min.)	Op - resistant Tr - usually not resistant
4. Growth rate in logarithmic phase of growth	Growth of Tr variants more rapid than Op variants
5. Butyric acid and isocaproic acid	Op variants produced more butyric and isocaproic acids than the Tr variants

butyric type fermentation and sporulation. Whether or not a
similar relationship between butyric acid metabolism and
sporulation exists in the *C. botulinum* strains exhibiting Op
and Tr variants studied by us will require further investigation.

The Op - Tr variation as described is not limited to *C.*
botulinum types A and B. Similar variations have been observed in strains of *C. botulinum* type F and *Clostridium bi-*
fermentans (M. Dezfulian, 1980, unpublished data) and *Bacillus*
caldolyticus (5). As in the case of *B. caldolyticus,* the Op -
Tr variation in *C. botulinum* types A and B cannot be attributed to somatic mutation because of the high incidence of its
occurrence, and we have insufficient information at this time
to speculate on the mechanisms involved in the phenomenon.

III.   PRODUCTION OF PHENYL-SUBSTITUTED FATTY ACIDS

We recently reported further studies of the production of
phenyl-substituted fatty acids by clostridia (M. Dezfulian, G.
L. Lombard, R. J. Landry and V. R. Dowell, Jr., 1981.

Submitted for publication). Two hundred and nine strains representing 38 species of *Clostridium* were examined for the production of hydrocinnamic acid and phenylacetic acid with a gas liquid chromatography procedure described by Dezfulian and Dowell (1). Routinely, peptone-yeast extract-glucose (PYG) broth (6) is used by the CDC Anaerobe Section for cultivation of organisms to be tested for volatile and nonvolatile acids by gas liquid chromatography. In this study, we also tested chopped meat glucose (CMG) broth (6), Lombard-Dowell (LD) broth with 0.1% glucose (7), Mueller-Hinton (MH) broth (BBL), Schaedler broth (BBL) supplemented with vitamin K1 (10 µg/ml) and hemin (5 µg/ml), and enriched thioglycollate (THIO) broth (6) cultures for acid products. We also tested the effects of added phenylalanine on production of phenyl-substituted acids and the effects of varying the incubation period from 30 min to 16 hr during methylation of nonvolatile acids in regard to detection by gas liquid chromatography.

Production of hydrocinnamic acid and phenylacetic acid by *C. botulinum* and related organisms in PYG medium is shown in Table 2. Smith (8) divided *C. botulinum* into four groups on the basis of cultural and serological characteristics, as follows:

Group   I.   Type A and proteolytic strains of types B and F.

Group   II.   Nonproteolytic strains of types B and F and all type E strains.

Group III.   Strains of types C alpha, C beta and type D.

Group   IV.   The proteolytic, but nonsaccharolytic, type G strains.

In Table 3, we show how these groups can be differentiated on the basis of hydrocinnamic acid and phenylacetic acid production using data derived from our study. We have also included data on *Clostridium sporogenes* and "E-like" organisms in Table 3 to show their relationships to Group I and Group II, respectively.

The effect of various culture media on hydrocinnamic acid production by two strains of *C. botulinum* type A is shown in Table 4. The quantities of HCA produced by the two strains ranged from 0.3 mEq/100 ml in LD plus 0.1% glucose to 1.2 to 1.4 mEq/100 ml in CMG medium.

We found that supplementing either CMG medium or LD medium plus 0.1% glucose with additional phenylalanine (0 to 10 mg/ml) resulted in a dramatic increase in HCA production by various strains of *C. botulinum* (type A and proteolytic type B) up to 5 mg phenylalanine/ml. Beyond that level of phenylalanine, HCA production did not increase further. Results obtained with a representative strain of *C. botulinum* type A in response to added phenylalanine are shown in Table 5.

TABLE 2. *Hydrocinnamic acid and phenylacetic acid production by C. botulinum and related organisms in PYG medium*

Organism	Number strains tested	Number producing HCA	Number producing PAA
C. botulinum type A	35	35	0
C. botulinum type B (proteolytic)	43	43	0
C. botulinum type B (nonproteolytic)	5	0	0
C. botulinum type C	3	0	0
C. botulinum type D	3	0	0
C. botulinum type E	3	0	1
C. botulinum type F (proteolytic)	5	5	0
C. botulinum type F (nonproteolytic)	3	0	0
C. botulinum type G	7	0	7
C. sporogenes	14	14	0
"E-like "Clostridia	2	0	0

HCA = hydrocinnamic acid; PAA = phenylacetic acid

TABLE 3. Production of hydrocinnamic acid and phenylacetic
         acid by C. botulinum of Groups I, II, III and IV
         as discussed by Smith (10) and related organisms

C. botulinum toxin type and related species		HCA production	PAA production
Group I	A, proteolytic B and F, C. sporogenes	+	-
Group II	Nonproteolytic B and F and type E "E - like" organisms	-	-+
Group III	C alpha, C beta and D	-	-
Group IV	G	-	+

HCA = hydrocinnamic acid; PAA = phenylacetic acid
+ = consistently positive; - = consistently negative;
-+ = usually negative, an occasional strain may be
     positive.

TABLE 4. Hydrocinnamic acid production by two strains of
         C. botulinum type A in various media

Medium	Hydrocinnamic acid detected in 48h cultures (milliequivalents per 100 ml)	
	Strain a - 15	Strain a - 28
Chopped meat glucose	1.2	1.4
Lombard - Dowell with 0.1% glucose	0.3	0.3
Mueller-Hinton	1.0	1.2
Peptone-yeast extract - glucose	0.7	0.8
Schaedler	0.5	0.6
Enriched thioglycollate	0.8	1.0

TABLE 5. *Hydrocinnamic acid production by a strain of C. botulinum type A (a 13) in PYG medium containing varying concentrations of added phenylalanine*

Phenylalanine concentration (mg/ml)	0	2.5	5.0	10.0
Hydrocinnamic acid detected (μg/ml)	19	95	130	128

Ten species of *Clostridium* other than *C. botulinum* produced HCA in PYG medium. Those strains which produced HCA included *C. sporogenes, C. difficile, C. novyi* type B, *C. ghoni* and *C. putrificum*. Production of HCA by the others was variable. Phenylacetic acid was produced by *C. subterminale, C. clostridiiforme, C. cochlearium, C. glycolicum, C. hastiforme, C. irregularis* and *C. propionicum* (Table 6).

There was no significant increase in the quantity of HCA detected by gas liquid chromatography when the methylation time was increased beyond the usual 30 min of incubation at 55°C (1). Incubation periods between 30 min and 16 hr gave comparable results.

IV. DEVELOPMENT OF A SELECTIVE MEDIUM FOR ISOLATION OF *C. BOTULINUM* FROM HUMAN FECES

On the basis of previous studies of the susceptibility of *C. botulinum* to various antimicrobials (1, 9), Dezfulian et al. (10) developed a selective medium for isolation of *C. botulinum* from human feces. The medium, CB1 agar, contains cycloserine (250 μg/ml), sulfamethoxazole (76 μg/ml) and trimethoprim (4 μg/ml) in a base of CDC modified McClung Toabe egg yolk agar (6).

Growth of various species of bacteria on CB1 medium is shown in Table 7. Bacteria not growing on CB1 agar, but showing growth on modified McClung Toabe egg yolk agar included: 3 strains each of *C. butyricum, C. difficile, C. innocuum, C. paraputrificum, C. septicum, C. tertium, Bacteroides fragilis, Escherichia coli* and *Proteus vulgaris;* 2 strains each of *C. limosum, C. sphenoides, C. subterminale, Eubacterium limosum, Propionibacterium acnes, Providencia stuartii* and *Staphylococcus aureus;* 1 strain each of *C. ramosum, Bacteroides distasonis, Bifidobacterium eriksonii, B. ovatus, B. thetaiotaomicron; B. uniformis, B. vulgatus, Eubacterium lentum, E. moniliforme, Citrobacter freundii, C. diversus, Bacillus cereus* and *B. subtilis;* 4 strains

TABLE 6. *Production of hydrocinnamic acid and phenylacetic*
acid by cultures of various Clostridium species
in PYG medium.

Species	Number of strains tested	Number producing HCA	Number producing PAA
C. absonum	1	0	0
C. aurantibutyricum	1	0	0
C. beijerinckii	1	0	0
C. bifermentans	4	3	0
C. butyricum	4	0	0
C. cadaveris	4	0	0
C. carnis	1	0	0
C. celatum	1	0	0
C. clostridiiforme	1	0	1
C. cochlearium	1	0	1
C. difficile	13	13	0
C. fallax	1	0	0
C. ghoni	1	1	0
C. glycolicum	1	0	1
C. haemolyticum	3	1	0
C. hastiforme	1	0	1
C. histolyticum	3	1	0
C. indolis	1	0	0
C. innocuum	4	0	0
C. irregularis	1	0	1
C. lentoputrescens	1	0	0
C. limosum	1	0	0
C. malenominatum	1	0	0
C. novyi type A	4	0	0
C. novyi type B	2	2	0
C. paraperfringens	1	0	0
C. paraputrificum	1	0	0
C. perfringens	4	0	0
C. propionicum	1	0	1
C. putrificum	1	1	0
C. ramosum	1	0	0
C. septicum	4	0	0
C. sordellii	4	0	0
C. sphenoides	1	0	0
C. subterminale	4	0	4
C. symbiosum	1	0	0
C. tertium	4	1	0
C. tetani	3	1	0

HCA = hydrocinnamic acid; PAA = phenylacetic acid

of *Proteus mirabilis,* and 5 strains of *Streptococcus fae-
calis.*

Quantitative studies revealed comparable recovery of *C.
botulinum* types A, B, F, and G on CB1 agar with that obtained
on modified McClung Toabe egg yolk agar. Type G colonies were
more difficult to recognize on CB1 medium than the other types
because of the lack of lipase production by type G.   Isolating
C. botulinum types A, B and F from seeded fecal samples was
easily done with CB1 medium.   Preliminary results of a current
evaluation of the medium by Hatheway and associates (C. L.
Hatheway, personal communication, March 1981) indicate that
it is very useful in isolating *C. botulinum* from fecal specimens and is especially useful in the rapid laboratory confirmation of infant botulism, which so far has been caused by *C.
botulinum* type A or proteolytic strains of types B and F.
Using the CB1 agar, it is possible to isolate and presumptive-
ly identify the causative organism from the feces of an infant
with botulism within 24 to 48 hr after the medium is inoculated.   Only a limited number of lipase-positive clostridia
(members of the *C. botulinum C. sporogenes* group) grown on CB1
agar (Table 7), and they are easily distinguished from other
species of *Clostridium* which grow on the medium.

TABLE 7.   *Growth of various bacteria on CB1 medium and CDC
modified McClung Toabe egg yolk agar*

Species	Number of strains tested	Number growing on:	
		CB1 medium	EYA medium
C. botulinum type A	14	14	14
C. botulinum type B (proteolytic)	21	21	21
C. botulinum type E	3	1	3
C. botulinum type F (proteolytic)	7	7	7
C. botulinum type G	3	3	3
C. bifermentans	3	3	3
C. cadaveris	3	3	3
C. perfringens	2	2[a]	2
C. sordellii	3	3	3
C. sporogenes	2	2	2

[a]*Indicates partial inhibition of growth.*

V. PRACTICAL IDENTIFICATION OF *C. BOTULINUM* ISOLATES

Some of the key characteristics which allow differentiation of *C. botulinum* from other clostridia include relationship to oxygen, microscopic features, endospore production, and lipase activity on egg yolk or CB1 agar, catalase, indole, indole derivative(s), glucose fermentation, casein hydrolysis, volatile and nonvolatile acid products and toxin production. In addition to CB1 agar, which allows presumptive identification of lipase-positive colonies as members of the *C. botulinum* - *C. sporogenes* group, the identity of *C. botulinum* isolates can be confirmed with a limited number of media as shown in Table 8.
As soon as single colony isolates of lipase-positive organisms are obtained on CB1 agar or modified McClung Toabe egg yolk agar, the following media are inoculated:
(a) 3 blood agar plates to check the purity of isolate and its relationship to oxygen (one plate is incubated in

TABLE 8. *List of media and differential characteristics for identification of C. botulinum*

Medium	Characteristics
1. Blood agar[a] incubated in air, candle extinction jar, anaerobic system	Relationship to oxygen, colony characteristics, microscopic features, endospores
2. Quadrant plate: LD agar	Catalase, indole, indole derivatives
LD glucose agar	Glucose fermentation
LD milk agar	Casein hydrolysis
LD egg yolk agar	Lecithinase, lipase, proteolysis
3. PYG medium with added phenylalanine (5 mg/ml)	Volatile and nonvolatile acid products
4. Chopped meat glucose starch medium	Toxin production, toxin neutralization tests

[a]*Only a segment of the medium in a plate is required to check the ability of an isolate to grow in a given atmosphere.*

air, one in a candle extinction jar, and one in an anaerobic system; (b) 1 quadrant plate containing LD, LD egg yolk, LD milk, and LD glucose agars; (c) 1 tube of PYG medium with added phenylalanine (5 mg/ml); and (d) 1 tube of chopped meat glucose starch medium.
The quadrant plate, PYG medium, chopped meat glucose starch medium and the one plate of blood agar are incubated in an anaerobic system for 48 hr at 35°C. After incubation, the cultures are removed from anaerobic conditions and the characteristics listed in Table 8 are determined as described in previous publications (1, 11). We are currently evaluating this procedure for isolating and identifying *C. botulinum*. A detailed description of the results of this study will be presented in another communication when the study is completed.

In summary, we conclude that the information derived from the studies described in this report have been useful to us in developing practical procedures for isolating and identifying *C. botulinum* and related organisms. The information should also be useful in further characterization and taxonomic classification of *C. botulinum*, which at present is a very heterologous group of microorganisms.

REFERENCES

1. Dezfulian, M., and V. R. Dowell, Jr. *J. Clin. Microbiol.* *11*, 604 (1980).
2. Ciccarelli, A. S., D. N. Whaley, L. M. McCroskey, D. F. Gimenez, V. R. Dowell, Jr., and C. L. Hatheway. *Appl. Environ. Microbiol. 34*, 843 (1977).
3. Emeruwa, A. C., and Hawirko, R. Z., *J. Bacteriol. 118*, 29 (1972).
4. Emeruwa, A. C., Hawirko, R. Z., Halverson, H., and Suzuki, J., *J. Bacteriol. 120*, 74 (1974).
5. Cook, W. R., and Ramalgy, R. F., in "Spores VII" (G. Chambliss, and J. C. Vary, eds.), p. 171. American Society for Microbiology, Washington (1978).
6. Dowell, V. R., Jr., Lombard, G. L., Thompson, F. S., and Armfield, A. Y., "Media for Isolation, Characterization and Identification of Obligately Anaerobic Bacteria." U.S. Department of Health, Education and Welfare, Public Health Service, Center for Disease Control, Atlanta, Ga. (1977).
7. Mena, E., Thompson, F. S., Armfield, A. Y., Dowell, V. R., Jr., *J. Clin. Microbiol. 8*, 28 (1978).
8. Smith, L. DS., "Botulism: The Organism, Its Toxins, and The Disease," p. 15. Charles C. Thomas, Springfield, Ill. (1977).

9. Swenson, J. M., Thornsberry, C., McCroskey, L. M., Hatheway, C. L., and Dowell, V. R., Jr., *Antimicrob. Agents Chemother.* *18,* 13 (1980).

10. Dezfulian, M., McCroskey, L. M., Hatheway, C. L., and Dowell, V. R., Jr., *J. Clin. Microbiol.* *13,* 526 (1981).

11. Dowell, V. R., Jr., and Lombard, G. L., "Presumptive Identification of Anaerobic Nonsporeforming Gram Negative Bacilli." U.S. Department of Health, Education and Welfare, Public Health Service, Center for Disease Control, Atlanta, Ga. (1977).

BACTERIAL TOXOIDS: PERSPECTIVES FOR THE FUTURE

M. Carolyn Hardegree

Division of Bacterial Products
Bureau of Biologics
Food and Drug Administration
Bethesda, Maryland

Toxin-mediated bacterial diseases of man have been prevented by use of passively administered antitoxin or by active
immunization with mixtures of toxin and antitoxin, or toxoids
(1-4).
Although there are many toxin-producing bacteria, only a
few biologics for passive or active immunization have been licensed for use in man in the U.S. Other products, not to be
discussed in this presentation, have been licensed for veterinary use. The first of these former products were the antitoxins prepared in horses (Table I). Subsequently, specific
immune human globulins were prepared (5-6). Table II lists
some of the antitoxic globulins which may be useful for prophylaxis or therapy. Of these, only Tetanus Immune Globulin
is now licensed.
A selected group of toxoids is shown in Table III. This
list includes toxoids which are licensed or which have been
used experimentally in man in recent years as well as an experimental toxoid which can be anticipated for clinical trial in
the future.

TABLE I. Selected Equine Antitoxins Licensed in U.S.

Diphtheria Antitoxin
Tetanus Antitoxin
Gas Gangrene Antitoxins
Botulinum Antitoxins
    Types A and B
    Type E
    Types A, B and E

ISBN 0-12-447180-3

TABLE II. Specific Immune Globulins Directed
Against Bacterial Toxins

Tetanus Immune Globulin[a]

Diphtheria Immune Globulin[b]
Botulinum Immune Globulin

Pseudomonas Immune Globulin[c]

---

[a]Licensed.
[b]Cited in literature.
[c]Anticipated.

Immunogens used to induce heterologous antitoxins were often prepared by modifying the toxins, so that the toxicity,
but not the immunogenicity or antigenicity, was destroyed.
These modifications included heat-inactivation and treatment
of the toxin with chemicals, such as iodine trichloride or
formaldehyde (1-2).
    The toxoids administered to animals for the preparation of
antitoxins have most frequently consisted of culture filtrates
inactivated by formalin (1-2). Toxoids used to immunize man
have generally been more purified. All U.S. licensed toxoids
have been inactivated with formaldehyde.
    Much of the progress made since the late 1800's in the
prevention of disease caused by bacterial toxins has been
either as a direct or indirect extension of the information
available for diphtheria and tetanus toxins.

TABLE III. Selected Bacterial Toxoids

Tetanus Toxoid[a]
Diphtheria Toxoid
Staphylococcus Toxoid

Botulinum Toxoid[b]
Cholera Toxoid
C. welchii Toxoid

Pseudomonas Exotoxin A Toxoid[c]

---

[a]Licensed.
[b]Experimental -- used in man.
[c]Experimental.

TABLE IV. *Types of Immunogens for Prevention of Toxin Mediated Diseases*

Inactivated Toxins

   Crude culture filtrates
   Partially purified
   Highly purified

Polypeptides

   Produced by bacteria
    Chains
    Fragments
    Subunits

   Synthetic

Proteins Obtained by Genetic Manipulation

   Purified cross reacting mutant proteins
   Live mutant bacteria
   Recombinant DNA products

Toxins, Toxoids or Polypeptides as Carriers

   Conjugated to hormones
   Conjugated to carbohydrates
   Conjugated to toxins/lectins/
     polypeptides/antibodies/drugs

The following is a review of selected aspects of the development of toxoids which have been used for both routine and experimental immunization of man and recent studies which may be pertinent to the anticipated development of new bacterial products. The types of immunogens to be discussed are shown in Table IV.

INACTIVATED TOXINS

Although *Corynebacterium diphtheriae* establishes itself as a mucosal or skin infection, the toxin produced by the organism exerts its effect distally as well as locally. Probably because of systemic distribution of the toxin, circulating diphtheria antitoxin was shown to be highly

effective in preventing the effects of the toxin. Following
the development of safe toxoids, immunization was widely
recommended (1). The toxoid was often combined with
aluminum adjuvants and with other antigens. A significant
reduction in the incidence of clinical diphtheria was
associated with the widespread acceptance of immunization
(1,7). It was several years after the development of this
successful immunogen that the toxin was purified and even
longer before its structure and molecular action were
determined (7-8). As attempts to inactivate purified
diphtheria toxin with formaldehyde were made, it became
apparent that toxoids could revert to a toxic state (9). The
addition of amino acids, especially lysine, during toxoiding
were reported to promote the preparation of stable toxoids
(10).

Clostridium tetani, like C. diphtheriae, establishes
itself as a local infection at its site of entry in the
tissue. The toxin then exerts its effects distally (2,11).
Circulating antitoxin was shown to be highly effective in
preventing systemic manifestations of the disease and
universal immunization was recommended. It, too, was often
combined with adjuvants and other antigens. This toxoid is
considered capable of inducing long lasting immunity (2). As
with diphtheria, the ability to produce an effective
immunogen was not dependent on knowledge of the structure and
function of tetanus toxin. The structure of tetanus toxin
(12-16) and some parameters of its action only recently have
been partially established (17-18). The molecular actions
are still to be defined. Tetanus toxoid has also been
reported to undergo reversion to its toxic state (19).

Other bacterial toxoids have been used experimentally.
Recently a toxoid prepared from the β toxin of C. welchii
(perfringens) was reported to prevent the necrotizing
enterocolitis known as pig-bel in New Guinea (20). The
parenteral administration of this vaccine prevented an
enteric disease.

Other papers in this symposium will discuss the
preparation and use of Botulinum Toxoids in detail. These
toxoids differ from those of tetanus and diphtheria in that
their use is restricted to specific populations (21). These
toxoids are not licensed but are distributed for controlled
use. Like diphtheria, botulism is a systemic disease
resulting from the entry of toxin from a mucosal surface or
rarely from the skin (22). Like tetanus and diphtheria an
immunogenic toxoid can be expected to induce sufficient
circulating antitoxin to prevent disease. However,
consideration of the induction of immunity to this neurotoxin
at the mucosa may be justified as is now being considered for

the enterotoxin of *Vibrio cholerae* (23). Parenteral immunization with a whole cell cholera vaccine is known to be effective, although the effectiveness is limited in duration (24).

Following the recognition of cholera as a toxin-mediated disease, it was suggested that parenteral administration of purified cholera toxoids to man would be effective in preventing cholera. Studies in animals showed that fluid output could be prevented by antitoxin; therefore toxoids were prepared (25). As had been shown earlier for diphtheria toxoid, the ability of one type of cholera toxoid which had been inactivated by formalin to undergo partial reversion to toxicity was shown both *in vivo* and *in vitro* (25). Subsequently glutaraldehyde was used to prepare a stable toxoid (25-26). Glutaraldehyde has also been used to prepare diphtheria, tetanus and pseudomonas toxoids (27-28). Unfortunately, the clinical trials using inactivated cholera toxin did not demonstrate cholera toxoids to be effective for a significant period (29).

Other approaches to immunization against cholera with purified antigens have been suggested. These include the administration of naturally occurring "toxoid" choleragenoid (30), the use of oral administration of antigens, such as toxoid, or toxin (23), isolated subunit B (31), or live mutant bacteria (30). Studies demonstrating protection against cholera toxin should also be relevant to the heat labile enterotoxin of *E. coli,* an immunologically related toxin (8) also active at the mucosal level.

It is to be noted that recent studies (23) showing that parenteral administration of antigens may actually cause either enhancement and immunosuppression of local gut antibody indicate that modulation of immune responses may not always be in the manner desired. Although the most effective way to induce immunity to cholera is yet to be defined, the information obtained during this period of intensive investigation of cholera toxin and toxoid contributed significantly to the understanding of the structure and function of bacterial toxins in general.

Exotoxin A may be a virulence factor for *Pseudomonas aeruginosa* (8). Antitoxin has been associated with increased survival of the patients infected with this organism (32). Thus a toxoid may be a useful product in the future. Preliminary reports on the preparation of toxoids have been presented (28,33-36). It is to be noted that formalin inactivation in the absence of lysine may lead to pseudomonas toxoids which retain their enzymatic activity (34-36).

For the preparation of new immunogens alternate methods
to formalin inactivation of intact toxins may therefore be
indicated.

POLYPEPTIDES

The recognition that bacterial toxins are often not
single chain molecules after release by the bacteria may lead
to such alternate methods for the preparation of immunogens
for use in man.

Almost simultaneously with the observation that
diphtheria toxin could be nicked to form Fragment B and
Fragment A, a fragment for binding and a fragment with
enzymatic activity (7-8), it was established that cholera
toxin was comprised of subunit B and subunit A, a subunit for
binding and a subunit with enzymatic activity (36). The
concept that toxins are comprised of binding and active
portions was rapidly extended to other toxins (8,12-16,18,22,
37). However the active site has not been identified for
toxins such as tetanus and botulinum.

It is also recognized that some of the chains can be
readily cleaved enzymatically to form fragments (13-16,22,38,
39). It has been shown for most of these toxins that
distinct antibodies can be induced to each of these subunits,
chains, and fragments and that these antibodies directed
toward different parts of the molecules may vary in their
neutralizing capacities (13-15,22,37,39-42). The ability to
form antibodies to some of these fragments may depend on the
animal species of origin of the antitoxin (13), whether the
protein had been treated with formalin (41,43-44) or the
presence of adjuvant (45). If we are to consider the use of
subunits or fragments as vaccines, it will be necessary to
determine that the antibodies will be protective or
therapeutic.

The experimental use of subunits as immunogens has begun.
Cholera subunit B has been prepared on a large scale (46) and
clinical studies are now in progress to evaluate the
parenteral and oral administration of this product (31).

Tetanus toxin can be used to illustrate how fragments may
be used. Like some botulinum toxins (18,22) it has been
shown that tetanus toxin exists intracellularly as a single
polypeptide chain (12-13), but in the extracellular culture
filtrate it exists in a nicked, dichain form allowing its
separation into heavy and light chains (13-14). Similar
findings have been reported for botulinum toxins (18). The
heavy chain of tetanus toxin can be further cleaved by

enzymes to form a fragment identified as β_1 (13) or C (14).
Data are available to show that the site of the toxin which
binds to ganglioside is located in the heavy chain (47-49).
It has been reported that both equine and human antitoxins
contain precipitating antibodies to these fragments (13). In
contrast, equine but not human antitoxins have been reported
to contain precipitating antibodies to the light chain (13).
Studies are now in progress in our laboratory to determine if
this is a general phenomenon for human antitoxins. The role
or need for light chain antibodies in either prophylaxis or
in treatment has yet to be defined. However Helting et al.
reported that anti-light chain antibody had neutralizing
capacity for tetanus toxin (14). Other workers have stated
that botulinum anti-light chain antibody is poor in its
neutralizing capacity for toxin type C_1, while anti-heavy
chain is highly effective against type C and cross neutralizes type D (42).

Our own studies show that radiolabeled Fragment C of
tetanus toxin will bind to both brain and thyroid membranes
and that it will undergo retrograde axonal transport (49).
It is not known whether this binding is to the specific
receptor necessary for the putative presynaptic action of
tetanus toxin.

As one approach to decreasing the reactions sometimes
seen with toxoid, it has been proposed that fragments of
tetanus toxin be considered as immunizing agents. Schwick et
al. have shown that Fragment B and Fragment C were similar to
tetanus toxoids in their ability to immunize guinea pigs and
mice. Because large quantities of Fragment B were reported
to cause unusual neurological signs and death of mice, this
Fragment was not considered suitable for use in man by these
workers. The administration of Fragment C as a booster
injection in man has been initiated (50). Sato et al. (39)
have reported that an aberrant systemic-type illness was
observed in mice after the local injection of tetanus toxin
which had been incompletely neutralized by an antibody that
had been induced by another enzymatically derived fragment.
Therefore the immune response directed against fragments,
etc., must be carefully evaluated for its ability to prevent
the disease under study.

One of the most significant new developments may be the
preparation of synthetic antigens. Audibert al al. recently
reported that antibodies to diphtheria toxin were induced by
immunizing animals with synthetic oligopeptides (51). The
amino acids of these peptides included those in the loop of
the 14 amino acids which are subtended by the disulfide
bridge near the NH_2 terminus of the toxin. The synthesis of

these peptides was based on knowing the complete sequence of
Fragment A and for the amino terminal stretch of Fragment B.
The synthetic peptide was covalently linked to BSA prior
to injection for immunization. Binding and neutralizing
antibodies were found. In addition, binding antibodies were
reported to be obtained using the tetradecapeptide coupled to
the synthetic branched, co-polymer, multi-poly-DL-alanyl
poly-α-lysine. These investigators reported that muramyl
dipeptide (MDP) could also be used as the adjuvant. They
have proposed the possibility of developing a completely
synthetic antidiphtheria vaccine. As these workers suggest,
once the sequence of other toxins is known it may be possible
to utilize this type of immunogen on a wide scale.

PROTEINS DERIVED BY GENETIC MANIPULATION

     Another approach to the preparation of antigens has been
that of genetic manipulation of the bacteria. Some investigators have proposed induction of local immunity to cholera
toxin by use of mutant strains of V. cholerae which can be
administered orally as live vaccines. Such strains would
provide a source of protective but non-toxic antigens. A
strain which is reported to produce subunit B, but not active
subunit A, has been administered to man under experimental
conditions (30,52).
     The power of the application of such approaches to the
production of non-toxic, cross reacting proteins was
illustrated when mutant strains of C. diphtheriae, capable
of making proteins immunologically cross reactive with
diphtheria toxin, were identified (40). Many such mutants
now exist (41). The potential for these CRM proteins as
immunogens was recently reemphasized by Porro et al. (44).
The original observations (40) which showed the need for
formalin as a stabilizer for CRM 197 protein, if not as an
inactivating substance, were confirmed. These mutant
proteins can be utilized to analyze the immune response of
man and animals and to study the effects of inactivating
agents on the quality and quantity of antibodies induced (40,
41,44). Modification of the CRM protein with formaldehyde
was shown to alter the ratio of the anti A to anti B
antibodies (40,41,44) and it has been suggested that formalin
treatment of the proteins may modify the avidity of the
antibody induced to these proteins.
     A mutant of Pseudomonas aeruginosa (CRM 66), which
produces a non-toxic protein immunologically cross reactive
with exotoxin A, has recently been described (53). Its

potential use as a vaccine strain is yet to be defined. This
protein lacks the enzymatic activity of the native toxin A in
a manner analogous to CRM 197 of *C. diphtheriae*. CRM
proteins can be expected to be isolated from other bacteria.
To date recombinant DNA technology has primarily been
limited to production of *E. coli* enterotoxins (54). It can
be predicted that this powerful tool will be used to prepare
intact toxins, peptides or cross reacting proteins in
appropriate systems under appropriate environmental safe-
guards. For example, the observation by Laird et al. (55)
that tetanus toxin production is associated with the presence
of a plasmid makes recombinant DNA studies potentially useful
if such studies could be performed under the applicable
guidelines.

TOXOIDS AS CARRIER MOLECULES

Toxoids and toxins are also being used experimentally as
immunogenic carriers for other antigens. One such antigen
has been the β subunit of human chorionic gonadotropin (hCG)
or synthetic oligopeptides unique to hCG (56). These
vaccines are being evaluated by several investigators for the
prevention of pregnancy (57-58). Tetanus toxoid has
generally been used as the protein carrier to which the
hormone is complexed. A few women have recieved these
products and are being evaluated (58).
The need to alter the immunogenicity of polysaccharides
so that they will provide an adequate level of antibody in
infants and children has resulted in the development of other
types of conjugated proteins. Toxins and toxoids have been
given to laboratory animals as carriers of "T-cell
independent" polysaccharide antigens to modify the immune
response and make it "T-cell dependent" (59-62).
It has been shown that linkage of meningococcal capsular
polysaccharides to tetanus toxoid modified the antibody
response to the polysaccharides (61-62) and that the antibody
response to the toxoid was comparable to the normal tetanus
toxoid response (61).
Schneerson et al. have shown that the introduction of a
spacer, adipic anhydride, between the capsular polysaccharide
of *H. influenzae* type B and diphtheria toxin (59-60), or
other proteins enables binding of the two large molecules.
The binding of the polysaccharide to a protein carrier
increases the immunogenicity of the polysaccharide. The
toxicity of the diphtheria toxin was significantly reduced by
coupling procedure. It is not known whether this toxoid
retained its immunogenicity for induction of antitoxin.

Other types of hybrid molecules of toxins, lectins, hormones and monoclonal antibodies have been prepared (64). Although these have not been recommended generally for use as antigens it can be anticipated that hybrids of toxin fragments and subunits will be considered as immunogens and as carriers in the future.

GENERAL COMMENTS

Additional toxins are likely to be identified as agents responsible for the pathogenesis of other diseases. It will be desirable to produce new types of toxoids or immunizing agents for these new as well as the known toxins such as botulinum toxin. As this is considered there are several factors which should be emphasized.

Procedures which have been used to modify the toxicity of tetanus and botulinum toxins were recently reviewed (18). Many of these procedures decrease the immunogenicity significantly. As discussed earlier even formaldehyde may modify the antigenicity of the proteins. Additionally, the inclusion of lysine may alter the type of modification achieved with formalin (10,35). The procedure used in the preparation of the hybrid molecules may also serve as detoxifying agents (59). As new procedures for detoxification of toxins or for conjugation are considered it will be necessary to carefully evaluate not only the ability of the agent to provide a stable, non-toxic molecule which does not revert to toxicity but it will be necessary to show that the final immunogen will be effective in providing neutralizing antibodies and will not give an aberrant immune response. In addition, products suitable for prophylaxis may not be suitable for the preparation of hyperimmune globulins for therapy.

In addition to being effective, the biologics must be safe when they are administered to man. This will require careful study as new procedures are used.

Although many types of adjuvants have been used experimentally only aluminum compounds have been used in licensed toxoids in the U.S. The need for substances which may enhance or prolong the immune response to toxoids is apparent. Adjuvants may not always increase the desired type of immune response. For example they may facilitate the formation of classes of antibodies not considered necessary for protection. Adjuvants must be carefully evaluated for both their acute and long term safety. The combination of the adjuvants with the immunogen may provide different safety considerations (65).

Relyveld has suggested that use of glutaraldehyde for the preparation of toxoids may increase the immunogenicity in such a way that adjuvants are not required (27). Studies in children with this type of product are now in progress. It is to be noted that the anti-cholera toxin response in man following administration of glutaraldehyde toxoid was not markedly increased by the addition of adjuvant (25). Thus adjuvants may not always be needed.

It can be expected that there will be increased interest in additional enterotoxins. As attempts are made to induce local immunity to these toxins the effect of parenteral administration of the antigen on the mucosal immunity must be carefully studied.

As the potential use of various new products are considered we must remain aware that toxoids, unlike most drugs, are administered to healthy individuals to prevent, not to treat, disease. Thus the benefit/risk ratio must be very high. Toxoids must be safe as well as effective. In the development of new types of toxoid vaccines, the potential for the induction of a toxin-mediated disease presenting with unexpected signs and symptoms or adverse reactions must be considered.

REFERENCES

1. Wilson, G.S., and Miles, A., *in* "Topley and Wilson's Principles of Bacteriology, Virology and Immunity," p. 1800. Williams and Wilkins, Baltimore, (1975).
2. Wilson, G.S., and Miles, A., *in* "Topley and Wilson's Principles of Bacteriology, Virology and Immunity," p. 2225. Williams and Wilkins, Baltimore, (1975).
3. Wilson, G.S., and Miles, A., *in* "Topley and Wilson's Principles of Bacteriology, Virology and Immunity," p. 2258. Williams and Wilkins, Baltimore, (1975).
4. Smith, L.DS., *in* "Botulism-The Organism, Its Toxin, The Disease" (A. Ballows, ed.), p. 177. Charles C. Thomas, Springfield, IL, (1977).
5. Hardegree, M.C., and Cox, C.B., *in* "Immunoglobulins: Characteristics and Uses of Intravenous Preparations" (B.M. Alving and J.S. Finlayson, eds.), p. 127. U.S. Department of Health and Human Services (1979).
6. Finlayson, J.S., Immune Globulins, *in* "Seminars in Thrombosis and Hemostasis, *Vol. VI,* p. 44, (1979).
7. Pappenheimer, A.M., Jr., *Ann. Rev. Biochem. 46,* 69 (1977).

8. Collier, R.J., and Mekalanos, J.J., *in* "Multifunctional Proteins" (H. Bassuringer and E. Schmincke-Ott, eds.), p. 261. John Wiley and Sons, New York, (1980).

9. Linggood, F.V., Stevens, M.F., Fulthorpe, A.J., Woiwod, A.J., and Pope, C.G., *Brit. J. Exp. Path. 44,* 177 (1963)

10. Scheibel, I., and Christensen, P.E., *Acta Path. Microbiol. Scandinav. 65,* 117 (1965).

11. Mellanby, J., and Green, J., *Neuroscience 6,* 281 (1981).

12. Craven, C.J., Dawson, D.J., *Biochem. Biophys. Acta 317,* 277 (1973).

13. Matsuda, M., Yoneda, M., *Biochem. Biophys. Res. Comm. 77,* 268 (1977)

14. Helting, T.B., Zwisler, O., *J. Biol. Chem. 252,* 187 (1977).

15. Matsuda, M., Hara, T., Yoneda, M., *Jap. J. Med. Sci. Biol. 31,* 215 (1978).

16. Bizzini, B., *Microbiol. Rev. 43,* 224 (1979).

17. Habermann, E., *in* "Handbook of Clinical Neurology" (P. J. Vinker and G.W. Bruyn, eds.), p. 491. North-Holland, New York, (1978).

18. Das Gupta, B.R., Sugiyama, H., *in* "Perspectives in Toxinology" (A.W. Bernheimer, ed.), p. 87. John Wiley and Sons, New York, (1977).

19. Akama, K., Ito, A., Yamamoto, A., and Sadahiro, S., *Jap. J. Med. Sci. Biol. 24,* 181 (1971).

20. Lawrence, G., Shann, F., Freestone, D.S., and Walker, P.D., *Lancet i,* 227 (1979).

21. Metzger, J.F., and Lewis, G.E., Jr., *Rev. Infect. Dis. 1,* 689 (1979).

22. Sugiyama, H., *Microbiol. Rev. 44,* 419 (1980).

23. Pierce, N.F., *in* "The Mucosal Immune System" (F.J. Bourne, ed.), Proc. of Symposium held September 9-11, 1980. Bristol, U.K. (in press).

24. Benenson, A.S., *in* "Symposium on Cholera" (H. Fukumi and Y. Zinnaka, eds.), Proc. of the 12th Joint Conference U.S.-Japan Cooperative Medical Science Program, p. 228, Sapporo, (1976).

25. Craig, J.P., *in* "Symposium on Cholera" (H. Fukumi and Y. Zinnaka, eds.), Proc. of the 12th Joint Conference U.S.-Japan Cooperative Medical Science Program, p. 259, Sapporo, (1976).

26. Rappaport, R.S., Bonde, G., McCann, T., Rubin, B.A., and Tint, H., *Infect. Immun. 9,* 304 (1974).

27. Relyveld, E.H., New Developments with Human and Veterinary Vaccines *in* "Prog. in Clin. and Biol. Research," *Vol. 47,* (A. Mizrahi, I. Hertman, M.A. Klingberg, A. Kohn, eds.), p. 51, Alan R. Liss, Inc., New York, (1980).

28. Leppla, S.H., Martin, O.C., and Pavlovskis, O.R. Ann. Meeting Amer. Soc. Microbiol. B96, p. 24 (1978).

29. Curlin, G.T., Levine, R.L., Aziz, K.M.A., Rahman, A.S.M. M., and Verivez, W.F., in "Symposium on Cholera" (H. Fukumi and Y. Zinnaka, eds.), Proc. of the 12th Joint Conference U.S.-Japan Cooperative Medical Science Program, p. 276, Sapporo, (1976).

30. Honda, T., and Finkelstein, R.A., Proc. Natl. Acad. Sci. USA 76, 2052 (1979).

31. Svennerholm, A.M., Sack, D.,Bardhan, P.K., Jertborn, M., Holmgren, J., in "Symposium on Cholera" (S. Kuwahara and Y. Zinnaka, eds.), Proc. of the 16th Joint Conference U.S.-Japan Cooperative Medical Science Program (in press).

32. Pollack, M., and Young, L.S., J. Clin. Invest, 63, 276 (1979).

33. Abe, C., Takeshi, K., Homma, J.Y., and Kato, I., Jap. J. Med. Sci. Biol. 32, 88 (1979).

34. Pollack, M., in "Seminars in Infectious Disease" Vol. VI. Bacterial Vaccines (J.B. Robbins, J.C. Hill and G. Sadoff, eds.), Thieme-Stratton, Inc., New York (1981) (in press).

35. Cryz, S.J., Jr., Friedman, R.L., Pavlovskis, O.R., and Iglewski, B.H., Infect. Immun. 32, 759 (1981).

36. Cryz, S.J., Jr., Pavlovskis, O.R., and Iglewski, B.H., in "Seminars in Infectious Disease" Vol. IV. Bacterial Vaccines (J.B. Robbins, J.C. Hill and G. Sadoff, eds.), Thieme-Stratton, Inc., New York (1981) (in press).

37. Holmgren, J., and Lönnroth, I., in "Cholera and Related Diarrheas" (O. Ouchterlony and J. Holmgren, eds.)., 43rd Nobel Symposium, p. 88. Stockholm, (1978).

38. Kozaki, S., Miyazaki, S., and Sakaguchi, G., Jap. J. Med. Sci. Biol. 31, 163 (1978).

39. Sato, H., Ito, A., Yamakawa, Y., and Murata, R., Infect. Immun. 24, 958 (1979).

40. Pappenheimer, A.M., Jr., Uchida, T., and Harper, A.A., Immunochem. 9, 891 (1972).

41. Cryz, S.J., Jr., Welkos, S.L., and Holmes, R.K., Infect. Immun. 30, 835 (1980).

42. Oguma, K., Syuto, B., Iida, H., and Kubo, S., Infect. Immun. 30, 835 (1980).

43. Rittenberg, M.B., Pinney, C.T., Jr., and Iglewski, B.H., Infect. Immun. 14, 122 (1976).

44. Porro, M., Saletti, M., Nencioni, L., Tagliaferri, L., Marsili, I., J. Infect. Dis. 142, 716 (1980).

45. Kameyama, S., Yamauchi, K., Uasuda, S., and Kondo, S., Jap. J. Med. Sci. Biol. 33, 67 (1980).

46. Tayot, J.L., Holmgren, J., Svennerholm, L., Lindblad, M., and Tardy, M., *Eur. J. Biochem. 113,* 249 (1981).

47. Helting, T.B., Zwisler, O., and Wiegandt, H., *J. Biol. Chem. 252,* 194 (1977).

48. van Heyningen, S., *FEBS Lett. 68,* 5 (1976).

49. Morris, N.P., Consiglio, E., Kohn, L.D., Habig, W.H., Hardegree, M.C., and Helting, T.B., *J. Biol. Chem. 255,* 6071 (1980).

50. Schwick, H.G., Helting, T.B., and Zwisler, O., New Developments with Human and Veterinary Vaccines *in* "Prog. in Clin. and Biol. Research," Vol. 47. (A. Mizrahi, I. Hertman, M.A. Klingberg, A. Kohn, eds.), p. 143, Alan R. Liss, Inc., New York, (1980).

51. Audibert, F., Jolivet, M., Chedid, L., Alouf, J.E., Boquet, P., Rivaille, P., and Siffert, O., *Nature 289,* 593 (1981).

52. Levine, M.M., Black, R.E., Clements, M.L., Nalin, D.R., Cisneros, L., and Finklestein, R.A., *in* "Volunteer Studies in Development of Vaccine Against Cholera and Enterotoxigenic *E. coli* Diarrhea: A Review. Nobel Conference 3. Acute Enteric Infection in Children." Elsevier-North Holland (in press).

53. Cryz, S.J., Jr., Friedman, R.L., and Iglewski, B.H., *Proc. Natl. Acad. Sci. USA 77,* 7199 (1980).

54. Elwell, L.P., and Shipley, P.L., *Ann. Rev. Microbiol. 34,* 465 (1980).

55. Laird, W., Aaronson, W., Silver, R.P., Habig, W.H., and Hardegree, M.C., *J. Infect. Dis. 142,* 623 (1980).

56. Task Force of Immunological Methods for Fertility Regulations. *Clin. Exp. Immunol. 33,* 360 (1978).

57. Ramakrishnan, S., Das, C., Dubey, S.K., Salahuddin, M., and Talwar, G.P., *J. Reproduct. Immunol. 1,* 249 (1979).

58. Nash, H., Talwar, G.P., Segal, S., Luukkainen, T., Johansson, E.D.B., Vasquey, J., Coutinko, E., and Sundaram, K., *Fertil. and Steril. 34,* 328 (1980).

59. Schneerson, R., Barrera, O., Sutton, A., and Robbins, J.B., *J. Exp. Med. 152,* 361 (1980).

60. Schneerson, R., Robbins, J.B., Barrera, O., Sutton, A., Habig, W.H., Hardegree, M.C., and Chaimovich, J., New Developments with Human and Veterinary Vaccines *in* "Prog. in Clin. and Biol. Research,", *Vol. 47,* (A. Mizrahi, I. Hertman, M.A. Klingberg, A. Kohn, eds.), p. 77, Alan R. Liss, Inc., New York, (1980).

61. Beuvery, E.C., Miedema, F., van Delft, R.W., and Nagel, J., *in* "Seminars in Infectious Disease" Vol. IV. Bacterial Vaccines (J.B. Robbins, J.C. Hill and G. Sadoff, eds.)., Thieme-Stratton, Inc., New York (1981) (in press).

62. Jennings, H.J. and Lugowski, C., *in* "Seminars in Infectious Disease" Vol. IV. Bacterial Vaccines (J.B. Robbins, J.C. Hill and G. Sadoff, eds.), Thieme-Stratton, Inc., New York (1981) (in press).

63. Uchida, T., Mekada, E., and Okada, Y., *J. Biol. Chem.* *255*, 6687 (1980).

64. Gilliland, D.G., Steplewski, Z., Collier, R.J., Mitchell, K.F., Chang, T.H., and Koprowski, H., *Proc. Natl. Acac. Sci.* *77*, 4539 (1980).

65. Edelman, R., *Rev. Infect. Dis.*, *2*, 370 (1980).

CLINICAL EVALUATION OF BOTULINUM TOXOIDS

James H. Anderson, Jr.[1,2]

Medical Division
U.S. Army Medical Research Institute of Infectious Diseases
Fort Detrick, Maryland

George E. Lewis, Jr.

Pathology Division
U.S. Army Medical Research Institute of Infectious Diseases
Fort Detrick, Maryland

I. INTRODUCTION

Since the time of the original description of the etiology and pathophysiology of botulism, prophylaxis has concentrated on avoidance of exposure to the causative toxins. Only a relatively small number of researchers have been concerned with the problems of inducing active immunity to botulinum toxins. A toxin of *Clostridium botulinum* was initially toxoided in 1924 (1) and the first experimental immunization of man was reported in 1934 (2). Production of antitoxin in guinea pigs by alum-precipitated toxoid was demonstrated in 1936 (3). The toxoids for use in humans were produced by

[1]*Present address: Department of Clinical Investigation, Brooke Army Medical Center, Fort Sam Houston, Texas.*

[2]*The opinions or assertions contained herein are the private views of the authors and are not to be construed as reflecting the views of the Department of the Army or the Department of Defense.*

BIOMEDICAL ASPECTS OF BOTULISM

growing highly toxigenic strains in culture media, removal of
bacterial cell material by centrifugation and purification of
the toxin by chemical means. The toxins produced were then
sterilized by filtration. Initially, type E toxin was treated
with trypsin to activate the toxin, however, subsequent
workers demonstrated that such activation decreased the antigenicity of the toxoid in experimental animals and in humans
(4). Formaldehyde was added and the mixture incubated at $37^{\circ}C$
until detoxification was completed as demonstrated by animal
testing. The toxoid was then adsorbed on aluminum phosphate
and 0.01% thimerosal added as a preservative (5).

There are certain problems associated with these traditional methods of toxoid production. Excessive amounts of
formaldehyde produce a toxoid with reduced antigenicity and
obviously too little formaldehyde results in incomplete inactivation. The quantity of formaldehyde necessary to cause
complete inactivation of toxin is dependent upon the total
protein concentration of the mixture to be toxoided and not
solely upon the toxin content. The toxoiding process is also
dependent upon pH, incubation temperature and duration of
reaction. The kinetics of toxoiding do not appear to be uniform for all toxin types. Therefore, toxoiding procedures
have been developed for each toxin type (5).

A. *Pentavalent Toxoids*

The pentavalent (ABCDE) toxoid currently in use was prepared in 1958 by Parke, Davis and Company (Parke Davis) under
contract to the US Army. Detectable antibody titers are consistently produced only after an initial series of three
toxoid injections and a subsequent annual booster. The
immunogenicity of this toxoid with respect to types B and D
toxins has been less than desirable.

However, the most common objections to the currently used
toxoid are the high rate of local reactogenicity of a moderate
to severe degree and the intense local pain experienced by
many individuals immediately after immunization with this product. Because of the undesirable characteristics, there have
been numerous calls since the 1960's for a new improved
toxoid. In 1974 the Center for Disease Control (CDC, now the
Centers for Disease Control) seriously considered terminating
distribution of this pentavalent botulinum toxoid.

In the early seventies, the Michigan Department of Public
Health (MDPH) under contract to the CDC began the production
of multiple lots of monovalent toxoids (A thru E) under the
direction of Dr. Charles Hatheway. The toxoid production procedures were very similar to those employed in the manufacture

TABLE I. C. BOTULINUM STRAINS USED IN PRODUCTION OF TOXOIDS

Type A	Hall strain
Type B	"Beans" strain
Type C	Onderstepoort strain C 1 d
Type D	Onderstepoort strain D 6 f
Type E	Dolman VH strain

of the Parke, Davis and Company toxoid. The *Clostridium botulinum* organisms were provided by Fort Detrick and were of the same strains used in the manufacture of the pentavalent toxoid by Parke, Davis and Company (Table I).

With the permission of the CDC which in 1978 held the Investigational New Drug application for the Parke, Davis and Company toxoid, the US Army Medical Research and Development Command awarded a contract to the Michigan Department of Public Health to bottle and test for safety and efficacy in animals three lots of pentavalent toxoid. These lots were released to the US Army Medical Research Institute of Infectious Diseases (USAMRIID) for reactogenicity and immunogenicity testing in human volunteers.

Two toxoid lots contain approximately one-half the amount of residual formaldehyde present in the other lot. MDPH Lot A-2 and Lot B-2 contain only 0.022% residual formaldehyde compared to MDPH Lot B-1 which contains 0.039%. The Parke, Davis and Company toxoid contains 0.034% residual formaldehyde. It was the hypothesis of those who produced these toxoids, and our hypothesis as well, that this reduction in formaldehyde content would reduce the intense local pain following immunization and perhaps reduce the incidence of reactogenicity.

After complete compliance with FDA regulations for packaging and testing, the toxoid in the final container was evaluated in both the CDC and USAMRIID laboratories. Tests for identity, potency and safety were satisfactory.

Animal immunogenicity studies conducted in 1978 in guinea pigs allow comparison of the Parke, Davis and Company pentavalent toxoid (Lot 1B1-F3) and the Michigan Department of Public Health toxoids (Lots A-2 and B-1). These studies are summarized in Table II and demonstrate a slight superiority of the MDPH toxoids with respect to the induction of neutralizing antibody to toxin types A, B, C and D. The type E response was below specification in the MDPH toxoids, but produced a 30 to 70% survival rate in immunized guinea pigs challenged with the type E toxin with no unimmunized animals surviving the challenge (6,7).

TABLE II. Guinea Pig Potency Testing of Pentavalent Botulinum Toxoids[a]

Toxoid	Neurotoxin Type	50% Endpoint	Antitoxin Titer IU/ml	Specification[b] (IU/ml)
Parke Davis	A	1:2.5	0.080	0.03
	B	< 1:1	< 0.008	0.01
	C	1:5	0.055	0.40
	D	1:1	0.023	0.12
	E	1:3.5	0.100	0.035
MDPH Lot A-2 (Low formaldehyde)	A	> 1:32	> 0.160	0.03
	B	1:1.26	0.010	0.01
	C	1:8	0.180	0.40
	D	1:8.95	1.140	0.12
	E	1:2.44	0.019	0.035
MDPH Lot B-1	A	> 1:32	> 0.160	0.03
	B	< 1:1	< 0.008	0.01
	C	1:9.2	0.207	0.40
	D	1:10.1	1.280	0.12
	E	< 1:1	< 0.008	0.035

[a] After Hatheway (6,7).

[b] Cardella, M. A., and Wright, G. G. (1964). "Specifications for Manufacture of Botulism Toxoid, Adsorbed, Pentavalent, Types ABCDE" (Technical Study 46). U.S. Army Biological Laboratories, Fort Detrick, Frederick, Maryland.

B. *Human Volunteer Studies Design*

A volunteer study was conducted at USAMRIID which is outlined in Table III. In the first group, four volunteers from the professional staff of USAMRIID who were already actively immunized with the Parke, Davis and Company pentavalent toxoid, were given 0.1 ml of toxoid from either MDPH Lot A-2 or B-1. These volunteers were observed for 21 days with no local reactions or adverse effects. In the second group, six nonimmune volunteers received one immunization with 0.05 ml (or 1/10 the normal dose) of either the Parke, Davis and Company toxoid, or Lot A-2 or B-1 of the MDPH toxoids. Again there were no local or systemic reactions nor adverse effects during 21 days of observation. The third group of volunteers, also nonimmune, received one injection of either the Parke Davis, MDPH Lot A-2 or MDPH Lot B-1 toxoid in the normal dose of 0.5 ml. These individuals were monitored for 21 days with only reports of mild erythema at the site of injection in some volunteers. There were no moderate or severe local or systemic reactions in any of the volunteers.

At this point 36 nonimmunized laboratory workers volunteered to participate in a full series immunization study evaluating the two MDPH Lots and the Parke Davis toxoid as a control. The accepted efficacy of toxoid administration made a saline control unnecessary. Each individual received 0.5 ml

TABLE III. *Initial MDPH Botulinum Toxoid Testing*

Group	Number	Protocols
1	4 (immune)	0.1 ml subcutaneously of MDPH Lot A-2 or MDPH Lot B-1
2	6 (nonimmune)	0.05 ml subcutaneously of Parke Davis, MDPH Lot A-2 or MDPH Lot B-1
3	6 (nonimmune)	0.5 ml subcutaneously of Parke Davis, MDPH Lot A-2 or MDPH Lot B-1
4	36 (nonimmune)	0.5 ml subcutaneously on Days 0, 14 and 84 of either Parke Davis, MDPH Lot A-2 or MDPH Lot B-1

of toxoid deep subcutaneously on days 0, 14 and 84 in a double blind study. The immunization schedule is the standard one used for "at risk" individuals receiving the Parke Davis toxoid. All individuals completed the three injection series.

C. Reactogenicity

The incidence of reactions following immunization is interesting. There was no significant difference discernible in the immediate pain on immunization among any of the groups including the low formaldehyde group MDPH Lot A-2. Local reactions were observed and recorded immediately and at 24, 48 and 72 hours in all volunteers and as needed after 72 hours in individuals who experienced any reaction.

After making measurements in two diameters perpendicular to each other, local reactions were graded by the CDC standard criteria for reactions:

None	No reaction
Mild	Erythema only; edema or induration which is measurable but 30 mm or less in any one diameter
Moderate	Edema or induration measuring greater than 30 mm and less than 210 mm in any one diameter
Severe	Any reaction measuring more than 210 mm in any one diameter or any reaction accompanied by marked limitation of motion of the arm or marked axillary node tenderness

The reaction rates in the USAMRIID study are summarized in Table IV. For each of the three toxoids evaluated, the reaction rates for each of the injections in the series is shown. There were 12 volunteers in the Parke Davis group; 13 received MDPH Lot A-2 and 11 were immunized with MDPH Lot B-1. MDPH Lot A-2 is the low formaldehyde toxoid. There were no severe reactions in any group and no volunteer missed work or was unable to perform his or her normal tasks. There were 7 moderate reactions in the MDPH Lot A-2 group and 5 in the MDPH Lot B-1 group. It should be noted that each of the individuals experiencing a moderate reaction after the third injection had also reacted similarly after the second so that in reality only 7 individuals experienced moderate reactions. The Parke Davis group had an unusually low rate of reactions and perhaps a better comparison could be made between the MDPH recipients and all individuals receiving the Parke Davis toxoid during the 1979-80 reporting period of the CDC (8).

Table V illustrates reaction rates of the recipients of the MDPH toxoids (both groups combined) in the USAMRIID study

TABLE IV. Incidence of Local Reactions in Human Volunteer Immunization Study[a]

Toxoid	Injection #	None or mild	Moderate	Severe	Total
Parke Davis[b]	1	11	1	0	12
	2	12	0	0	12
	3	12	0	0	12
	Subtotal	35 (97%)	1 (3%)	0 (0%)	36
MDPH Lot A-2[c,e]	1	13	0	0	13
	2	9	4	0	13
	3	10	3	0	13
	Subtotal	32 (82%)	7 (17.9%)	0 (0%)	39
MDPH Lot B-1[d]	1	11	0	0	11
	2	8	3	0	11
	3	9	2	0	11
	Subtotal	28 (85%)	5 (15%)	0 (0%)	33

[a] USAMRIID
[b] Pentavalent (ABCDE) botulinum toxoid, Parke, Davis and Company.
[c] Botulinum toxoid adsorbed pentavalent (ABCDE), Michigan Department of Public Health Lot A-2.
[d] Botulinum toxoid adsorbed pentavalent (ABCDE), Michigan Department of Public Health Lot B-1.
[e] Low formaldehyde toxoid.

TABLE V. Incidence of Local Reactions to Immunization (Initial Series) with Pentavalent Botulinum Toxoid[a]

Toxoid	Injection #	None or mild	Moderate	Severe	Total
MDPH[b]	1	24	0	0	24
	2	17	7	0	24
	3	19	5	0	24
	Subtotal	60 (83%)	12 (16%)	0 (0%)	72
Parke Davis[c]	1	87	7	0	94
	2	83	10	0	93
	3	71	7	1	79
	Subtotal	241 (90%)	24 (9%)	1 (0.4%)	266 (loss of 16)[d]

[a] Data from USAMRIID and CDC.

[b] Combined USAMRIID data for MDPH Lot A-2 and MDPH Lot B-1.

[c] Data reported by CDC for Parke Davis pentavalent toxoid 1979-1980 (8).

[d] Immunization not given and/or data not reported.

and the reaction rates reported to the CDC of all individuals receiving the Parke Davis toxoid. There were no severe reactions in the MDPH groups but one severe reaction in the Parke Davis group. The moderate reaction rate with the MDPH toxoid was 16% while the Parke Davis group had 9% moderate reactions. There are two explanations for this apparently adverse comparison. The first is that as an experimental study each of the USAMRIID volunteers was observed more frequently than in the standard CDC protocol and each volunteer is also in a subset of individuals hyperimmunized to multiple antigens. Additionally, 16 immunization experiences were lost from second and third immunizations in the CDC figures - which if previous reactions were the explanation for discontinuing the series it could be anticipated that they would have also had reactions with second and third immunization, thus making a truer incidence of reactions to the Parke Davis toxoid 14% which is not significantly different from the MDPH rate.

D. *Immunogenicity*

The immunogenicity of the toxoids is of course of prime importance. Thus far neutralizing antibody titers to toxin types A, B and E have been measured and are illustrated in Table VI. There were no statistically significant differences among any of the toxoids, for induction of antibody to type A neurotoxin although the mean titers for the groups receiving the MDPH toxoids were twice that of the Parke Davis group mean titer. There was a significant difference in type B antibody response. A mean titer of 0.10 IU/ml was elicited in MDPH Lot A-2 recipients as was a mean titer of 0.09 IU/ml in the MDPH Lot B-1 volunteers. Both of the MDPH toxoid group mean titer responses, while not different from each other, were clearly superior to the Parke Davis toxoid group mean response of 0.02 IU/ml with statistically significant differences at a p value of less than 0.01 (one-way analysis of variance, least significant difference).

The type E response to the MDPH toxoids was not significantly different from that induced by the Parke Davis toxoid.

These results demonstrate the superiority of the MDPH toxoids as type B immunogens in this initial clinical trial. Unfortunately, use of the MDPH toxoids did not reduce the rate of reactogenicity, even with the use of low formaldehyde toxoid. One must remember that the MDPH toxoids are a product of the technology of the 1960's. The pentavalent toxoid preparation contains only about 10% type A neurotoxoid and similar values are predicted for the other neurotoxin

TABLE VI. Titer Response to Initial Botulinum Toxoid Series[a]

Neutralizing Antibody Type	Toxoid	N	Geometric Mean Titer IU/ml (95% CI)[b]	Statistical Significance[c]
A	Parke Davis[d]	12	0.18 (0.07-0.51)	
	MDPH[e] Lot A-2	13	0.46 (0.15-1.41)	
	MDPH Lot B-1	11	0.35 (0.18-0.67)	
B	Parke Davis	12	0.02 (0.01-0.05)	
	MDPH Lot A-2	13	0.10 (0.05-0.21)	$p < 0.01$ $p < 0.01$
	MDPH Lot B-1	11	0.09 (0.05-0.19)	
E	Parke Davis	12	0.04 (0.02-0.10)	
	MDPH Lot A-2	13	0.03 (0.02-0.04)	
	MDPH Lot B-1	10	0.03 (0.02-0.04)	

[a] USAMRIID study.

[b] 95% confidence interval of the geometric mean titer.

[c] One-way analysis of variance with the least significant difference procedure, using the $\log_{10}$ IU/ml of neutralizing antibody at 14 days after completion of initial series.

[d] Pentavalent (ABCDE) Botulinum Toxoid, Parke, Davis and Company.

[e] Toxoid, Adsorbed, Pentavalent (ABCDE), Michigan Department of Public Health.

types (9,10). This lack of purity clearly indicates a continued need to develop new and improved toxoids using modern
technology as our understanding of immunology, biochemistry,
physiology, and the toxoiding kinetics of the botulinum toxins
increases.

II. MONOVALENT TOXOIDS

Another important area with which USAMRIID has been concerned has been the production of botulinum immune plasma of
human origin (11). As discussed in another chapter, one problem has been the relatively low concentration of antitoxin
generated in human plasma relative to the equine product.
This is particularly true with respect to the type B antitoxin
response in humans.

It had been suggested in animal studies that the use of a
monovalent toxoid would elicit a higher response than the same
amount of antigen contained in a multivalent preparation. A
modification of this hypothesis was examined in the USAMRIID
plasmapheresis program for the collection of botulinum immune
plasma of human origin. Under contract to the U. S. Army
Research and Development Command, the Michigan Department of
Public Health bottled one lot of the monovalent B toxoid produced at the same time as the B toxoid that was used in the
pentavalent MDPH toxoids discussed previously. The MDPH monovalent B toxoid underwent the same rigid safety testing outlined for the MDPH pentavalent toxoids. A research protocol
with fully informed consent was then conducted with volunteers
in the USAMRIID botulism immune plasma program. These volunteers, who had been immunized and received 8 to 12 annual
boosters of botulinum toxoids prior to 1970, were given a
booster immunization with the Parke Davis pentavalent toxoid
in 1979. Their type B titer antibody response measured in
international units at four weeks after booster immunization
is illustrated on the left hand section of Figure 1. Twelve
months later, these same individuals received another booster
of the Parke Davis pentavalent toxoid and, in the opposite
arm, a 0.5 ml dose of the MDPH monovalent B toxoid. The
volunteers uniformly reported much less immediate pain with
MDPH monovalent B toxoid. Local reactions in the volunteers
were no greater in frequency than in the pentavalent series
presented previously; it is interesting to note that the
three individuals who did have moderate reactions had
approximately equal reactions to both the pentavalent and
monovalent B toxoids. The 1980 B titer response, again four
weeks following immunization, is illustrated on the right hand
side of Figure 1. Individual responses for both points are

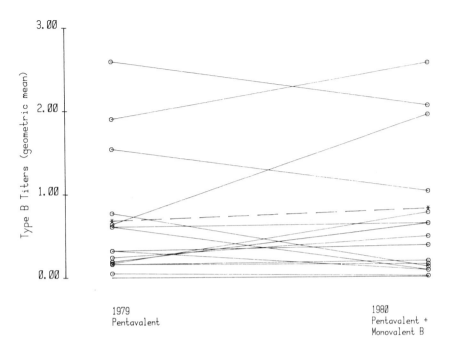

FIGURE 1.   Type B titers (geometric mean) 4 weeks following booster immunization with Parke Davis pentavalent toxoid (1979) and with Parke Davis pentavalent and MDPH monovalent B toxoids (1980).

connected by a solid line. The broken line is the mean titer response of the 16 individuals. The increase in B titer compared to that elicited from pentavalent toxoid alone is not statistically significant. Excluded from this, however, is one individual whose 1979 B titer was 1.14 IU/ml, who had a 1980 titer response of 6.40 IU/ml. Although the mean response is not dramatically positive, additional studies must be done in terms of numbers and timing of immunizations.

USAMRIID has also received a MDPH type E monovalent toxoid produced at the same time as the MDPH monovalent B toxoid. Currently, laboratory evaluations are underway as is an initial human study. It is anticipated that this monovalent toxoid might have value in some "at risk" populations where type E botulism is prevalent, such as the Alaskan natives.

III. CONCLUSION

Botulinum toxoids are entering a new era. In the past
toxoids have been used for animals and limited human protection of a generalized nature. Reactogenicity has always been
a major problem. Purity of toxoids has been far less than
ideal. Failure to significantly reduce reaction rates by
modification of the toxoid (e.g., reduced formaldehyde content) reflects our lack of knowledge in the past. In the
decade since the last toxoids were produced our understanding
of both the biochemical nature of the toxins of *Clostridium
botulinum* and human immunology has increased substantially.
The future has promise of purer toxoid preparations which may
induce fewer adverse reactions. Unique applications of monovalent and multivalent toxoids have recently resulted in a new
therapeutic agent, Botulism Immune Plasma (Human), for the
treatment of botulism. Specific prophylaxis for "at risk"
populations may result from the use of monovalent toxoids.
Although currently used in a relatively small group of individuals, the newer botulinum toxoids may play a major role in
the protection (and indirectly in the treatment) of larger
numbers of people.

ACKNOWLEDGMENTS

The authors would like to express their sincere gratitude
to Dr. Charles Hatheway (CDC) for the detailed information on
antibody titer responses from his laboratory. We would like
to give special credit to the tremendous effort, devotion and
expertise of Robert W. Wood (USAMRIID) in producing the technical data in this report.
The volunteers were U.S. Army personnel or civilian
United States Government employees. These tests were
governed by principles, policies, and rules for medical
volunteers as established by Army Regulation 70-25 and the
Declaration of Helsinki. The study was conducted as part of
a long-term program for the investigation of mechanisms of
vaccine efficacy and host reponses to infectious diseases.

REFERENCES

1. Cardella, M. A., *in* "Botulism" (K. H. Lewis and K.
    Cassel, eds.), p. 152. U. S. Public Health Service,
    Cincinnati, (1964).
2. Velikanov, I., *Klin. Med. 12*, 1802 (1934).
3. Melnik, M. L., and Starobinetz, G. M., *Ann. Inst. Metch.
    4*, 33 (1936).
4. Kondo, H., Kondo, S., Murata, R., and Sakaguchi, G., *in*
    "Toxic Microorganisms" (M. Herzberg, ed.), U. S. Dept. of
    Interior, Washington, D.C., (1970).
5. Smith, L. D. S., *in* "Botulism", p. 152. Thomas, Spring-
    field, Ill., (1977).
6. Hatheway, C., *Personal Communication* (G.E.L.), (1978).
7. Hatheway, C., *Progress Report #12:BB-IND 161 Pentavalent
    (ABCDE) Botulinum Toxoid*. Center for Disease Control,
    Atlanta, (1978).
8. Boutwell, J. H., *Progress Report #14:BB-IND 161 Penta-
    valent (ABCDE) Botulinum Toxoid*. Center for Disease
    Control, Atlanta, (1980).
9. Boroff, D. A., Meloche, H. P., and DasGupta, B. R.,
    Infect. Immun. 2, 679 (1970).
10. Siegel, L. S., and Metzger, J. F., *Appl. Environ. Micro-
    biol. 38*, 606 (1979).
11. Metzger, J. F., and Lewis, G. E. Jr., *Rev. Infect. Dis.
    2*, 689 (1979).

PRODUCTION, PURIFICATION AND TOXOIDING OF
CLOSTRIDIUM BOTULINUM TYPE A TOXIN

Peter Hambleton, Brian Capel, Nigel Bailey
Nicholas Heron, Alan Crooks and Jack Melling

Vaccine Research and Production Laboratory
C.A.M.R., Porton Down, Salisbury
Wiltshire, U.K.

Chun-Kee Tse and J. Oliver Dolly

Department of Biochemistry
Imperial College of Science and Technology
London, U.K.

I. INTRODUCTION

The anaerobic spore-forming Gram-positive bacillus *Clostridium botulinum* elaborates toxins that are among the most powerful neuroparalytic poisons known. In man the neuroparalytic illness, botulism, may result from the ingestion of food contaminated with preformed toxin, from colonization of wounds by *Cl. botulinum,* or in the case of infant botulism from the absorption of toxins formed *in vivo* by *Cl. botulinum* organisms that colonize the infant intestine (1). Consequently, there are various groups of scientific workers who use *Cl. botulinum* as a test organism, are involved in diagnosing the illness and detecting toxins or use the toxins in the course of their research. It is people in such groups who may need to be protected against possible intoxication, by active immunization with chemically inactivated toxins (toxoids).

In addition to active immunization botulinum toxoids are also of value as a means of providing antisera for passive therapy and for use in ELISA assay systems for the detection and assay of toxins.

Address correspondence to Dr. Melling.

BIOMEDICAL ASPECTS OF BOTULISM

247

Although this paper concentrates on Type A toxin, similar production and purification methods have been applied by us to Type B and Type E toxins with a view to establishing a standard process for preparing these products for use in vaccine production.

II.   MATERIALS AND METHODS

A.   *Bacterial Growth and Production of Toxin*

Clostridium botulinum type A NCTC 2916 was used and stock suspensions of viable spores in Robertson's meat broth stored at -20° were used as starting inocula. The organisms were grown in a medium that contained proteose peptone No 3 (Difco Laboratories, Detroit, Michigan, USA), 20g/l; yeast extract (Difco Labs), 10g/l; N.Z. amine A (Humko Sheffield Chemical, Lyndhurst, N.J. USA). 10g/l and Sodium mercaptoacetate (BDH Chemicals Ltd, Poole, Dorset, UK), 0.5g/l. The pH of the medium was adjusted to 7.3 with 3M NaOH prior to autoclaving (15 psi, 15 min). Subsequently glucose solution (50%w/v), was added aseptically to the medium to a final concentration of 1%(w/v). For toxin production 100ml of complete medium was inoculated with 1 ml of spore suspension, incubated for 24h at 34°, and the resulting bacterial suspension used to inoculate a 1 l. culture that, after incubation for 24-48 h, was used to seed a 20 l culture. Such large cultures were grown at 34° in a cabinet-enclosed fermenter (6), with minimal stirring. Period-ically the head-space of the culture vessel was flushed with oxygen-free nitrogen gas.

B.   *Toxicity Determinations*

Toxin samples were serially diluted in 0.2% (w/v) gelatine, 0.07M Na_2HPO_4, pH 6.5. Groups of 4 Porton mice (20g) were injected (i.p.) with samples of diluted toxin (0.5ml per animal) and the mouse lethal dose 50 (MLD_{50}) estimated.

C.   *Protein Determinations*

Protein estimations were carried out using a modified Folin method (12) with bovine serum albumen as a standard.

D. *Immuno Double Diffusion Tests*

Gels (1.5mm deep) of 1% (w/v) agarose (Miles Laboratories
Ltd) were cast on glass microscope slides and 3.0mm diam. holes
cut using a template. Samples (5μl) of toxin and horse antitoxin (type A) were placed in adjacent wells and allowed to
diffuse towards each other for up to 2 days at 4°.

E. *Purification of Toxic Components*

The method used to purify toxic components is a modification
of those described previously. (3,13).

Stage 1. The pH value of a 20 l culture incubated for 48h
was adjusted automatically to 3.5 with 3N H_2SO_4, the culture
being stirred during the addition of acid to the fermenter to
ensure efficient mixing. The resulting precipitate was recovered with a continuous flow centrifuge (40,000 rpm, Carl
Padberg Zentrifugenbau GMBH, 7630 Lahr, W. Germany). Recovery
of the acid precipitated toxin and subsequent purification
steps were performed in Class III biological safety cabinets
of the types described by Melling and Allner (6).

Stage 2. Acid precipitated toxin from a 20 l. culture (55-
60g) was extracted with sodium phosphate buffer (200ml, 0.2M,
pH 6.0) for 1 h at room temperature. The acid paste did not
readily disperse in buffer but was rapidly and efficiently
resuspended using a Colworth Stomacher homogenizer (Seward
Laboratories). Care was taken to maintain the pH of the
suspension at 6.0 throughout the extraction by adding 1M NaOH
as necessary. The extract was clarified by centrifuging
(20,000g, 10min, 4°) and the sediment re-extracted with
phosphate buffer.

Stage 3. The clarified extracts were pooled and treated
with ribonuclease (100μg/ml, 34°, 3h; 5 x crystalized, C.P.
Laboratories Ltd. Bishops Stortford, Herts. UK).

Stage 4. Ammonium sulphate was added to 60% saturation
and precipitated toxin centrifuged (20,000g, 10min),
redissolved in sodium citrate buffer (50-100ml, 0.05M, pH 5.5)
and dialysed against the same buffer at 4° to remove residual
ammonium sulphate.

Stage 5. At this stage toxin preparations contained a
brown pigment that bound tightly to DEAE-ion exchange materials
causing blockage of the chromatographic columns used in the
next stage [6]. Most of the pigment was removed by adding

about half a volume of swollen DEAE-Sephadex A50 or DEAE-
Sephacel (Pharmacia (Gt Britain) Ltd), and allowing the mixture
to stand, with occasional mixing, for several hours. The gel
was subsequently removed by centrifuging.

Stage 6. The clear extract was loaded onto a column (90 x
8cm) of DEAE-Sephacel previously equilibrated with 0.05M
citrate buffer, pH 5.5. Toxin was eluted with the equilibration
buffer and fractions from the first protein peak eluted having
a $^{260}/_{280}$ nm absorbance ratio of 0.54-0.58 were pooled.

Stage 7. Ammonium sulphate was added to 60% saturation the
precipitate recovered after centrifuging, dissolved in 0.03M
sodium phosphate buffer (pH 6.8) and dialysed against the same
buffer to remove residual ammonium sulphate.

Stage 8. Some preparations of the partially purified
haemagglutinin-neurotoxin complex recovered after ion-exchange
chromatography *[stage 7]* were contaminated with low molecular
weight proteins that could be removed by gel filtration.
Conjugate toxin was loaded onto a column (2.2 x 70cm, 265cm^3
bed volume) of Sephacryl S-300 (Pharmacia (Gt Britain) Ltd)
previously equilibrated with 0.05M citrate buffer pH 5.5, 0.15M
NaCl and eluted with the same buffer. The bulk of toxic
activity eluted was associated with components with molecular
weights of >500,000.

F. *Preparation of Neurotoxin*

The haemagglutinin component of the conjugate toxin was
selectively removed using an affinity chromatographic method
(10).
Haemagglutinin-free toxin prepared by affinity
chromatography could be further purified by DEAE ion-exchange
chromatography using a method previously described for the
preparation of haemagglutinin-free toxin (9).

G. *Polyacrylamide gel electrophoresis*

Components of toxin samples were separated by electrophoresis on gradient pore polyacrylamide gels (4-30% acrylamide,
PAA 4/300, Pharmacia). For analysis of subunit structure,
toxin samples were denatured by heating in electrode buffer
containing SDS (1% w/v) with or without β-mercaptoethanol (5%,
V/V) at 100° for 5-10 min.

H. *Inactivation of Toxins*

Samples of complex toxin (10^8 MLD_{50}/ml) or purified neurotoxin (2 x 10^5 MLD_{50}/ml) in 200mM sodium succinate (pH 5.5)
were inactivated by adding neutralized formalin (0.6%, V/V)
and incubating at 34°.

III. RESULTS AND DISCUSSION

A. *Growth of* Cl.botulinum *and Production of Toxin Stirred
Fermenter Cultures*

The growth of *Cl.botulinum* type A NCTC 2916 and the
appearance of toxin in a typical culture is shown in Table I.
Following a short lag phase (1-4h) growth was exponential for
12-14h. The optical density of the culture remained maximal
for a further 30h and thereafter decreased as lysis of
vegetative cells occured.

TABLE I. *Growth and Toxin Production of
          Type A NCTC 2916 in a Stirred Fermenter*

Culture Age (h)	Optical Density (540nm)	Total bacteria no/ml	pH	Toxicity MLD_{50}/ml
0	0.1	4 x 10^7	7.3	10^4
4	0.15	5 x 10^7	7.0	1.5 x 10^4
6	1.1	1.2 x 10^8	6.6	3 x 10^4
10	3.1	4.2 x 10^8	6.0	2.5 x 10^5
14	3.8	9.5 x 10^8	5.9	5 x 10^5
22	4.8	1.2 x 10^9	5.5	8 x 10^5
31	4.9	Not done	5.3	10^6
50	4.9	Not done	5.6	10^6
71	1.3	Not done	5.7	10^6
95	0.4	Not done	5.8	10^6

Toxin levels increased exponentially with growth up to a
maximum of about 10^6 mouse LD_{50}/ml and remained at this level
even during the period of culture lysis. The pH of the
cultures was not controlled during growth and fell during the
exponential phase, reaching a final value of about 5.3 after
24-36h growth. Siegel and Metzger (4) obtained similar yields
of toxin in stirred fermenter cultures although they reported

that control of the culture pH was necessary to maintain the toxicity in cultures aged 28h or over. These workers also reported that culture lysis was apparently not required for maximum toxin concentrations in the culture fluid. In the present study culture filtrates taken during the late exponential phase, when little or no culture lysis might have been expected to occur, were found to contain at least 50% of the toxicity of the whole culture confirming Siegel and Metzger's observations. This contrasts somewhat with previous observations that toxin is liberated from *Cl.botulinum* type A only by autolysis. This inconsistancy is not readily explained but it may be due partly, for example, to the difficulty of obtaining representative samples from static cultures or to the fact that better mixing of cells and nutrients occurs in stirred as opposed to static cultures. Differences in the composition of growth medium or even the bacterial strains may contribute to the discrepancy.

B.   *Purification of Type A Haemagglutinin-neurotoxin Complex*

TABLE II.   The Effect of pH Value on the Solubilization by 0.2M Phosphate Buffer of Acid-precipitated Cl.botulinum *Type A toxin*

pH	*% of acid-precipitated toxin extracted*
5.0	*0.15*
5.5	*0.6*
6.0	*>90.0*
6.5	*25.0*
7.0	*6.0*
7.5	*2.5*

Acid precipitation has been used as a preliminary step in the recovery of type A toxin from bacterial cultures for over 40 years (7,8,13,14). Subsequent solubilization of acid-precipitated type A Toxin has been attempted with water (7) and $CaCl_2$ solutions (3,8), but in our hands $CaCl_2$ extractions gave very variable recoveries of toxin. Kozaki, Sakaguchi and Sakaguchi (15) re-extracted acid-precipitated type B toxin with 0.2M phosphate buffer, pH 6.0. We found consistently that type A toxin was more efficiently extracted with 0.2M phosphate buffer, pH 6.0, than with $CaCl_2$ solutions but that efficient extraction (>90%) was only achieved if the pH value was maintained within the range 6.0–6.5 during extraction. Considerably less toxin was recovered if the pH was outside this range (Table II).

A typical purification of the haemagglutinin-neurotoxin conjugate is shown in Table III. Ribonuclease treatment of toxic extracts before ion-exchange chromatography is considered essential since on occasions toxic material not so treated was found to become tightly bound to DEAE-resins and could not effectively be recovered.

TABLE III. Purification of Cl.botulinum Type A Hemagglutinin-neurotoxin Complex

Stage	Procedure	Protein (mg)	Total Mouse LD_{50}	MLD_{50}/mg protein	Recovery % stage	Recovery % overall
			Toxicity			
1	Whole culture (20 l).	–	10^{10}	–	100	100
2	Precipitation at pH 3.5, adjusted with 3N H_2SO_4.	4600	$7.5x10^9$	$1.6x10^6$	75	75
3	Extraction with 0.2M phosphate buffer at pH 6.0.	1300	$6.8x10^9$	$5.2x10^6$	91	68
4	Ribonuclease treatment (100µg/ml, 34°, 3h).	1300	$6.8x10^9$	$5.2x10^6$	100	68
5	Precipitation at 60% saturation (at 25°) of ammonium sulphate.	–	$6.5x10^9$	–	96	65
6	DEAE-Sephadex A50 batch preabsorption.	860	$5.0x10^9$	$5.8x10^6$	77	50
7	DEAE-Sephacel ion-exchange chromatography at pH 5.5.	195	$4.8x10^9$	$2.5x10^7$	96	48
8	Precipitation at 60% saturation (at 25°) of ammonium sulphate.	195	$4.8x10^9$	$2.5x10^7$	100	48

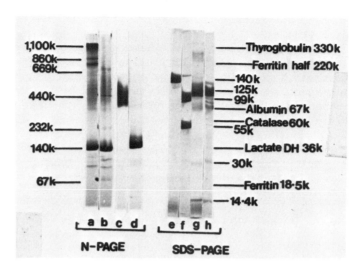

FIGURE 1. Native (N) and SDS gradient pore PAGE of Cl.
botulinum *type A toxic components. Track a, haemagglutinin-*
neurotoxin complex (TABLE III, stage 8); b, neurotoxin from
affinity gel (TABLE IV, stage 1); c, high toxicity component
from DEAE-chromatography (TABLE IV, stage 2a); d, low toxicity
component from DEAE-chromatography (TABLE IV, stage 2b); e,
high toxicity component (SDS-non-reduced); f, high toxicity
component (SDS-reduced); g, low toxicity component (SDS-non-
reduced); h, low toxicity component (SDS-reduced).

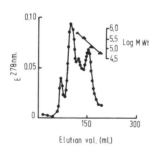

FIGURE 2. Gel filtration of Cl.botulinum type A
haemagglutinin-neurotoxin complex on Sephacryl S-300. Proteins
were eluted with 0.05M sodium citrate, 0.15M NaCl, pH 5.5.
Protein markers with known molecular weights (thyroglobulin,
ferritin, aldolase and bovine serum albumen) were gel filtered
under similar conditions on the same column. E^{287nm}*,* ● *;*
molecular weight, ▲ *.*

C. *Characterisation of Type A Haemagglutinin-neurotoxin Complex*

The specific toxic activity of conjugate type A toxin obtained (2.5×10^7 LD_{50}/mg protein) is similar to that reported by other workers (3.0–3.7×10^7 LD_{50}/mg protein; 3,16) and up to 48% of the original toxicity of the culture could be recovered.

Gradient pore PAGE of haemagglutinin-neurotoxin complex showed (Fig 1) that it comprised several high molecular weight species (>500,000 Daltons) together with a component of about 140,000 Daltons. Such preparations often contained low molecular weight components not reported present in crystalline toxins prepared by other workers (3,16). This may reflect the high resolving power of the gradient-pore gels or might be in part a consequence of the gels being run at pH 8.4 at which some dissociation of complex toxin might be assumed to have occured. The apparent greater homogeneity of an earlier crystalline toxin preparation (16) might also relate to differences in the purification process. Thus, the combination of alcohol precipitation and crystallization from ammonium sulphate might have tended to select a particular toxic fraction.

The presence of low molecular weight materials in preparations of complex toxin, as shown by gradient-pore PAGE, did not interfere with subsequent purification of type A neurotoxin. However, low molecular weight contaminants could be effectively removed by gel exclusion chromatography on Sephacryl S-300. Fig.2 shows a typical elution profile for such a separation.

Affinity chromatography using p-amino-phenyl-β-D-thio-galactopyranoside as ligand, was used (10) to obtain haemagglutinin-free neurotoxin preparations from complex type A toxin. Table IV shows that 76% of the toxic activity bound to the affinity absorbant was recovered. A single, sharp, peak of haemagglutinin-free toxin was eluted (Fig 3) that had a specific toxicity of 4.5×10^7 LD_{50}/mg protein. On gradient pore PAGE this material gave a sharp band of 140,000 Daltons and a diffuse band in the region of 3.5×10^5 Daltons (Fig 1).

The two components eluted from the affinity gel were subsequently separated by DEAE-Sephadex chromatography (Fig 4). The first peak eluted (at 140 mM Cl^-) appeared on native gradient-pore PAGE analysis to be identical with the diffuse band observed in the toxin obtained after affinity chromatography (Fig 1). This material had a high toxicity (Table IV; 8.3×10^7 LD_{50}/mg protein) and on PAGE analysis in the presence of SDS gave a single sharp band at a molecular weight of 140,000 Daltons (Fig 1). Faint bands with molecular weights of ca. 30,000 were observed when gels were loaded with high levels of protein. SDS-PAGE analysis in the

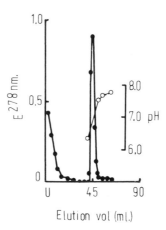

FIGURE 3. Affinity chromatography of Cl.botulinum type A
toxin. Haemagglutinin-neurotoxin complex (TABLE III, stage 8)
was bound to p-aminophenyl-β-D-thiogalactopyranoside linked to
Sepharose-4B in 50mM phosphate buffer, pH 6.3. Haemagglutinin-
free neurotoxin was eluted with 100mM sodium phosphate, 1M NaCl
pH 7.9. E^{278nm}, ● , pH, ○.

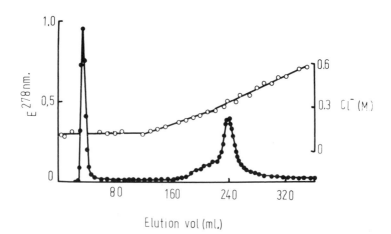

FIGURE 4. DEAE ion-exchange chromatography of Cl.
botulinum type A neurotoxin. Toxin from affinity chromatography (TABLE IV, stage 1) was loaded onto a DEAE-Sephacel
column (55 x 1cm) equilibrated with 0.15M Tris-HCl, pH 8.0.
Proteins were eluted with a linear (0-1.0M) gradient of NaCl
in 0.15M Tris/HCL, pH 8.0. E^{278nm}, ● ,[Cl⁻],○.

presence of β-mercaptoacetate showed that this component had
two subunits with molecular weights of approximately 55,000
and 99,000 Daltons (Fig 1). This material appears to
correspond to the neurotoxin described previously (10,17).

TABLE IV.   Purification of Cl.botulinum Type A Neurotoxin
Components.[a]

Stage	Procedure	Protein (mg)	Toxicity		Recovery	
			Total Mouse LD_{50}	MLD_{50}/mg protein	stage	overall
1	Affinity chromato-graphy.	44.8	$2x10^9$	$4.5x10^7$	76	37
2	DEAE-chromatography-Cl^- gradient elution.					
	a) First peak	14.3^b	$1.2x10^9$	$8.3x10^7$	60	23
	b) Second peak	23.7^b	$1.4x10^6$	$5.9x10^4$	0.1	<0.1

[a] Starting material was a portion (93mg, $2.7 \times 10^9 MLD_{50}$) of the
product from stage 8 TABLE IV.
[b] Values multiplied by a factor of 1.3 to calculate % recovery
of toxicity since only 75-80% of material from stage 1 was
further purified.

The second peak (Fig 4) eluted at 350mM Cl^- corresponded
to the sharp band (about 140,000 Daltons) observed on native
gradient-pore PAGE-analysis of the affinity gel-purified toxin.
This component had a relatively low toxicity (Table 5;
5.9×10^4 LD_{50}/mg protein) and gave three sub-units on SDS-
PAGE in both reducing and non-reducing conditions with
molecular weights of 125,000, 30,000 and 14,000 Daltons
respectively (Fig 1). This component may not have been
described previously although Moberg and Sugiyama (10) did
describe the presence of components in their affinity-purified
neurotoxin with molecular weights of about 130,000, thought to
represent less than 1% of the total protein of their
preparation.
        The subunit patterns of the two components and their
markedly different toxicities suggest that they may be distinct
molecular species. In addition the two components differ antigenically. In agarose gel double diffusion tests against a
horse anti-toxin the type A haemagglutinin-neurotoxin complex
gave (Fig 5) two precipitin lines; a defined line corresponding

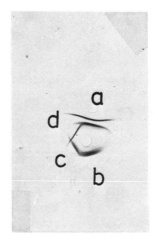

FIGURE 5. *Agarose gel double diffusion of* Cl.botulinum
type A toxic components. Centre well horse anti-type A serum.
Outer wells; a, haemagglutinin-neurotoxin complex; b, affinity
gel purified toxin (TABLE IV, stage 1); c, high toxicity
component (TABLE IV, stage 2a); d, low toxicity component
(TABLE IV, stage 2b).

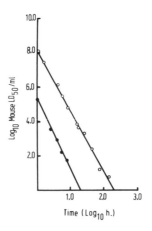

FIGURE 6. *Formaldehyde inactivation of* Cl.botulinum *type A*
complex toxin(○) and purified neurotoxin(●). Toxoiding was
carried out as in Materials and Methods.

to the haemagglutinin and a more diffuse line corresponding to the neurotoxin. Haemagglutinin-free toxin eluted from the affinity gel gave a single, diffuse, line identical to the inner line given by the complex toxin. The two toxic components separated by the subsequent DEAE-chromatography of the affinity gel eluate each gave single precipitin lines that had reactions of partial identity with the neurotoxin line of the complex toxin but which were themselves antigenically distinct (Fig 5). These data imply that the two components are indeed distinct molecular species. The trace components (130,000 molecular weight) present in the affinity-purified neurotoxin of Moberg and Sugiyama (10) may have given rise to a second precipitin line observed when high levels of toxin were tested in double diffusion tests against anti-crystalline toxin serum but it is not possible to draw conclusions as to whether or not this trace component is similar to the low toxicity component isolated in the present study.

D. *Preparation of Toxoids of Cl.botulinum Type A*

Formaldehyde inactivation of type A complex toxin prepared as described above (see Materials and Methods) resulted in loss of toxicity (Fig 6), similar to that observed previously (11). Formaldehyde inactivation of purified neurotoxin appears not to have previously been described. In this study the formaldehyde inactivation of neurotoxin, prepared by a combination of affinity and ion-exchange chromatographic methods, was found to have similar kinetics to that of the inactivation of complex toxin (Fig 6). Indeed, there was no statistical difference in the slopes of the two inactivation curves.

Insufficient neurotoxoid has yet been prepared for its efficacy as a potential vaccine to be assessed. An advantage of a neurotoxoid vaccine could be that it might elicit minimal side effects, since less foreign protein might need to be administered. On the other hand it is not certain that the antigenicity of a neurotoxoid would necessarily be sufficient to induce an adequate level of anti-toxin formation. Nor is it known whether the stability of a neurotoxoid would be similar to that of inactivated complex toxin. A further use of neurotoxoids could be in the production of monoclonal antibodies for use in immunoassays for neurotoxin.

ACKNOWLEDGEMENT

We are grateful to Professor E J Schantz for gifts of crystalline toxin and for his freely given help and advice to one of us (JM) when this work began.

REFERENCES

1. Arnon, S.S., Midura, T.F., Clay, S.A., Wood, R.M. and Chin.J. *J.amer.med. Assoc. 237* 1942 (1977).
2. Bonventre, P.F. and Kempe, L.C. *Appl. Microbiol. 7,* 372 (1959).
3. Sugiyama, H., Moberg, L.J. and Messer, S.L. *Appl. environ. Microbiol. 33,* 963(1977).
4. Siegel, L.S. and Metzger, J.F. *Appl. environ. Microbiol. 38,* 606 (1979).
5. Hambleton, P., Tse, C.K., Capel, B.J., Dolly, J.O. and Melling. J. in *"Proceedings of the World Congress Food-borne Infections and Intoxications Berlin (West)",* Paul Parey, Berlin, (1981). *In press.*
6. Melling, J. and Allner, K. in *"Essays in Appl. Microbiol"* (J.R. Norris and M.H. Richmond, eds) John Wiley & Sons Inc. (1981). *In press.*
7. Lamanna, C., McElroy, D.E. and Eklund, H.W. *Science, 103,* 613 (1946).
8. Duff, J.T., Wright, G.G., Klerer, J., Moore, D.E. and Bibler, R.H. *J. Bacteriol. 73,* 42 (1957).
9. DasGupta, B.R. and Boroff, D.A. *J. biol. Chem. 243,* 1065 (1968).
10. Moberg, L.J. and Sugiyama, H. *Appl.environ.Microbiol. 35,* 878 (1978).
11. Wright, G.G., Duff, J.T., Fiock, M.A., Devlin, H.B. and Soderstrom, R.L. *J. Immunol. 84,* 384 (1960).
12. Lowry, O.H., Rosebrough, N.J., Farr, A.L. and Randall, R.J, *J. biol.Chem.193,* 265 (1951).
13. Tani, S. *Compt.rend.soc.Biol. 114,*237 (1933).
14. Sommer, H. *Proc. soc. exptl. biol. Med. 35,* 530 (1936).
15. Kozaki, S., Sakaguchi, S. and Sakaguchi, G. *Infect. Immun. 10* 750 (1974).
16. Schantz, E.J. in *"Botulisum"* (K.H. Lewis and K.Cossel Jr. eds). P 91, U.S. Dept. Health, Education and Welfare. Pub. 999-FB-1. (1964).
17. DasGupta, B.R., Boroff, D.A. and Rothstein, E. *Biochem. Biophys.res.Commun.22* 750 (1966).

APPROACHES TO THE PROPHYLAXIS, IMMUNOTHERAPY,
AND CHEMOTHERAPY OF BOTULISM

George E. Lewis, Jr.

Pathology Division
U.S. Army Medical Research
Institute of Infectious Diseases
Fort Detrick, Frederick, Maryland

Botulism therapy, despite the availability of heterologous polyvalent botulinal antitoxins and substantial advances in the quality of intensive care, is still unsatisfactory. Over 17 years ago, Dr. C. S. Petty discussed the hazards of utilizing heterologous (equine) antitoxins, and the advantages of its future replacement with homologous, human-derived immune globulin for the treatment of patients poisoned with botulinal toxin (1).

The time lag between exposure and/or symptoms of botulism may be as short as a few hours, or as long as several days. Most often, by the time a diagnosis of botulism is made, toxin has reached a substantial number of nerve terminals and has induced an often thought to be irreversible blockade of acetylcholine release, sufficient in magnitude to produce noticeable muscular paralysis. Treatment with any antitoxin at this advanced stage of disease will not reverse or provide relief from the existing paralysis, but should, if administered in sufficient quantity, neutralize all free toxin. In addition, use of the heterologous (equine) antitoxin currently available introduces the life-threatening risk of eliciting immediate adverse reactions in sensitized recipients and of inducing delayed serum sickness reactions.

This report presents and discusses numerous approaches to the prophylaxis, immunotherapy and chemotherapy of botulism.

Problems posed by the use of heterologous (equine) antitoxin and the desire to reverse existing botulinal toxin-induced paralysis may be approached in a number of ways (Table I).

TABLE I.   Approaches to the Prophylaxis, Immunotherapy
and Chemotherapy of Botulism

---

1. Homologous (human) immune globulin
2. A variety of heterologous (i.e., bovine) antitoxins
3. Improved monomeric equine immune globulin
4. Monoclonal, homologous (human) antibody
5. Cross-reacting materials, nontoxins
6. Chemically and enzymatically altered toxins
7. Antagonistic chemotherapy (i.e., aminopyridines)
8. Combined approaches

First, the use of homologous (human) plasma or immune globulin in the treatment of patients poisoned by ingestion of
preformed botulinal toxin would surely eliminate a vast majority of the immediate and delayed adverse reactions induced in
the recipients of equine-derived antitoxin (2, 3).   A
human-derived product should have an effective toxin-neutralizing half-life that is considerably longer, 21-28 days, than
that experienced with the use of heterologous products of
equine origin, 5-7 days (4, 5).   A longer half-life would be
particularly advantageous in cases of toxico-infection, where
both toxin-producing organisms and preformed toxin have been
ingested, and the ingested organisms continue to produce toxin
in the gut (6).

In infant botulism patients, in which the bowel is colonized by toxin-producing Clostridium botulinum, neurotoxin is
often present for many weeks in the gut (7).   These infants
may benefit from both a very low rate of adverse reactions and
from the extended period of neutralizing activity expected
from homologous immune globulin.   If the provision of an extended period of toxin-neutralizing activity is indeed a concern, then less homologous immune globulin, having toxin-neutralizing activity equivalent to or even considerably less
than a heterologous antitoxin, could be administered initially
to obtain and maintain the desired prolonged period of protection.

Treatment of wound botulism patients with homologous immune globulin, rather than with heterologous antitoxins,
should provide similar benefits, particularly if the infecting
organism were to be resistant to the more commonly used antibiotics, i.e., penicillin, and a slow and prolonged release of
toxin is anticipated.

In each of these instances, the ingestion of preformed
toxin, toxico-infection and infant and wound botulism, the
prolonged maintenance of substantial circulating levels of the

administered homologous immune globulin should preclude the necessity for subsequent antibody treatment.

It is generally accepted that with botulism, a short incubation period is usually indicative of exposure to a larger quantity of toxin, followed by a rapid progression of signs and symptoms; these events herald the onset of a severe and often fatal disease. Because of physician and/or patient unwillingness to risk inducing an unwarranted adverse reaction to heterologous proteins, equine-derived antitoxin is most often withheld until definitive signs or symptoms of botulism are evident. In instances where the exposure has been clearly defined prior to the development of clinical signs, this apprehension to the administration of equine-derived antitoxin would be negated if homologous material were available. Thus, in many instances, the severity of potential illness could be reduced and the development of both signs and symptoms possibly mediated by the prophylactic use of homologous immune globulin. The risky "wait and see" period would be eliminated and early prophylaxis could begin as soon as homologous immune globulin had been obtained.

A program for the production and collection of botulism immune plasma (human) has been in effect for the past 3 years, utilizing over 80 human volunteers (9). Each individual had previously received 7-11 immunizations with a pentavalent (ABCDE) botulinum toxoid, but none had received the toxoid for 7-8 years prior to a first reimmunization booster. After boosting, volunteers entered a plasmapheresis program in which each donated plasma twice weekly for 15 consecutive weeks. Many of the initial donors were again boosted and plasmaphe-resed one year after the reimmunization. Over 2,000 liters of botulism immune plasma (human) were collected and stored as single, donor units of fresh, frozen plasma. The anamnestic responses, as measured by serum neutralizing titers, induced by the first booster reimmunization of the first group of 24 donors are presented in Table II.

A 52-liter lot of this human plasma was processed by the Michigan Department of Public Health in accordance with Cohn method #6 and #9 procedures, to produce an experimental pilot lot of intravenous quality immune globulin. This product was designated Botulism Immune Globulin (Human), lot #1. The neutralizing titers for toxin types A, B and E of this product and of the plasma pool from which it was derived are presented in Table III.

The less than desirable activity of the immune globulin (only about 10 international units/ml) to type B is indicative of the low type B titer in the original plasma pool. Titers to all three toxins are much less than are available in commercial equine antitoxins.

TABLE II. Group Response of 24 Donors to a Booster Reimmunization with Pentavalent Botulinum Toxoid[a]

Toxin type tested against	Geometric mean titer[b]		P
	Before	After	
A	0.82	8.98	< 0.001
B	0.06	0.52	< 0.001
E	0.16	2.30	< 0.001

[a] Pentavalent (ABCDE) botulinum toxoid, IND-161.

[b] Titer expressed as international units/ml serum. (Adapted from ref. 4).

TABLE III. Toxin Neutralizing Titers of an Experimental Pool
of Botulism Immune Plasma (Human) and the Corresponding Experimental Lot of Botulism Immune Globulin (Human)

Toxin type tested against	Neutralizing titer (IU/ml)		Concentration increased titer/ml (X)
	Plasma pool	Immune globulin	
A	11.5	> 250	22
B	0.5	> 10	20
E	3.2	> 80	25

Although the stable production of large and standard quantities of homologous immune globulin for the prophylaxis and
treatment of botulism is highly desirable, the difficulties in
recruiting, repeatedly immunizing, plasmapheresing and obtaining large pools of high-titer plasma from varied populations
of volunteers over prolonged periods of time may render such a
goal unattainable. Indeed, once this unique supply of human
donors is exhausted, other less time-consuming, less expensive
and less invasive means of producing high quality and safe
antitoxin must be developed. In an earlier effort to prevent
second-dose reactions and to conserve available homologous
antitoxin, Habermann and Bernáth proposed the use of human-
derived antitoxin only after the use of equine antitoxin (10).
    A second approach to therapy of botulism and the avoidance
of adverse reactions induced by heterologous antitoxins has
been proposed (11). The production of botulinal antitoxins of

bovine origin warrants consideration, in that treatment of
patients with bovine-derived botulinal antitoxin, sequential
to the use of equine-derived material, could afford a lesser
degree of reactogenicity in patients not sensitized to bovine
serum proteins. The use of a bovine antitoxin initially would
prevent adverse reactions to equine proteins and avoid possible sensitization of a patient to them. By utilizing a variety of large domestic animals, large quantities of standard-
ized antitoxin could be produced continually. Modern chromatographic techniques are available for the purification and
production of high quality monomeric heterologous immune globulins. One such technique involves the chromatography of
silicone dioxide-treated equine plasma on QAE-Sephadex for the
purification of large quantitites of antilymphocyte globulin
(12). The resulting product is a monomeric IgG, low in anti-
complementary activity, free of both plasmin and prekallikrein
activator activity and with an incidence of adverse reactions
of less than 5%.

A third approach would be to use hybridoma techniques to
select and produce a homologous monoclonal antibody specific
fo: each immunologically distinct botulinal toxin. More
id :alistically, a single monoclonal antibody specific for at-
ta :hment or toxic site antigens, possibly common to all the
botulinal neurotoxins, would be highly desirable. Once the
desired clone(s) is isolated, the costs and risks of antibody
production should be considerably less than those incurred
from more conventional methods.

If and when such antibodies are developed, it should provide the clinician and researcher with a variety of distinct
advantages, not the least of which would be an inexhaustible
supply of highly purified and specific monomeric antibody
having a negligible risk of reactogenicity and, hopefully, a
long metabolic half-life. For prophylactic and therapeutic
use, antibodies derived from human, rather than mouse or rat,
lymphocytes would be highly desirable. To date, there have
been no reports of stable hybridomas totally of human origin.
In the future, human hybridomas may become the main source of
antibody specific for therapeutic use and could be selected to
react with any of the botulinal toxins.

A fifth approach would involve the identification of
cross-reacting materials and their use as competitors for presynaptic attachment sites. This approach of competitive
blocking of receptor sites on target cells has received considerable attention with diphtheria toxin (13, 14). The development of nontoxic botulinal neurotoxins would offer yet another approach to prophylaxis and treatment of botulism. Botulinal neurotoxins, chemically or enzymatically altered so as
to be nontoxic, but still possessing intact attachment sites,
theoretically could compete with circulating neurotoxin for

attachment sites on presynaptic nerve terminal membranes (15). The usefulness of such an approach remains to be explored, since, after administration of these altered proteins, the patient would still be left with the problem of disposing of larger quantities of the toxic forms of circulating botulinal neurotoxin. The subsequent use of antitoxin would seem necessary to complement this form of therapy.

Lastly, the implementation of combined therapeutic approaches is most attractive and has already been practiced with very limited success in four patients poisoned with type E botulinal toxin (16). Both intra- and extravascular tissues may be sujected to antitoxin sufficient in quantity to neutralize all free and unbound toxin, thus preventing progression of paralysis resulting from the binding of additional toxin. However, the administration of antitoxin cannot be expected to reverse the toxin-induced paralysis, nor can it be expected to neutralize toxin internalized within nerve terminals (17). By the time signs and symptoms of botulism appear, toxin has reached synaptic areas and caused an irreversible blockade of transmitter release. For this reason, numerous chemotherapeutic approaches have been sought to antagonize or reverse existing botulinal toxin-induced paralysis (16-19).

A somewhat ideal, practical approach would be to combine the use of homologous immune globulin for the purpose of binding all immediately available unbound toxin and any toxin that may be released from the gut, or recycled at the cellular level during the course of disease, with the use of antagonistic chemotherapy capable of overcoming the neurotoxin-induced blockade of evoked acetylcholine release (6-8, 16).

Used in this manner specific immune globulin would bind to free toxin and thus prevent the attachment and uptake of additional toxin. The damaged nerve terminal, in conjunction with the administered antagonistic drug, would have to deal only with overcoming the paralytic effects of bound and internalized toxin. The addition of an antagonistic compound such as 4-aminopyridine (4-AP), or preferably 3,4-diaminopyridine (3,4-DAP), would facilitate an influx of additional Ca^{++} into the damaged nerve terminal and in turn allow for evoked release of acetycholine (8, 20-22). This would occur within an environment void of free toxin available for attachment and uptake, and thus negate the induction of additional paralysis.

The clinician and patient could deal exclusively with supportive measures and the rejuvenation of damaged nerve terminals. Possibly, the patient could be titrated with 3,4-DAP without concern for coping with additional toxin-induced damage to already debilitated nerves and without risking damage to previously nonpoisoned nerve terminals.

Evaluation and management of a patient in whom aminopyridine alone is used would be difficult, because of the uncertainty that an unsatisfactory response was due to the binding and uptake of additional free toxin, rather than a failure on the part of the drug to antagonize the paralysis existing at the time of drug administration.

Drugs, such as selected aminopyridines, could be useful in a number of advanced clinical situations. The actual prevention of the development of clinical signs and symptoms of botulism may even be possible. In rapidly developing emergencies, such drugs in the proper dosages could be used as a "quick fix," allowing for improved respiration, mobility and possible stabilization of the patient until he or she can be placed in a respirator or can acquire appropriate medical assistance.

A single dose of 4-AP is known to antagonize for a transient period of time the neuromuscular paralysis produced in rats by type A botulinum toxin (21). Experimentally, 3,4-DAP has been shown to be effective in prolonging survival of mice poisoned with a lethal dose of type A botulinum toxin (23). Table IV presents data from a study in which mice were poisoned with type A botulinal toxin. At 16 hours after poisoning, when 15 of the poisoned mice had died of respiratory paralysis, the remaining partially paralyzed and dying mice were treated intraperitoneally with 3,4-DAP at a dose of 1 or 4 mg/kg body weight. Treatment improved muscle tone, restored mobility, and induced alertness for periods lasting 2-3 hours. A series of retreatments at 3-hour intervals relieved paralysis to a lesser degree with each usage. This compound is also effective, when administered intravenously (i.v.) at 1 mg/kg body weight, for temporarily restoring muscle tone,

TABLE IV. *Effectiveness of 3,4-DAP in Prolonging Survival of Mice Poisoned with Type A Botulinal Toxin*

Number of mice			3,4-DAP (mg/kg)
Poisoned	Treated[a]	Surviving 48 hr (%)	
20	14	8 (57)	4
20	15	4 (27)	1
20	16	2 (12)	Placebo[b]
10	0	0 (0)	None

[a]15 poisoned mice died before treatment was begun at 16 hours after poisoning. Mice were treated every 3 hours for 48 hours.

[b]Phosphate buffered saline.

respiration and stimulating mobility in moribund cynomolgus
monkeys poisoned i.v. with type A toxin (unpublished data).
Another possible approach would be the use of certain
aminopyridines at low but continuous dosage to wean a paralyzed patient from respiratory support and thus reduce the
risk of nosocomial infection and substantially shorten the
duration of costly intensive care.

Unfortunately, many basic questions must be investigated
as to the efficacy of using any of the aminopyridines to sup-
plement the conventional treatment of botulism. Numerous
side-effects accompany the use of 4-AP. At low dosages (less
than 1 mg/kg), anxiety, insomnia, restlessness and perioral
paresthesia occur. These signs may be accompanied by a rise
in cystolic blood pressure and a decrease in cerebral blood
flow. At dosages of 1 mg/hr or greater, convulsive phenomena
may occur (16).

By definition, type-specific monovalent and polyvalent
botulinal antitoxin and immune globulin preparations unequivo-
cally neutralize any or all of the eight immunologically distinct botulinal neurotoxins employed to stimulate their production. However, both the basic neuromuscular and clinical
studies available attest to the effectiveness of 4-AP and 3,4-
DAP as antagonists of the paralysis induced by only two types,
A and E, of the eight neurotoxins. Unfortunately, the action
of only one of these, type A, has been thoroughly studied in
mammalian neuromuscular preparations by physiologists using
modern techniques.

Numerous approaches to the prophylaxis, immunotherapy and
chemotherapy of patients suffering from botulism are currently
under study; additional approaches will be explored in the
near future. All botulism patients, regardless of route of
poisoning or stage of illness, should incur a degree of benefit from the use of a homologous botulism immune globulin.
However, the necessity of using humans for the production of
such a product severely limits the quantity of high-titer product that can be produced. The implementation of a variety of
large domestic animals as factories for antitoxin production
may solve the problems of supply and quality, but may only
partially eliminate detrimental immune reactions in human recipients. The development and testing of competitive nontoxic
cross-reacting materials and chemically altered nontoxic botulinal toxins is certainly interesting and should be pursued.

Some of the most promising and potentially applicable
long-term approaches to prophylaxis, immunotherapy and chemotherapy of botulism may be: (a) production by modern methodo-
logy of new high-quality monomeric heterologous antitoxins
free of aggregates and fragments and inducing essentially no
adverse reactions in recipient patients, (b) the development
of a hybridoma of totally human origin capable of producing

therapeutic quantities of monoclonal antibody possessing specific neutralizing activity for all botulinal toxins, (c) the
development and evaluation of clinically safe compounds that
are antagonistic to botulinal toxin-induced paralysis, and (d)
the routine implementation of combined therapy utilizing both
monoclonal antibody and chemotherapeutic agents to neutralize
circulating unbound toxins and to reverse existing toxin-
induced paralysis.

ACKNOWLEDGMENTS

The outstanding technical assistance of Robert M. Wood is
gratefully acknowledged.

The volunteers were civilian United States Government
employees. These tests were governed by the principles, policies, and rules for medical volunteers as established by Army
Regulation 70-25 and the Declaration of Helsinki. The study
was conducted as part of a long-term program for the investigation of mechanisms of vaccine efficacy and host responses
to infectious diseases.

In conducting the research described in this report, the
investigator adhered to the "Guide for the Care and Use of
Laboratory Animals," as promulgated by the Committee on Care
and Use of Laboratory Animals of the Institute of Laboratory
Animal Resources, National Research Council. The facilities
are fully accredited by the American Association for Accreditation of Laboratory Animal Care.

The views of the author do not purport to reflect the
positions of Department of the Army or the Department of
Defense.

REFERENCES

1. Petty, C. S., in "Botulism" (K. Lewis and K. Cassell,
   Jr., eds.), p. 177. U.S. Government Printing Office,
   Washington (1964).
2. Merson, M. H., Hughes, J. M., Dowell, V. R., Taylor, A.,
   Barker, W. H., and Gangarosa, E. J., *J.A.M.A.* 229, 1305
   (1974).
3. Black, R. E., and Gunn, R. A., *Am. J. Med.* 69, 567 (1980).
4. Smolens, J., Vogt, A. B., Crawford, M. N., and Stokes,
   J., Jr., *J. Pediatr.* 59, 899 (1961).

5. Lewis, G. E., Jr., and Metzger, J. F., *in* "Natural Toxins" (D. Eaker and T. Wadström, eds.), p. 601. Pergamon Press, Oxford (1980).
6. Piven', I. N., Golosova, T. V., and Sidorova, A. V., *Probl. Gematol. Pereliv. Krovi 20(11)*, 46 (1975).
7. Arnon, S. S., *Annu. Rev. Med. 31*, 541 (1980).
8. Sellin, L. C., *Med. Biol.*, in press (1981).
9. Metzger, J. F., and Lewis, G. E., Jr., *Rev. Infect. Dis. 1*, 689 (1979).
10. Habermann, E., and Bernáth, S., *Med. Microbiol. Immunol. 161*, 203 (1975).
11. Sinel'nikov, G. Ye., Preger, S. M., and Muzafarova, N. Kh., *Zh. Mikrobiol. Epidemiol. Immunobiol. 55(1)*, 123 (1978).
12. Condie, R. M., *in* "Immunoglobulins: Characteristics and Uses of Intravenous Preparations" (B. M. Alving and J. S. Finlayson, eds.), DHHS Publicaton No. (FDA)-80-9005, p. 179. U.S. Government Printing Office, Washington (1979).
13. Ittelson, T. R., and Gill, D. M., *Nature 242*, 330 (1973).
14. Zanen, J., Muyldermans, G., and Beugnier, N., *FEBS Lett. 66*, 261 (1976).
15. DasGupta, B. R., and Sugiyama, H., *Biochem. Biophys. Res. Commun. 93*, 369 (1980).
16. Ball, A. P., Hopkinson, R. B., Farrell, I. D., Hutchinson, J. G. P., Paul, R., Watson, R. D. S., Page, A. J. F., Parker, R. G. F., Edwards, C. W., Snow, M., Scott, D. K., Leone-Ganado, A., Hastings, A., Ghosh, A. C., and Gilbert, R. J., *Q. J. Med. 48*, 473 (1979).
17. Simpson, L. L., *J. Pharmacol. Exp. Therap. 212*, 16 (1980).
18. Puggliari, M., and Cherington, M., *J.A.M.A. 240*, 2276 (1978).
19. Messina, C., Dattola, R., and Girlanda, P., *Acta Neurol. (Napoli) 34*, 459 (1979).
20. Lundh, H., and Thesleff, S., *Eur. J. Pharmacol. 42*, 411 (1977).
21. Lundh, H., Leander, S., and Thesleff, S., *J. Neurobiol. Sci. 32*, 29 (1977).
22. Durant, N. N., and Marshall, I. G., *J. Physiol. (London) 280*, 21p (1978).
23. Lewis, G. E., Jr., Metzger, J. F., and Wood, R. M., *in* Abstracts, 20th Interscience Conference on Antimicrobial Agents and Chemotherapy, 22-24 September, abstract 449. New Orleans, La. (1980).

Epidemiologic Characteristics of Botulism in the
United States, 1950-1979

Roger A. Feldman
J. Glenn Morris, Jr.
Robert A. Pollard

Bacterial Diseases Division
Center for Infectious Diseases
Centers for Disease Control
Atlanta, Georgia

INTRODUCTION

This 30-year review of epidemiologic information about
botulism, a relatively uncommon illness, is possible only
because the distinctive clinical picture, the limited availability of antitoxin therapy, and the possible association
with commercial products has resulted in the reporting of
probable cases of botulism to local, state and federal author-
ities in the United States. Using this information, it has
been possible to confirm some earlier observations (1) and,
in addition, to indicate areas for future study of the epidemiology of botulism.

MATERIALS AND METHODS

In this review, we have divided information about botulism outbreaks and cases into 4 categories: foodborne, vehicle undetermined, wound, and infant botulism. The foodborne
category includes those outbreaks with which a vehicle was
epidemiologically associated. In the category "vehicle undetermined," investigation during the outbreak did not identify
a specific vehicle. Wound botulism cases are those in which
an antecedent wound was associated with clinical botulism,

ISBN 0-12-447180-3

and cases of infant botulism are those in which neurological
signs and symptoms characteristic of botulism were found in
an infant in association with the identification of toxin
and/or organisms from stool specimens.

Data concerning clinical cases, outbreaks, ages, deaths,
and laboratory confirmation were collected from 3 primary
sources. The line listings of K. F. Meyer (2) were a major
source of data for the 1950s. Limited information was available concerning ages of patients in the decade 1950-59. Laboratory data for the decade 1950-1959 were predominantly from
state health departments. In the later decades, more information was available from reporting to the Centers for Disease
Control (CDC), unpublished information from state health departments, and published case reports. Much of the laboratory data in the decade 1970-1979 came from state health departments and was confirmed at CDC or was developed by CDC
laboratories. If health departments reported a case of botulism, even without laboratory confirmation, these reports are
included in the final tabulations. Cases were assigned to the
state in which the exposure to the vehicle occurred.

A. *Foodborne Botulism*

In the period 1950-1979, 215 outbreaks (566 cases) of
foodborne botulism were reported to the CDC (foodborne outbreaks). Ninety-four outbreaks (275 cases) were reported in
the period 1970-1979, an increase over the 56 outbreaks (147
cases) reported during the 1960s and the 65 outbreaks (144
cases) reported in the period 1950-1959. There was an average
of 2.6 cases per outbreak (range, 1-57 cases); 45% of outbreaks involved only 1 case. There was no significant change
in the number of cases per outbreak over the 30-year period.

Toxin types were known in 161 (75%) of the outbreaks; 87
(54%) were due to *Clostridium botulinum* type A, 41 (25%) to
type B, 32 (20%) to type E, and 1 to type F (Table 1). Foodborne outbreaks were reported from 37 of the 50 states, with
cases occurring most frequently in states along the Pacific
coast and in the Northwest (Figure 1). In keeping with the
observed geographic distribution of botulinal spores (3), 85%
of the type A outbreaks occurred in states west of the Mississippi; and 63% of the type B outbreaks occurred east of the
Mississippi; 54% of the type E outbreaks occurred in Alaska.
Fifty percent of type A and B outbreaks occurred in the last
four months of the year; 77% of type E outbreaks occurred
from May to October.

Home-canned or home-processed foods accounted for 92% of
the foodborne outbreaks. The most commonly implicated single

TABLE 1. *Percent Distribution of Botulism by Toxin type[a] within Epidemiologic Category, United States, 1950-79*

Epidemiologic category	Number[a]	Percent distribution by toxin type			
		A	B	E	F
Foodborne	161	54	25	20	1
Undetermined Vehicle	42	71	26	2	0
Wound	12	67	33	0	0
Infant	121	54	45	0	1

[a]Excludes outbreaks with unknown toxin type: 54 for foodborne; 77 for undetermined vehicle; 7 for wound; and 1 for infant.

vehicles were beets and green beans, which were responsible for 8.4% and 7.9% of the outbreaks, respectively; fish of all types accounted for 16% of the outbreaks. Sixty-four percent of the outbreaks in which fish was implicated involved *C. botulinum* type E, with 9% due to type B and 27% due to type A (Table 2); there was a significant association between type E botulism and fish-related outbreaks (p <.0001, Fisher's exact test, two-tailed). Outbreaks involving green beans were significantly more likely to occur in the southeastern states (p=.029, Fisher's exact test, two-tailed) and to involve *C. botulinum* type B (p=.032). It was not possible to show a significant association between other vehicles and toxin type, geographic region, or time period.

The median age of patients with foodborne botulism was 37 years. The highest attack rate was in the 30-39 year-old age group; the lowest was in children under the age of ten (Table 3). Males and females were equally represented (49.3% and 50.7% of patients, respectively). Patients with type B botulism had a median age of 30 years, which was significantly less than the median age of 39 years in type A patients (p=.002, Mann-Whitney U test) or the median age of 40 years in type E patients (p=.0008, Mann-Whitney U test).

One hundred forty-two (25%) of the 566 foodborne botulism patients died of their disease. The case-fatality rate showed a steady decline over the 3 decades, from 47% in 1950-1959 to 28% in 1960-1969 and 12% in 1970-1979 (chi-square due to linear trend=59.39). The median age of patients who died was 45 years; patients who survived had a significantly lower median age of 35 years (p=.001, Mann-Whitney U test). With the exception of the 0-9 year age group, the age-specific case-fatality rate shows a steady increase with age

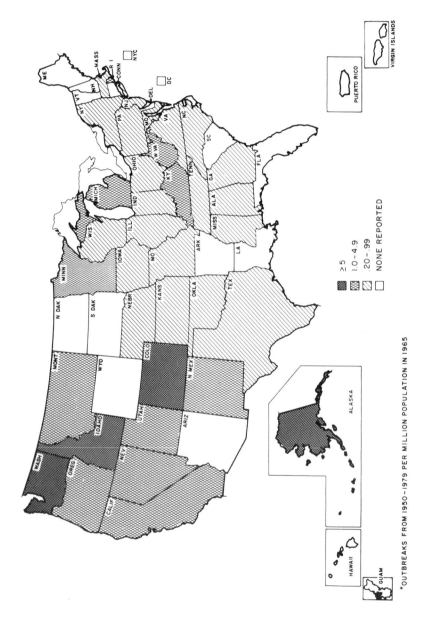

*OUTBREAKS FROM 1950–1979 PER MILLION POPULATION IN 1965

≥ 5

1.0 – 4.9

.20 – .99

NONE REPORTED

FIGURE 1. Foodborne botulism rates*, by state, United States, 1950–1979.

TABLE 2. *Food Products Associated with Botulism Outbreaks, 1950–1979*

Toxin type	Vegetables	Fish and Fish products	Fruits	Condiments[a]	Beef	Pork	Poultry	Other	Total
A	38	9	2	19	2	0	1	16	87
B	22	2	2	7	0	1	1	6	41
E	0	21	0	0	0	0	0	11	32
F	0	0	0	0	0	0	0	1	1
Unknown	35	3	4	5	1	1	0	5	54
Total	95	35	8	31	3	2	2	39	215

[a]Includes outbreaks associated with tomato relish, chili peppers, chili sauce, and salad dressing.

TABLE 3. Age-specific Attack Rates[a], Cases of Foodborne
Botulism and Cases of Undetermined Vehicle, 1950-1979

| | | Undetermined |
Age	Foodborne	vehicle
0-9	0.22	0.10
10-19	0.71	0.19
20-29	1.31	0.30
30-39	1.71	0.49
40-49	1.24	0.53
50-59	1.06	0.73
60-69	1.27	0.52
>70	0.89	0.50
All ages	0.97	0.36

[a]Per 10 million population per year (based on 1965 estimated
population); age distribution of patients of unknown age assumed to be similar to those of known age.

(chi-square due to linear trend=17.61). Of patients with
type B disease, 8.8% died; this was significantly less than
the 24.3% of type A patients who died (p=.0003, Fisher's
exact test, two-tailed) and the 30.6% of type E patients who
died (p <.0001, Fisher's exact test, two-tailed). At a 99%
confidence level, toxin type rather than age was the variable
associated with an increased risk of death (multiple linear
logistic regression).

B. Botulism - Undetermined Vehicle

One hundred nineteen outbreaks (210 cases) of botulism
for which no vehicle could be identified (vehicle undetermined) were reported to CDC. The percentage of total botulism outbreaks in adults that were classified as vehicle undetermined remained fairly constant during the 30-year period, changing from 40% in 1950-1959 to 35% of the total in
1970-1979. There was an average of 1.8 cases in each outbreak (range, 1-7 cases), which was significantly fewer than
the number of cases in foodborne outbreaks (p <.0001, Mann-
Whitney U test). There was no significant change in the number of cases per outbreak over the 30-year period.

A toxin type was identified in only 35% of outbreaks;
during the first 2 decades of the 30-year period, there was a
clear association between an inability to identify a vehicle
in an outbreak and an inability to determine the toxin type

(p <.0001, Fisher's exact test, two-tailed). Of the 42 outbreaks in which a toxin type was identified (Table 1), 30
(71%) were due to *C. botulinum* type A, and 11 (26%) were due
to type B; only 1 outbreak was due to type E, which represents
a significant decrease from the percentage of foodborne outbreaks attributed to type E (p=.004, Fisher's exact test, two-
tailed). Cases were reported from 37 states (Figure 2); 77%
of the type A outbreaks occurred in states west of the Mississippi, and 91% of the type B outbreaks occurred in states
east of the Mississippi.

The median age of patients in outbreaks of undetermined
vehicles was 43.5 years, which was significantly greater than
the median among patients in foodborne outbreaks (p=.029,
Mann-Whitney U test). The highest attack rate was in the 50-
59 year-old age group (Table 1). There was no significant
difference in ages by toxin type.

Fifty (24%) of the patients died. The case-fatality rate
showed a slight decline during the 30-year period, dropping
from 29% in 1950-1959 to 20% in 1970-1979. Of patients with
type A disease, 21.6% died, compared with 23.1% of patients
with type B disease. The median age of individuals who died
was 43 years, compared with a median age of 44.5 years for
survivors. The highest case-fatality rate was in individuals
aged 0-9 years (50%), with the next highest rate in persons
>70 years; there was no clear increase in the rate with age,
in contrast to that in patients in foodborne outbreaks.

C. Wound Botulism

Between 1950 and 1979, 19 cases were reported to CDC.
Seventeen (89%) of the 19 cases were reported in the 1970s.
The toxin type was known in 12 cases. Eight cases were due to
C. botulinum type A, and 3 to type B; in 1 case, type A toxin
was found in serum, while type B organisms were cultured from
the wound. Six cases were reported from California, 3 from
Washington, and 2 cases each from Idaho, Nebraska, and Texas;
single case reports came from Maryland, New Jersey, Pennsyl-
vania, and West Virginia. The highest rates were in the West
(Figure 3).

The median age of wound botulism patients was 24 years,
significantly less than the median age for other adult botulism patients (p=.0004, Mann-Whitney U test). Sixteen (84%)
of the 19 were male, a significant change from other adult
botulism patients (p=.009, Fisher's exact test, two-tailed).
Two wound botulism patients died; both had cases of *C.
botulinum* type A.

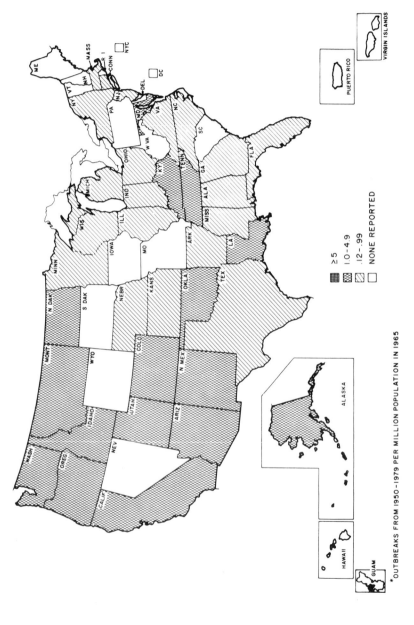

* OUTBREAKS FROM 1950-1979 PER MILLION POPULATION IN 1965

FIGURE 2. Vehicle-of-undetermined origin botulism rates*, by state, United States, 1950-1979.

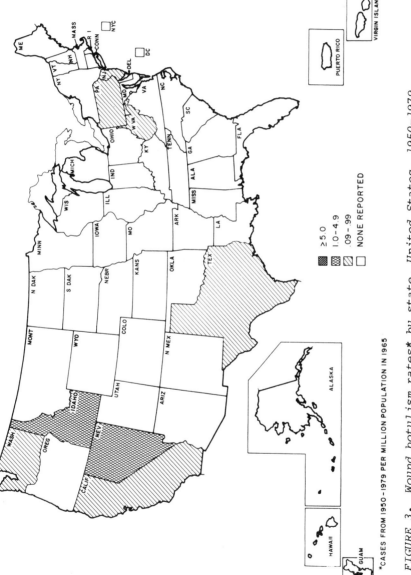

*CASES FROM 1950-1979 PER MILLION POPULATION IN 1965

≥ 5.0
1.0 – 4.9
.09 – 99
NONE REPORTED

FIGURE 3. Wound botulism rates* by state, United States, 1950-1979.

D. *Infant Botulism*

One hundred twenty-one cases of infant botulism were reported to CDC from 1975 through the end of 1979 (Figure 4).
Cases were reported most frequently from California (58 of
121 cases), although the case rate per 100,000 live births was
highest in Utah (10.3 cases/100,000 live births, 1976-1979)
(Figure 5). The number of cases was somewhat greater in the
fall, with 62% of cases occurring in the last 6 months of the
year; excluding 1975 and 1976, 58% of cases occurred in the
last 6 months of the year.

Sixty-five (54%) of cases involved *C. botulinum* type A; 55
(45%) involved type B (Table 1); and one case was due to *C.
botulinum* type F. Type B cases occurred more frequently in
infants than in adults (p=.009, Fisher's exact test, two-tailed). As in adult cases, the geographic distribution of cases
by toxin type correlated roughly with the distribution of botulinal spores in the environment (3), with 66% of cases west
of the Mississippi caused by *C. botulinum* type A and 88% of
cases east of the Mississippi by type B.

Cases occurred most frequently in infants in the second
month of life (Figure 6); 97.5% of cases were in infants under
6 months of age. Infants with type B botulism tended to be
younger than those with type A, although the difference was
not statistically significant (p=.08, Mann-Whitney U test).
Three deaths were reported in association with infant botulism
cases. All three deaths involved type A patients; these infants were 4, 8, and 16 weeks of age.

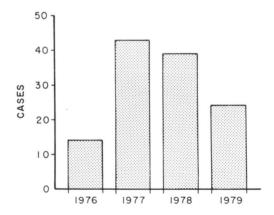

*Figure 4. Number of cases of infant botulism reported to
CDC, United States, 1976-1979.*

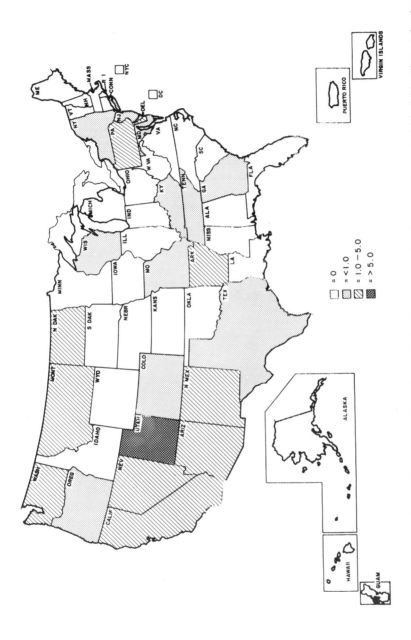

FIGURE 5. Number of cases of infant botulism reported to CDC, per 100,000 live births, by state, 1976 – 1979.

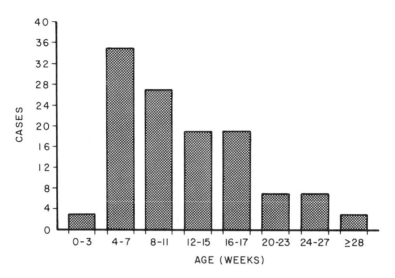

Figure 6. Age distribution of infant botulism cases reported to CDC, United States, 1976-1979.

DISCUSSION

 The data used in this 30-year review, especially those for the first decade, often lacked information concerning ages, deaths, vehicles, and toxin types. Diagnostic competence has increased significantly during this 30-year period, especially following use of identification of toxin in stool specimens as a method of laboratory confirmation (4). In addition, during the last 15 years, reports of requests for antitoxin were used to learn about possible cases, which probably increased the percentage of minor cases reported. In spite of variations in completeness of reporting during this 30-year period, observations concerning foodborne botulism, including age-specific case-fatality ratios and distribution of toxin types, do not appear related to variations in data collection. Insufficient data were available concerning the vehicle-undetermined outbreaks in the first two decades to allow meaningful comparisons with all the data for foodborne outbreaks.

 For the foodborne botulism cases, the case-fatality ratios for the type B cases were lower than those for cases due to type A or type E. This difference may relate to a quantitative difference in the ingested dose of toxin or gastrointestinal absorption of toxin received by persons in type B as compared with type A or E outbreaks. Insufficient data are now available to study these possibilities. The difference may also relate to different characteristics of the toxins

themselves, such as binding at the nerve endings (5).
Although the median age of patients with Type B botulism is
less than that of patients with type A or E botulism, the
differences in case-fatality ratios for the different toxin
types do not appear related to age.

The description of infant botulism has increased interest
in the possibility that some cases in adults in the category
vehicle undetermined may have a pathogenesis similar to that
described for infant botulism (6). The reason vehicle-undetermined patients had a higher median age and were smaller in
number may relate to difficulties in obtaining a food history
from older patients in single case outbreaks and be primarily
a surveillance artifact. The higher percentage of males in
the vehicle-undetermined category is difficult to explain.
The fact that there was little change in the case-fatality
ratio in the 3 decades may result from the fact that the vehicle-undetermined outbreaks were generally less well investigated, either in the laboratory or clinically, were diagnosed later (7), and treated less optimally than the foodborne outbreaks. However, the possibility remains that some
of these cases resulted from absorption of toxin produced in
the intestinal tract.

The wound botulism cases occurred with greatest frequency
in the young male age group, a distribution similar to that
found for tetanus in adults before the use of toxoid (8). It
remains uncertain whether a wound botulism illness occurs that
is similar to neonatal tetanus. Since the illness could be
characterized almost only by respiratory paralysis, it could
easily be missed.

Major occurrences in the decade of the 1970s are the description of infant botulism and the associated attempts to
explain the limited age distribtuion, geographic distribution, and possible risk factors (9). From 1975-79, infant
botulism due to type B had its peak age of onset at an earlier age than that of cases due to type A, and a higher percentage of the total cases were due to type B than would be expected from the percentage of type B foodborne cases. Both
these observations are still unexplained. However, if most
infant botulism cases resulted from an exposure to spores, the
same findings would be seen if an additional group of cases
resulted from ingestion of group B spore-contaminated vehicles.

The annual number of cases of botulism in the United
States and the annual number of outbreaks have not declined
over this 3-decade period, suggesting that preventive measures have not been remarkably successful. Since 90% of the
cases are associated with home-canned or home-processed products, efforts on a federal level to control the problem are

best focused on education about home-canning and continued vigilance in the investigation of outbreaks associated with commercial products.

ACKNOWLEDGMENT

Data concerning botulism outbreaks have been received at the Centers for Disease Control from physicians and state epidemiologists from throughout the United States, and much additional information has been obtained from published sources. These data have been tabulated at frequent intervals, and an updated manual has been published by CDC that includes line lists of much of these data. We are indebted to the individuals who developed the original information, to those who maintained these line lists for the summarization of data, and to Katherine Greene, who assisted in updating the data for this summary.

REFERENCES

1. Gangarosa, E. J., Donadio, J. A., Armstrong, R. W., Meyer, K. F., Brachman, P. S., Dowell, V. R., *Am. J. Epidemiol.* *93*, 93 (1971).
2. Meyer, K.F., Eddie, B., "Sixty-five Years of Human Botulism in the United States and Canada." George Williams Hooper Foundation, University of California, San Francisco (1965).
3. Smith, L. DS., *Hosp. Lab. Sci. 15*, 74 (1978).
4. Dowell, V. R., McCroskey, L. M., Hatheway, C. L., Lombard, G. L., Hughes, J. M., Merson, M. H., *JAMA 238*, 1829 (1977).
5. Smith, L. DS., *Rev. Infect. Dis. 1*, 637 (1979).
6. Merson, M. H., Hughes, J. M., Dowell, V. R., Taylor, A., Barker, W. H., Gangarosa, E. J., *JAMA 229*, 1305 (1974).
7. Morris, J. G., Hatheway, C. L., *J. Infect. Dis. 142*, 302 (1980).
8. Fraser, D. W., *Am. J. Epidemiol. 96*, 306 (1972).
9. Arnon, S. S., *Ann. Rev. Med. 31*, 541 (1980).

BOTULISM IN ALASKA, 1947-1980

William L. Heyward
Thomas R. Bender

Alaska Investigations Division
Center for Infectious Diseases
Centers for Disease Control
Anchorage, Alaska

INTRODUCTION

The journals of early Arctic explorers contain numerous
accounts of foodborne outbreaks of fatal illness among Eskimo
families (1). However, it has only been in the last 30 years
that clinical and laboratory methods have been available to
confirm that some of these were outbreaks of botulism. In
this paper we summarize the epidemiologic and clinical findings of Arctic botulism in Alaska, a now well-recognized
"hazard of the North" (1).

MATERIALS AND METHODS

The records for all outbreaks of botulism from 1947
through 1980 reported by the Alaska Department of Health and
Social Services, the Alaska Area Native Health Service, Indian
Health Service, and the Alaska Investigations Division, Centers for Disease Control, were reviewed. Complete clinical
and laboratory information on patients in some of the early
outbreaks was not available. However, since the food source,
type of illness, and outcome were very suggestive of botulism,
these patients were included in the review.
Illness suggestive of botulism included persons with at
least three of the following signs or symptoms: nausea/vomit-
ing, dysphagia, diplopia, dilated fixed pupils, dry throat,
respiratory insufficiency, ptosis, constipation, diarrhea, and

BIOMEDICAL ASPECTS OF BOTULISM

285

ISBN 0-12-447180-3

urinary retention. Persons with these symptoms, in the presence of fever, altered mental status or asymmetric neurological deficits, were felt to have illness other than botulism.
Confirmed botulism was defined as a clinical illness compatible with botulism and Clostridium botulinum isolated in
culture or botulinal toxin identified in food, serum, or stool
specimens. Suspected botulism was defined as clinical illness
compatible with botulism, but without laboratory confirmation.
Laboratory tests were performed by the Bureau of Laboratories, Centers for Disease Control, Atlanta, Georgia, and the
Arctic Health Research Center, Fairbanks, Alaska.

RESULTS

Since 1947, 42 outbreaks of suspected or confirmed botulism have been investigated in Alaksa. Of 220 persons who had
eaten food suspected of being contaminated with botulinal
toxin, 81 had illness suggestive of botulism and 18 died (22%
case-fatality rate). No outbreaks occurred in the period
1961-1967. For the period 1947-1961, the case-fatality rate
was 46% (11 of 24 persons died). Since 1967, even though the
annual number of outbreaks of botulism has risen, the case-
fatality rate has been reduced to 12% (7 of 57 persons died)
(Fig. 1).

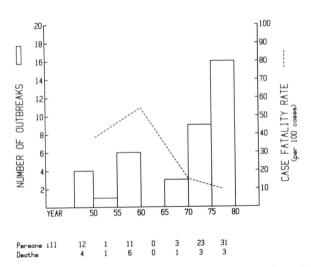

FIGURE 1.   Outbreaks of Botulism and Associated Case-
            fatality Rate in Alaska, 1947-1980.

All outbreaks have occurred among Eskimos, Indians, or Aleuts who lived in villages on the coast or along rivers near the sea. Botulism was diagnosed in patients of all age groups except children less than 5 years of age (range: 6 to 73 years), and was evenly distributed among males and females.

All outbreaks were associated with eating uncooked, dried, or fermented traditional Eskimo or Indian foods (Table I). Whale meat or muktuk (whale skin and blubber) were the most commonly incriminated foods and accounted for eight deaths. Of the foods involved, 60% had been prepared by fermentation (putrefaction), and 78% had been stored in airtight containers such as plastic bags, sealed jars, and barrels or had been covered with seal or whale oil. Plastic bags, which apparently provide a relatively anaerobic environment, have been closely associated with botulism caused by Alaskan Native foods in recent years (2). Five outbreaks have been associated with eating fermented salmon heads and eggs, whitefish, dried herring, and beaver tail that had been stored in plastic bags.

Botulism was confirmed by laboratory methods in 30 (71%) of the investigations. Botulinal toxin was detected in specimens (serum, vomitus, or stool) from 37 patients and in the suspected food in 20 outbreaks. Type E botulinal toxin was found in 22 (73%) of the confirmed outbreaks and accounted for nine deaths. Other outbreaks involved type A-5, type B-1, type A and B-1, and type F-1. No significant difference was

TABLE I. *Native Foods Involved in Confirmed Botulism Outbreaks in Alaska, 1947-1980*

Food	No. of outbreaks	Percentage
Sea mammal		
Whale (meat or muktuk[a])	6	30.0
Seal (meat or muktuk)	3	15.0
Fish		
Whitefish	3	15.0
Salmon	1	5.0
Salmon eggs	5	25.0
Herring	1	5.0
Freshwater mammal		
Beaver tail	1	5.0
Total	20	100.0

[a] *Skin and blubber.*

found in the mortality or the implicated foods among the botulinal toxin types.

Histories of symptoms and clinical findings were available
for 51 of 56 persons with laboratory-confirmed botulism. Many
of these patients had a diagnostic pentad of nausea/vomiting,
dysphagia, diplopia, dilated pupils, and dry throat. Forty-
eight of the 51 (94%) persons had at least three of these five
signs and symptoms. Of the three other patients, two had
respiratory insufficiency severe enough to require mechanical
ventilation without preceding gastrointestinal or other neurologic illness. The signs or symptoms in patients with botulism did not differ by the etiologic toxin type.

DISCUSSION

Botulism is an uncommon but persistent public health problem among Alaskan Natives. Spores of C. botulinum are ubiqui-
tous in Alaska, having been found in beach soil and in the
gills and gut contents of fish and marine mammals (3-5). Because the spores are so widespread and because of the food
preparation and storage methods used by the Alaskan Natives,
outbreaks will almost certainly continue to occur.

Immunization of high-risk persons with botulinal toxoid is
under consideration, but at present two approaches to the
problem are being emphasized: 1) the elimination of C. botulinum spores and toxin from food and 2) public health education of health care providers and Alaskan Natives about botulism and how to recognize it early. The former approach is
difficult, since subsistence hunting and fishing and the practice of eating fermented foods are integral parts of the
Alaskan Native culture. The factors contributing to the formation of botulinal toxin in the Native foods include preparing foods where they can easily be contaminated with botulinal
spores, fermenting foods in an anaerobic environment, and
eating these foods uncooked. In such a setting, botulism
could most easily be prevented by total avoidance of Native
foods, but this approach has not been practical, since these
foods are often the only ones available to, or desired by,
the people. Public health education measures since 1967
emphasizing careful cleaning of fish and meat, the dangers of
eating uncooked fermented foods and the potential hazards of
using plastic bags to hold fermented foods have not caused a
decline in the number of botulism outbreaks among Alaskan
Natives.

Therefore, the major emphasis in previous control efforts
has been directed toward public health education of health
care providers and Alaskan Natives about botulism and how to

recognize its symptoms early. Education of health care providers in Alaska has emphasized a careful history, a high level of suspicion, and that the diagnostic pentad of nausea/ vomiting, dysphagia, diplopia, dilated pupils, and dry throat occurs with great frequency among botulism cases. Systems for botulism surveillance, combined with the widespread availability of botulinal antitoxin, prompt supportive medical care, and continued education efforts, have been shown to reduce the fatality rate associated with botulism in this population (6). The decline in the case-fatality rate in the presence of a rise in the annual number of botulism outbreaks reflects the improved recognition of botulism and prompt therapy for this disease that have resulted from these public health efforts.

REFERENCES

1. Dolman, C. E., *Arctic 13*, 230 (1960).
2. Eisenberg, M. S., and Bender, T. R., *Alaska Med. 18*, 47 (1976).
3. Miller, L. G., Clark, P. S., and Kunkle, G. A., *Appl. Microbiol. 23*, 427 (1972).
4. Miller, L. G., *Can. J. Microbiol. 21*, 920 (1975).
5. Houghtby, G. A., and Kaysner, C. A., *Appl. Microbiol. 18*, 950 (1969).
6. Eisenberg, M. S., and Bender, T. R., *JAMA 235*, 35 (1976).

CLINICAL AND EPIDEMIOLOGICAL ASPECTS
OF BOTULISM IN ARGENTINA

Alberto S. Ciccarelli[1]

Cátedra de Microbiología
Facultad de Ciencias Médicas
Universidad Nacional de Cuyo
Mendoza, Argentina

Domingo F. Giménez[2]

Laboratorio de Alimentos
Universidad Nacional de San Luis
San Luis, Argentina

I. INTRODUCTION

Although botulism in Argentina is quoted by 1911 (1), the
first documented outbreak was recorded in 1922 (2). In the
recorded epidemics up to 1950, its diagnosis was made only on
clinical grounds; neither bacteriological nor toxicological
studies for laboratory confirmation were done.

In 1957, in La Plata city, the capital of the Province of
Buenos Aires, an outbreak traced to commercially processed pi-
mientos affected 21 persons and caused 12 deaths. For the
first time, type A botulinal toxin was recognized in samples

[1]*Supported by Grants 7-C-978 Res 3462/79 and 1600/80 from
Consejo de Investigaciones de la Universidad Nacional de Cuyo
(CIUNC), Mendoza, Argentina.*
[2]*Supported by Grant 7901 from Universidad Nacional de San
Luis and Secretaría de Ciencia y Técnica (SECYT), Ministerio
de Cultura y Educación, Argentina.*

of the suspected food by neutralization test in mice and a
strain of Clostridium botulinum type A was isolated from the
feces of one of the patients (3). Thereafter, only the serologic type A of this bacterium has been found responsible for
all the outbreaks where the agent or its toxin were identified.

The specific toxic food could not be identified in all the
reported outbreaks, but in most cases the source of the poisoning was epidemiologically traced to the food that the group
of involved persons had shared either in the same meal or
separately.

In spite of the conspicuous tradition of most of the rural
population in orcharding areas or preparing home-canned vegetables, the generous prevalence of toxigenic C. botulinum in
soil and the diversity of serological types found in this
country, botulism is an uncommon disease in Argentina. Although the medical profession is aware of this poisoning, perhaps a failure in some step of the reporting process might
have impeded the knowledge of the real magnitude of this
health problem.

Botulism recognized in Argentina belongs to the classical
foodborne poisoning. No cases of wound botulism or infant
botulism have been recorded to the present.

II. EPIDEMIOLOGY

During the 1922-1980 period, 36 outbreaks affecting 163
persons with 89 deaths have been reported. Table I shows, by

TABLE I. Botulism Outbreaks in Argentina, 1922-1980

Years	Outbreaks	Cases	Cases per outbreak	Cases per year	Deaths	Case fatality ratio
1922-1929[a]	4	22	5.5	2.2	19	86.4%
1930-1939	4	18	4.5	1.8	17	94.4%
1940-1949	0	0	-	0	0	-
1950-1959	3	29	9.7	2.9	17	58.6%
1960-1969	5	13	2.6	1.3	6	46.2%
1970-1979	17	77	4.5	7.7	29	37.7%
1980[b]	3	4	1.3	4.0	1	25.0%
Total	36	163	4.5	2.8	89	54.6%

[a] 8-year period.

[b] 1-year period.

decades, the number of outbreaks, cases, deaths, cases per
year and case fatality ratios. During the decade 1940-1949,
no outbreak was recorded. Furthermore, this blank period
actually expands through 15 years from 1936-1949. During the
period 1970-1979 an increasing trend started in outbreak recordings. A sharp increment is noted in this decade with an
average number of 1.7 outbreaks per year. In 1980, 3 outbreaks were recorded.

During the decade 1950-1959, an average number of 9.7
cases per outbreak was recorded. This is the highest observed
value and comes from a period with only 3 outbreaks, including
one with 21 cases in 1957. A similar situation occurred in
1970-1979, with an average number of 4.5 cases per outbreak
that includes one outbreak with 24 cases in 1974.

The case fatality ratio has been steadily decreasing from
its highest value of 94.4% for the decade 1930-1939 to the
lowest one, 25.0% in 1980.

An outstanding epidemiological feature is that Argentinian
soils are largely contaminated with proved human pathogenic
types (A, B, F) and potentially human pathogenic types (G and
subtype Af) of toxigenic $\underline{C}$. $\underline{botulinum}$, but only the serologic
type A has been identified or isolated from foods and clinical
materials. Table II shows outbreaks, cases, deaths and case
fatality ratios by toxin type.

A. *Geographic Distribution*

Another noticeable epidemiological feature is that botulism outbreaks appear polarized in two areas: Mendoza province (Mz) with 1,187,305 inhabitants and Buenos Aires province
(BA, including Buenos Aires City, the capital of the country,
with a total population of 13,704,037 inhabitants (Fig. 1).
Both areas are located between 32 and 40° south latitude.
This polarization has no adequate explanation. Nevertheless,
it is necessary to remark that the Province of Mendoza is the
most important producer of commercially processed vegetables
in Argentina. Also, its population has the inveterate habit
of preparing home-canned vegetables. Perhaps these facts --
high production, cheap prices during the season and a solid
tradition for preparing home-canned vegetables -- explain why
Mendoza records botulism outbreaks caused by home-processed
foods only. On the other hand, the Province of Buenos Aires,
including the City, with 49.2% of the total population of
Argentina (27,862,771 inhabitants), is the most important consuming area of the country. In this region, outbreaks caused
by foods from both origins, commercially and home-processed,
have been recorded.

TABLE II. Botulism Outbreaks, Cases and Deaths, by Toxin Type, Argentina, 1922-1980

Toxin type	Years							
	1922–1929[a]	1930–1939	1940–1949	1950–1959	1960–1969	1970–1979	1980[b]	Total
Toxin type A								
Outbreaks	0	0	0	2	4	11	3	21
Cases	0	0	0	25	12	60	4	101
Deaths	0	0	0	14	5	21	1	41
Case fatality ratio (%)	–	–	–	56.0	41.7	35.0	25.0	40.6
Toxin type unknown								
Outbreaks	4	4	0	1	1	6	0	15
Cases	22	18	0	4	1	17	0	62
Deaths	19	17	0	3	1	8	0	48
Case fatality ratio (%)	86.4	94.4	–	75.0	100.0	47.1	–	77.4
Total								
Outbreaks	4	4	0	3	5	17	3	36
Cases	22	18	0	29	13	77	4	163
Deaths	19	17	0	17	6	29	1	89
Case fatality ratio (%)	86.4	94.4	–	58.6	46.2	37.7	25.0	54.6

[a] 8-year period.
[b] 1-year period.

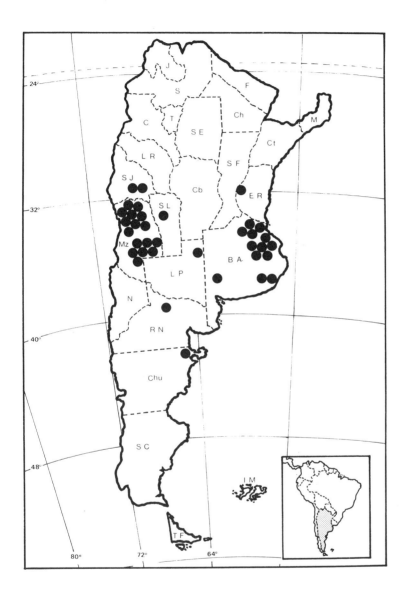

FIGURE 1. Geographic distribution of 36 botulism outbreaks recorded in Argentina, 1922-1980.

B. *The Food*

The type, origin and processing of foods incriminated in botulism outbreaks are shown in Tables III and IV. The

TABLE III. *Botulism Outbreaks Attributed to Commercially Processed or Home-Processed Foods, Argentina, 1922-1980.*

Years	Source of food			
	Home processed	Commercially processed	Unknown	Total
1922-1929[a]	4	0	0	4
1930-1939	4	0	0	4
1940-1949	0	0	0	0
1950-1959	1	1	1	3
1960-1969	2	1	2	5
1970-1979	8	3	6	17
1980[b]	1	1	1	3
Total (%)	20 (55)	6 (17)	10 (28)	36 (100)

[a] 8-year period.
[b] 1-year period.

TABLE IV. *Food Involved in 36 Botulism Outbreaks, Argentina, 1922-1980.*

Food	Outbreaks	
	No.	%
String beans	6	16.7
Peppers	5	13.9
Tomatoes (with other vegetables)	5	13.9
Cheese	3	8.3
Fish	3	8.3
Asparagus	2	5.6
Green peas + potatoes + carrots	1	2.8
Hearts of palm	1	2.8
Spinach	1	2.8
Octopus	1	2.8
Sausages	1	2.8
Peaches	1	2.8
Unknown	6	16.7
Total	36	100.0

percentage of outbreaks caused by preserved foods of vegetable origin (58.3%) is significantly higher than that recorded for those produced by foods of animal origin (22.2%).

An overall increase of outbreaks produced by commercially
processed foods has been recorded during the last decade.
Most of them have occurred in the Province of Buenos Aires
with foods of both origins, vegetable and animal.

C. The Agent

For most of the country, the prevalence of C. botulinum
in nature is not well known. Table V shows the results of
studies on the distribution of toxigenic C. botulinum in soil
samples from some areas of Argentina (4, 5, unpublished results). It is seen that there is a high prevalence of the
organism and a diversity of serological types, principally in
a dry and temperate region with similar ecological characteristics in the central western part of the county, located between 28 and 40° latitude south and from 64 to 72° longitude
west.

The highest percentage of soil samples positive for toxigenic C. botulinum was observed in Mendoza (42%) with 44% for
cultivated soils and 36% for virgin soils. Also, in this
Province was found the greatest variety of serologic types (A,
B, F), including the new type G and subtype Af.

III. CLINICAL AND LABORATORY OBSERVATIONS

The confirmation of botulism outbreaks through the identification and typing of the toxin and the isolation of the
agent from the suspected food and clinical materials, is given
in Table VI. During outbreaks occurring up to 1956, botulinal toxin was never investigated in Argentina and the diagnosis was made only on clinical grounds. In 1957, type A botulinal toxin was identified for the first time. Since then, an
increasing role of the laboratory in the epidemiology and
diagnosis of botulism in this country is appreciated.

TABLE V. Frequency of Argentine Soil Samples Positive for Toxigenic C. botulinum.

Province	Type of soil			Toxin type							
	Cultivated	Virgin	Total	A	B	A+B	Af	F	A+F	G	Und.[a]
Mendoza	97/220 (44)[b]	20/56 (36)	117/276 (42)	61 (52)	9 (8)	8 (7)	14 (12)	8 (7)	1 (1)	1 (1)	15 (13)
San Luis	48/104 (46)	14/75 (19)	62/179 (35)	51 (82)	4 (7)	2 (3)	3 (5)	1 (2)	0	1 (2)	0
Córdoba	26/65 (40)	2/6 (33)	28/71 (39)	9 (32)	12 (43)	4 (14)	0	1 (4)	0	0	2 (7)
Rio Negro	36/192 (19)	1/4 (25)	37/196 (19)	23 (62)	8 (22)	0	0	1 (3)	0	0	5 (14)
Total	207/581 (36)	37/141 (26)	244/722 (34)	144 (59)	33 (14)	14 (6)	17 (7)	11 (5)	1	2 (1)	22 (9)

[a] Toxin type undetermined.
[b] percentage.

TABLE VI. Laboratory Confirmation of Botulism Outbreaks, Argentina, 1922-1980

	Diagnosis					
	Laboratory confirmed		Clinical grounds or laboratory data unrecorded		Total	
Years	*No.*	*%*	*No.*	*%*	*No.*	*%*
1922-1950	0		9	100	9	100
1951-1956	0		0		0	
1957-1971	7	64	4	36	11	100
1972-1980	13	81	3	19	16	100
Total	20	56	16	44	36	100

Table VII summarizes the symptoms and signs recorded from 98 patients in 19 botulism outbreaks. These data, as well as part of the epidemiological observations have been compiled through the information received from medical officers, hospitals and private physicians.

IV. THERAPY

Up to the present, the specific therapy of botulism in Argentina has been based on the use of bivalent AB antitoxin. During 1972, the Argentinian Ministry of Public Health discontinued the local production of botulinal AB antitoxin. Since then, imported American, Canadian and Russian AB or ABE antitoxins have been used. The efficacy of these antitoxins deserves some considerations: (a) type A antitoxins from different foreign countries, as well as those that were prepared in Argentina, are made from either A 62 or A Hall toxigenic strain; (b) toxigenic A strains isolated from soil samples in this country (6) and from human outbreaks (data not published) have shown in serological cross-neutralization tests, a higher consumption (up to 6 times) of heterologous A antitoxin for its neutralization. This finding raises the immediate question, if the recommended doses for treatment are adequate when these antitoxins are employed in Argentina; (c) the human pathogenic A, B and F types and the potential human and animal pathogenic type G (7) and subtype Af (8) have been recognized in Argentine soils (9, 10). These facts imply that our population is at risk not only to type A and that an adequate botulinal antitoxin treatment should be started with a

TABLE VII. Outbreaks of Botulism in Which One or More
Persons were Affected by a Given Symptom or Sign, Argentina,
1922-1980

Symptoms/Signs	Type of toxin			%
	Type A	Und.[a]	Total	
Symptoms				
Blurred vision, diplopia, photophobia	9	8	17	89
Generalized weakness	6	6	12	63
Dysphonia	8	4	12	63
Dizziness or vertigo	6	6	12	63
Nausea and/or vomiting	4	5	9	47
Dysphagia	6	2	8	42
Constipation	1	6	7	37
Diarrhea	1	3	4	21
Abdominal pain, cramps, fullness	2	1	3	16
Sore throat	1	2	3	16
Urinary retention or incontinence	0	1	1	5
Signs				
Respiratory impairment	6	8	14	74
Specific muscle weakness/paralysis	6	8	14	74
Eye muscle involvement, including ptosis	6	6	12	63
Dilated, fixed pupils	4	5	9	47
Dry throat, mouth or tongue	2	6	8	42
Ataxia	3	2	5	26
Nystagmus	1	0	1	5
Somnolence	1	0	1	5

[a]Toxin type undetermined or unspecified.

tetravalent ABFG antitoxin until the serological type involved
is identified. Also, taking into account the serological variation of local type F toxins (11) similar to those recorded
for type A toxins, botulinal antitoxins to be used in Argentina should preferentially be prepared from local strains until the implication of this fact is cleared up through experimental work.

The progressive decrease of the case fatality ratio from
1922 to 1980, reflects better medical assistance to the patients, the recognition of outbreaks of less dramatic presentation and the increasing role of the laboratory in the

identification of the agent. The efficiency of the imported
antitoxins currently in use at the standard recommended doses
is not known and is, at present, being investigated in our
laboratory.

REFERENCES

1. Buzo, A., *Rev. Oral Cienc. Méd. (Bs. As.) 10,* 17 (1937).
2. Miyara, S., *9a. Renunión Soc. Arg. Patol. Reg. Comunic.
    151,* 776 (1935).
3. Bentotilla, M., Manzullo, A., and Martino, O. A., *Med.
    Panam. 10,* 149 (1958).
4. Giménez, D. F., and Ciccarelli, A. S., *Bol. Of. Sanit.
    Panam. 69,* 505 (1970).
5. Giulietti de Rigo, A. M., Thesis, Universidad Nacional de
    San Luis, Argentina (1973).
6. Ciccarelli, A. S., and Gimenez, D. F., *Rev. Latinoamer.
    Microbiol. 13,* 67 (1971).
7. Ciccarelli, A. S., Whaley, D. N., McCroskey, L. M., Gime-
    nez, D. F., Dowell, V. R., and Hatheway, C. L., *Appl.
    Environ. Microbiol. 34,* 843 (1977).
8. Giménez, D. F., and Ciccarelli, A. S., *Zbl. Bakteriol.
    Parasitenkd. Infektionskr. Hyg. Abt. 1 Orig. 240,* 215
    (1978).
9. Giménez, D. F., and Ciccarelli, A. S., *Zbl. Bakteriol.
    Parasitenkd. Infektionskr. Hyg. Abt. 1 Orig. 215,* 212
    (1970).
10. Giménez, D. F., and Ciccarelli, A. S., *Zbl. Bakteriol.
    Parasitenkd. Infektionskr. Hyg. Abt. 1 Orig. 215,* 221
    (1970).
11. Giménez, D. F., and Ciccarelli, A. S., *Medicina (Bs. As.)
    32,* 596 (1972).

DIFFERENT TYPES OF CLOSTRIDIUM BOTULINUM
(A, D, AND G) FOUND AT AUTOPSY IN HUMANS:
II. PATHOLOGICAL AND EPIDEMIOLOGICAL FINDINGS
IN TWELVE SUDDEN AND UNEXPECTED DEATHS

Ortrud Sonnabend

Department of Pathology
Kantonsspital St. Gallen
St. Gallen, Switzerland

Wolfgang Sonnabend

Institute of Medical Microbiology
St. Gallen, Switzerland

Little has been written regarding the necropsy diagnosis
of botulism. Although van Ermengem (1) and others (2-7) have
isolated Clostridium botulinum (C. botulinum) from necropsy
specimens of clinically and toxicologically proven cases, C.
botulinum was regarded as a nonpathogenic saprophyt and botulism was defined as an intoxication. Only when infant botulism
was recognized as a new entity, the possibility of a toxico-
infection was established (8,9).

In our autopsy study 882 cadavers out of a total of 6'905
were examined microbiologically between January 1975 and December 1980 for the presence of an infection. C. botulinum organisms and/or toxins were only found in twelve patients, who
died unexpectedly. In the other examined cadavers, where the
organ specimens were likewise thoroughly tested by aerobic and
anaerobic methods, no C. botulinum could be isolated. This paper deals with the comparison of pathological and epidemiological findings in these twelve individuals as well as the
symptoms preceding their deaths. The history of four of the
cases involving type A botulinal toxin is given in detail.

BIOMEDICAL ASPECTS OF BOTULISM

I. MATERIALS AND METHODS

The selection procedure of autopsies studied and the
microbiological methods applied are described in part I of
this paper. In all cases a complete necropsy was performed.
Paraffin sections of formalin fixed tissues were cut at six
microns and stained with hematoxylin and eosin and special
staining techniques. Toxicological examinations for poisons
and drugs were also performed from these twelve necropsies.

II. EPIDEMIOLOGICAL FINDINGS

The age distribution of the patients studied microbiologically at autopsy (1/1/1975 - 12/31/198o) is shown in table I.
882 patients, 116 of whom died suddenly and/or unexpectedly
with no cause obvious before autopsy, were thoroughly examined. Different botulinal toxins (A, D, and G) were identified
in the serum of twelve of the patients (table II). All these
cases were single cases. They were observed in the northeastern part of Switzerland within a range of 5o km, where the
Departments of Pathology and Forensic Medicine of the Kantonsspital St. Gallen are in charge of all autopsies. The cases
concerned nine males and three females. There were ten adults

TABLE I. *Age Distribution of Patients Studied*
          Microbiologically at Autopsy

	Total number of cases studied	Cases with sudden and/or unexpected deaths	Cases with botulinal toxin involved
0- 5 months	91	24	1
6-11 months	12	11	1
1- 9 years	27	12	0
10-29 years	61	15	3
30-49 years	128	25	3
50-69 years	291	21	3
>70 years	272	8	1
Total	882	116	12

TABLE II. Microbiological Findings in Twelve Patients with Identification of Botulinal Toxin

Case No.	1	2	3	4	5	6	7	8	9	10	11	12
Autopsy No.	SN87	SN562	SN769	SN611	SN143	GM56	GM140	GM77	GM73	SN599	GM99	GM63
Age (years)	27 wks	57	79	68	24	33	29	45	18 wks	26	44	55
Sex	f	m	f	f	m	m	m	m	m	m	m	m
Date of death	2/77	7/78	9/78	8/80	2/77	6/78	12/77	7/78	6/78	7/78	8/80	4/79
Time interval[a]	3	2	22	22	24	24	24	53	57	12	26	57
Toxin in serum	A	A	A	A	A	A	G	G	G	D	D	D
Organisms in												
Heart blood	O[b]	O	O	□O	□A + G	G	G	O	□O	D	□O	D
Spleen	O	O	O	O	□A + G	G	O	□G	O	D	□O	D
Lung	O	□O	O	□O	□A + G	□G	□G	□O	□O	D	□D	□O
Liver	O	O	O	O	□A + G	G	O	□O	O	D	□O	D
Kidney	O	O	O	□O	□A + G	O	O	□O	O	D	□O	O
Brain	O	O	O	□O	O	O	NA	O	O	D	O	D
Myocardium	NA[c]	NA	NA	NA	A + G	G	O	NA	NA	NA	NA	NA
Small intestine	O	O	O	NA	O	G	G	O	G	NA	D	O
Large intestine	O	O	O	NA	O	G	G	O	O	NA	O	O

[a] Hours. [b] O = no C. botulinum isolated. [c] Not available for testing. □ = other bacteria isolated.

between the ages of 24 and 79, and two infants of 18 and 27 weeks, respectively. The deaths occured in every season, but there seems to be a concentration during the summer months. Two cases occured in February, one in April, two in June, three in July, two in August, one in September and one in December. In no case the history could be traced to a contaminated food, since this study was not initiated as research project for botulism. The investigations of the samples took up a lot of time, and when the isolated strains were identified as C. botulinum of different types, remains of food, ingested by the patients, were no longer available for investigation.

III. CLINICAL AND PATHOLOGICAL FINDINGS

A. *Detailed History and Pathology of Four Cases without Isolation of Botulinal Organisms, but Identification of Botulinal Toxin Type A*

1. *Case Report 1.* A 27-week-old infant *(SN 87/77)* had diarrhea six days before death. The last two days she did not show any symptoms and seemed healthy. In the early morning the baby was found dead at home in her bed. At necropsy, performed three hours later, cultures taken from heart blood, spleen, lung, liver and brain were sterile. No virus could be isolated from different organs. The serum revealed no raised titers for viral infections. Histologically the lungs showed an increase of cellularity of the alveolar walls, alveolar hemorrhage, a generalized alveolar edema and dystelectasis. The mucosa of the small and the large intestine showed slight lymphatic hyperplasia. The findings at autopsy lead to the diagnosis of "cot death". Three years later the serum was tested for the presence of botulinal toxins and type A botulinal toxin was identified. This was only possible, because deep frozen serum was still available.

2. *Case Report 2.* A 57-year-old man *(SN 562/78)* was admitted to the hospital the day before he died. He came from abroad and had suffered for eight months from weakness and fatigability of the legs and the arms, and from intermittent abdominal pain. He also complained of decreased sexual ability. The clinical investigations from abroad four months ago did not reveal any cause. The possibility of a myopathy was discussed, but electromyographic studies were not done and the possibility of botulism was not taken into consideration.

Since the admission of the patient to our hospital was in the late Sunday afternoon, only a short orientating examination was made by a physician. The patient was found to be in good condition. Only in the middle of the abdomen a slight palpatory pain was noted. No muscle weakness of the extremities could be stated objectively. At 7.3o a. m. he was found dead in his bed.

Autopsy was performed 2 hours later. Cultures taken from heart blood, spleen, liver, kidney and brain were sterile. From the lung five aerobic and two anaerobic bacteria could be isolated, but not clostridia. C. botulinum was neither isolated from the gastric content nor from the content of small and large intestine. The main pathological findings were dilatation of the right ventricle with congestion of the internal organs. The lungs showed petechiae of the pleura and severe hemorrhagic edema. Microscopically the alveoli were focally filled with blood. No aspiration could be observed. The heart was scattered with petechiae of the epicardium. Histologically focal hyaline degeneration of muscle fibers and interstitial edema were noted. The coronary arteries had, according to age, very slight sclerosis. The ileum and the coecum contained brownish-red masses of liquid and foam and the mucosa of the colon showed superficial focal necrosis. The kidneys showed focal tubular necrosis. The cerebral cortex revealed significant satelitosis of the neurons. The glia cells had swollen nuclei with marginal chromatin. These nuclei were arranged in double or four-position.
Since the cause of death remained unclear even after autopsy, serum taken at necropsy under sterile conditions was tested for the presence of botulinal toxin several weeks after death. This serum had been stored at $- 30\,^{\circ}C$. Type A botulinal toxin was identified. The search for botulinal toxin in the deep frozen contents of stomach and ileum was negative.

3. *Case Report 3.* A 79-year-old women *(SN 769/79)* was found unconcious at home in the evening. On admission she was clear again and complained of severe dyspnea. The pulse was regular, 84/min. The body temperature was normal. The blood pressure was 12o/7o mm Hg. The liver and the spleen were enlarged, the abdomen was soft and painless. Sedimentation rate was elevated to 12o mm/hr. Severe leukopenia was stated in the peripheral blood. Thrombocytes were within normal range. Electrolyte studies and liver function tests were within normal limits. After admission the patient's condition worsened, the blood pressure dropped quickly to 7o/5o mm Hg and the periphery became cool with a marble-like skin. Somnolence was

noted again prior to death. The patient died 15 hours after
admission. Autopsy performed 22 hours later, after the cadaver
had been in storage at 4°C, failed to reveal any obvious cause
of death. A myocardial infarction was not found. There was no
coronary atherosclerosis. Though the clinicians had supposed
septicemia, no organisms were isolated from blood cultures
taken on admission. At necropsy heart blood and tissue specimens of spleen, lung, liver, kidney and brain were also sterile. No septic lesions or microthrombi were found in the
tissues. No botulinal organisms were isolated from the bowel.
Elevated serological titers could not be observed for respiratory, gastrointestinal or nervous system pathogens.

The main pathological macroscopic finding was congestion
of internal organs. The lungs showed histologically a dilatation of the alveolar capillaries and focal intraalveolar hemorrhage. The hypopharynx, the esophagus, and the rectum
showed focal small ulcerations of 1 mm in diameter. The bone
marrow was normal. The most striking histological findings
were fragmentation, focal hyaline degeneration and focal necrosis of myocardial fibers, as well as interstitial edema of
the myocardium. There was no cellular infiltration at all.
After the cultural investigations had not revealed any organisms, these histological changes recalled the observations
made three months before, in case no. 2, and lead to the examination of the serum for the presence of botulinal toxin.
Type A of C. botulinum was then detected by the mouse neutralization test. Unfortunately, the serum which was collected
15 minutes prior to death, and which revealed an elevated
creatinine phosphokinase (2'23o mU/ml) and an elevated lactic
dehydrogenase (454 mU/ml), was discarded. Therefore a comparison of toxin was not possible.

4. *Case Report 4.* Two months prior to death, a 68-year-old
women *(SN 611/8o)* had a subtotal gastrectomy because of an
adenocarcinoma of the stomach. Postoperatively a subphrenic
abscess developed and was successfully drained. The general
state of the patient improved steadily, and discharge was
taken into consideration when, two days prior to death, her
condition worsened suddenly, and fever and tachypnoe arose.
Laboratory tests were within normal limits one day prior to
death. During the last three weeks the patient had repeatedly
suffered from attacks of incomplete intestinal obstruction.
In addition, a constant tachycardia of unknown etiology between 120 and 140/min had been noted. It should be pointed out
that, at that time, late complications of the subphrenic abscess were not present. There was also no elevated body tempe-

rature that could explain this long-enduring tachycardia.

Even after autopsy, terminal illness and cause of death remained, to a certain degree, unclear. Necropsy was performed 22 hours after death. Only one circumscribed adhesion was found in the middle of the small intestine. Nevertheless the whole bowel showed a severe dilatation with abundant liquid and bad smelling content. The left and the right ventricle were dilatated. Histologically, an interstitial edema of the myocardium, a more eosinophilic cytoplasm and fragmentation of the myocardial fibers, and some focal necrotic areas were seen without any cellular infiltration. The kidney showed cloudy swelling of the tubules. Edema and terminal aspiration were noted in the lungs, from which four aerobic and two anaerobic bacteria were isolated. Terminal bacteremia occured with identification of E. coli in heart blood, lung, kidney and brain. Clostridia were not isolated. No septic lesions were noted in the tissues. Because of an error the intestinal contents were discarded and could not be tested for the presence of botulinal organisms or toxins. From the other tissues no C. botulinum was isolated. In the serum, however, type A of botulinal toxin was identified by the standard mouse assay.

B. Data of Five Cases with Isolation of C. Botulinum Type G and Three Cases with Isolation of C. Botulinum Type D

The data concerning the five cases with isolation of type G (no. 5 - 9) have already been published elsewhere in detail (1o). These patients all died at home, two of them showed symptoms similar to those of botulism; one for about 12 hours (no. 7), the other for about 72 hours (no. 6) preceding their deaths. One case was a sudden infant death syndrome concerning an 18-week-old baby. One patient (no. 8) died from pneumonia.

The three patients with isolation of C. botulinum type D died at home suddenly and unexpectedly. One of them (no. 1o) showed symptoms which can also be observed in clinically proven cases of botulism.

C. Symptoms Prior to Death

Patient no. 5, 9 and 11 did not show any symptoms prior to death. Nine of the twelve patients (no. 1 - 2, 5 - 9, 11 - 12) died in their sleep. Their deaths were completely unexpected and sudden, but the interviews with the patients' families

TABLE III. Symptoms and Signs Prior to Death in Twelve Patients with Identification of Botulinal Toxin

Case No.	1	2	3	4	5	6	7	8	9	10	11	12
Toxin type involved	A	A	A	A	A	A	G	G	G	D	D	D
Nausea, vomiting	O[a]	O	O	+	O	+	+++[d]	+	O	O	O	+
Generalized weakness	O	+[b]	++[c]	+	O	++	++	++	O	+++	O	+
Dizziness, vertigo	?[e]	O	?	O	O	+++	?	+	?	O	O	O
Dry mouth, thirst	O	O	O	O	O	+++	+++	O	O	+	O	O
Dysphagia, sore throat	O	O	O	O	O	?	?	?	O	+++	O	O
Dysarthria	O	O	O	O	O	?	?	+	O	+	O	O
Respiratory difficulty	?	?	+++	+++	?	?	?	+++	?	++	?	++
Abdominal pain	O	+	O	+	O	++	+	?	?	O	O	O
Constipation	O	(+)	O	+++	O	O	O	?	O	O	O	O
Diarrhea	++	O	O	O	O	O	O	?	O	O	O	O
Hypotension	?	?	+++	++	?	+	?	?	?	?	?	?
Somnolence	O	O	+	(+)	?	?	?	?	O	+	?	O
Tachycardia	?	O	O	++	?	?	?	?	?	+	?	?
Fever	O	O	O	+	?	?	?	?	?	++	?	?

Symbols mean: [a] None. [b] Slight. [c] Moderate. [d] Severe. [e] Information not available.

or physicians revealed some symptoms prior to their deaths.
These are listed in table III. Five patients suffered from
nausea and/or vomiting. Eight patients complained of distinct
weakness and lassitude. One of them (no. 6) had severe and one
(no. 8) had mild dizziness and vertigo. Exceptional thirst
which could not be quenched was observed in two patients (no.
6 and 7), while another one (no. 10) complained of dry mouth,
thirst, severe dysphagia, dysarthria, and sore throat. Severe
respiratory difficulty was observed in five patients (no. 3-4,
8, 10-11), substernal burning in one, abnormal perspiration in
two (no. 2 and 6). Four patients (no. 2, 4, 6-7) complained of
abdominal pain with severe constipation in one (no. 4). Diarrhea was observed six days prior to death in the 27-week-old
infant. Episodes of hypotension prior to death were noted in
three patients (no. 3-4, 6) and also preterminal somnolence
(no. 3-4, 10). Tachycardia occured in two persons (no. 4 and
10). Fever was observed in two patients.

D. *Pathological Findings*

The pathological findings of the twelve cases were rather
non-characteristic (table IV): one of the main macroscopic
findings were dilatation of the heart, with congestion of the
internal organs, and edematous dark red lungs which were observed in ten cases. In several cases this was thought to be
primarily due to an influenza pneumonia. The possibility of an
influenza-virus infection could be excluded, since no virus
was isolated from the lung specimens, no raised titers for
respiratorial infections were found, and no changes of the
bronchial epithelium were observed histologically. The macroscopic aspect was mainly due to severe congestion of the lung
with dilation of the alveolar capillaries, alveolar edema, and
hemorrhage, which seemed more pronounced in the lower than in
the upper lobes. The intrapulmonal congestion with hemorrhage
was similar to that in mice, that died after 0.6 ml of the patients' serum was given i. p. in the mouse toxin assay.
Histological evidence of severe aspiration was found in
three patients (no. 4, 8, and 11), slight aspiration was noted in one and only very small amounts of aspiration in four
patients. Other striking features were changes of the myocardium in six cases (no. 4-6, 10-12). Macroscopically it was soft
and loam-coloured. Epicardial petechiae were noted in three cases. Histologically there was an interstitial edema in all
cases with fragmentation of the myocardial fibers. Hyaline degeneration with more eosinophilic fibers and sometimes with

TABLE IV. *Macroscopic Pathological Findings in Twelve Patients with Identification of Botulinal Toxin*

Case No.	1	2	3	4	5	6	7	8	9	10	11	12
Toxin type involved	A	A	A	A	A	A	G	G	G	D	D	D
Severe congestion of internal organs	+[b]	+	O	+	+	+	+	+	+	+	+	+
Hemorrhagic edema of the lung on section	O[a]	+	+	O	+	+	+	(+)	+	+	+	+
Petechiae of the pleura	+	+	O	O	O	O	O	O	O	O	O	O
Pharyngitis/laryngitis	O	O.	O	O	O	O	O	O	O	+	O	O
Pneumonia	O	O	O	O	O	O	O	+	O	O	O	O
Soft, loam-coloured myocardium	O	O	O	+	+	+	O	O	O	+	+	+
Dilatation of the heart	+	+	O	+	+	+	O	+	+	+	+	+
Slight coronary sclerosis	O	(+)	O	O	O	+	O	+	O	O	+	+
Petechiae of epicardium	+	+	O	O	+	O	O	O	O	O	O	O
Focal ulcerations of the bowel mucosa	O	+	+	O	O	O	O	O	O	O	O	O
Severe dilatation of the small intestine	O	+	O	+	O	O	O	O	O	O	O	O

Symbols mean: [a] None. [b] Yes.

312

TABLE V. Histological Findings in Twelve Patients with Identification of Botulinal Toxin

Case No.	1	2	3	4	5	6	7	8	9	10	11	12
Toxin type involved	A	A	A	A	A	A	G	G	G	D	D	D
Lung: Hyperemic capillaries	+	(+)	+	+	+	+	+	+	+	+	+	+
Intraalveolar edema	+	+	+	+	+	+	+	+	+	+	+	+
Intraalveolar hemorrhage	O	+	++	O	++	+	+	+	(+)	+	(+)	+
Intraalveolar macrophages	+	(+)	(+)	O	+	+	+	+	++	+	+	+
Leucocytosis in vessels	+	+	O	O	O	O	+	+	+	+	++	O
Slightly increased interstitial cellularity	+	O	O	O	O	O	O	O	+	O	O	O
Purulent bronchopneumonia	O	O	O	O	O	O	O	+	O	O	O	O
Pulmonary aspiration	O	O	O	++	O	(+)	+	++	(+)	O	++	(+)
Interstitial edema of the myocardium	+	+	+	+	+	+	+	(+)	+	+	+	+
Hyaline degeneration of myocardial fibers	O	+	++	+	+	(+)	+	O	O	O	(+)	+
Fragmentation of myocardial fibers	O	+	+	+	+	+	+	+	O	(+)	+	+
Cloudy swelling of the tubules of the kidney	O	+	O	+	O	+	+	(+)	O	+	O	+

focal necrosis could be observed in eight cases. It should be
pointed out, that there was no coronary thrombosis, or severe,
or moderate coronary sclerosis. The bowel mucosa showed focal
ulcers in two patients. Severe dilatation of the small intestine was noted in two cases. Cloudy swelling of tubules of the
kidney was observed in seven patients.

IV. DISCUSSION

    Attempts to analyse bacteriological findings of C. botuli-
num organisms and/or toxins obtained from the routine culture
of postmortem specimens present some problems. There is the
question as to what role the agents played in the etiology and
pathogenesis of the patients' sudden and/or unexpected deaths.
There are, unfortunately, *no postmortem criteria for the diagnosis of botulism* other than presumptive diagnosis on epidemiological grounds, and demonstration of botulinal toxin from
a food source.
    Our cases are not associated with an outbreak of botulism
in which several persons were involved. There may be instances
in which a contaminated product results in only *a single case
of illness.* In 1977, we had such a situation with type B botulism in the western part of Switzerland, in which contaminated
food was ingested by a group of 15 persons, but only a two-
year-old girl developed manifest clinical botulism. In the
period 1976 - 1980, five cases caused by type A and type B,
respectively, have been reported from different parts of Switzerland. All of these cases were single cases of botulism. On
the other hand it may be difficult to diagnose botulism if
only a single case occurs. Even in outbreaks with typical
symptoms of botulism, it has been reported that the first
seven cases were misdiagnosed and three patients died before
botulism was recognized (11).
    Though they died suddenly and unexpectedly several of our
patients had *symptoms and signs* that can also be observed in
clinically proven cases of botulism. Gastrointestinal symptoms
like nausea, vomiting, abdominal pain are well known in Type B
or E botulism outbreaks (12). Dryness of mouth can be a prominent symptom in botulism which occurs early and can be particularly severe (11). Aspiration pneumonia is well known in
clinical botulism(13). Severe bilateral bronchopneumonia has
been found to be a complication in fatal cases of botulism
(14). Pharyngeal pain, sore throat, dysphagia, and the findings of a hyperemic swollen pharynx have led to the mistaken

diagnosis of streptococcal or viral pharyngitis in clinical
botulism (11)

Considering the history of our patients no. 3, 6 - 8, and
lo, the possibility of *food borne botulism* cannot be excluded,
since time between the first symptoms and death in outbreaks
of clinical botulism was reported as short as 11 hours (4).

Constipation is a frequent symptom in *infant botulism*. It
is generally accepted that botulinal toxin is produced in the
intestine in this condition. Two instances in adults have been
observed, where the same mechanism of toxin production was
supposed (15). Several investigators in the Soviet Union postu-
late a toxinfection in the adult, too (6, 16). Our patient no.
4 complained of severe constipation and suffered from a incomplete intestinal obstruction that lasted three weeks.

Case no. 1 and 9 were *sudden infant death syndromes (SIDS)*,
in one of which type G botulinum organisms were isolated from
the small intestine. It has been suspected that some cases of
SIDS could be due to a severe form of infant botulism (17).

We have no explanation for the sudden deaths of patient
no. 2, 5, 11 and 12. Patient no. 2 had suffered from symptoms
which have been described as late effects of botulism (18).
Wether the demonstration of botulinal toxin early after death
per se proves the diagnosis of botulism, still remains an un-
solved problem. Finally the possibility of *postmortem toxin
production* in the cadaver should be discussed. The possibility of postmortem invasion of tissues and blood by botulinal
organisms in case 1-4, and the thereupon following production
of toxin, cannot be taken into consideration. No C. botulinum
was isolated from any of these specimens, and the interval
between death and specimen collection was, especially in case
1 and 2, very short with two, and, respectively three hours.
How could type A toxin reach the circulation in these cases
other than before death?

Our conclusion is that according to the symptoms preceding
death and the pathological, bacteriological, and toxicological
findings at autopsy, case six, seven and ten appear to represent typical fatal cases of botulism. To get further information regarding the necropsy diagnosis of botulism, especially
in those cases that "began" in death (16), the importance of
taking cultures of blood, several tissues and the intestinal
content of all clinically proven cases of botulism undergoing
necropsy is quite evident. In every case of sudden unexpected
death *autopsy* should be made *as soon as possible after death*
and should *include microbiological examinations* to determine
infectious causes and *to detect botulinal toxin as a possible
reason.*

REFERENCES

1. van Ermengem, E., *Z. Hyg. Infekt. - Krh. 26*, 1 (1897).
2. Geiger, J. C., *Public Health Rep. 36*, 1663 (1921).
3. Dubovsky, B. J., and Meyer, K. F., *J. Infect. Dis. 31*, 501 (1922).
4. Stricker, F. D,. and Geiger, J. C., *Public Health Rep. 39*, 655 (1924).
5. Schneider, H. J., and Fisk, R., *J. Am. Med. Assoc. 113*, 2299 (1939).
6. Minervin, S. M., *in* "Botulism 1966" (Ingram, M., and Roberts, T., A., ed.), p. 336. Chapman and Hall Limited, London (1967).
7. Toyoda, H., Omata, K., Fukai, K., and Akai, K., *Acta Pathol. Jpn. 3o*, 445 (198o).
8. Pickett, J., Ber, B., Chaplin, E., and Brunsteller, M., *N. Engl. J. Med. 295*, 770 (1976).
9. Midura, T. F., and Arnon, S. S., *Lancet 2*, 934 (1976).
lo. Sonnabend, O., Sonnabend, W., Heinzle, R., Sigrist, T., Dirnhofer, R., and Krech, U., *J. Inf. Dis. 143*, (1981). *In press*.
11. Koenig, M. G., Spickard, A., Cardella, M. A., and Rogers, D. E., *Medicine 43*, 517 (1964).
12. Smith, L. DS., *in* "Botulism: the Organism, its Toxin, the Disease", p. 180. Charles D. Thomas, Bannerstone House, Springfield, Ill. (1977).
13. Koenig, M. G., Drutz, D. J., Mushin, M. D., Schaffner, W., and Rogers, D. E., *Am. J. Med. 42*, 2o8 (1967)
14. Horwitz, M. A., Marr, J. S., Merson, M. A., Dowell, V. R., and Ellis, J. M., *Lancet 2*, 861 (1975).
15. Chin, J., *Rev. Inf. Dis. 1*, 646 (1979).
16. Petty, B. S., *Am. J. Med. Sci. 249*, 345 (1965).
17. Arnon, S. S., Midura, T. F., Damus, K., Wood, R. M., and Chin, J., *Lancet 1*, 1273 (1978).
18. Maroon, J. C., and Bissonette, D., *J. A. M. A, 238*, 129 (1977).

CURRENT TRENDS IN THERAPY OF BOTULISM
IN THE UNITED STATES

J. Glenn Morris, Jr.

Bacterial Diseases Division
Center for Infectious Diseases
Centers for Disease Control
Atlanta, Georgia

I. INTRODUCTION

The case fatality rate for botulism in the United States has declined from approximately 70% in 1910-1919 (1) to 12% in 1970-1979 (2), a decrease due at least in part to improvements in therapy. Although a number of reports of botulism cases have been published, there has been little systematic analysis of current practices in treating the disease in this country. This study was undertaken to provide data on therapy administered in botulism cases occurring in the United States for the period 1979-1980; this included data on use of respiratory support, antitoxin, and drugs such as guanidine and antibiotics.

II. MATERIALS AND METHODS

A. *Adult Botulism*

Information on therapy was sought for all non-infant cases of botulism reported to the Centers for Disease Control (CDC) during 1979-1980; this includes 26 cases (20 outbreaks) of foodborne botulism, 5 cases of wound botulism, and 6 cases (6 outbreaks) of botulism of undetermined classification (cases of botulism occurring in individuals >1 year of age for which no vehicle can be identified (3)) (Table 1). Data

TABLE 1. Number of cases and therapy administered--botulism cases reported to CDC, 1979-1980

Category	No. of cases	No. of outbreaks	No. requiring respiratory support/No. for whom data available (%)	No. receiving antitoxin/No. for whom data available (%)	No. receiving Guanidine/No. for whom data available (%)
Foodborne	26	20	20/26 (77%)	20[a]/24 (83%)	2/16 (13%)
Classification undetermined (vehicle undetermined)	6	6	6/6 (100%)	5/6 (83%)	1/4 —
Wound	5	—	4/5 (80%)	4[a]/5 (80%)	0/4 —
Infant	90[b]	—	20/42[c] (48%)	—	—

[a] Patients receiving antitoxin do not correspond exactly with patients receiving respiratory support.
[b] 51 Non-California and 39 California infant botulism cases.
[c] Excludes California infant botulism cases.

were obtained from state epidemiologists, and, with the con-
currence of the state epidemiologist, from patients'
physicians. Completeness of reporting was variable, with
some data available on all patients and other data known for
only a few. Data on reactions to botulinal antitoxin were
also sought for patients who had received antitoxin but were
subsequently found not to have had botulism. A portion of
the data from 1979 has been published previously (4).

B. *Infant Botulism*

Information on therapy was sought for the 51 cases of
infant botulism reported to CDC from outside of the state of
California during 1979-1980 (Table 1). Data were obtained
using a specialized CDC surveillance questionnaire filled
out by state health department or CDC personnel. Surveillance questionnaires were completed, at least in part, for
43 infants.

III. RESULTS

A. *Adult Botulism*

Thirty (81%) of the 37 adult botulism patients required
respiratory support (Table 1). There was no significant
difference in the percentage of individuals requiring
respiratory support by disease category (foodborne, classification undetermined, or wound). Eighty-four percent of
adults with type A botulism required respiratory support,
compared with 62% of those with type B botulism (Table 2), a
difference which was not statistically significant (p=.32,
Fisher's exact test, 2-tail). Data on duration of respiratory therapy were available for 16 individuals. Median
duration of respiratory therapy was 44 days (range 3-150
days); in our sample it was not possible to show a difference
in duration of respiratory therapy by disease category or by
toxin type.

Twenty-nine (83%) of 35 adult botulism patients for whom
data were available had received trivalent (ABE) equine
antitoxin; all antitoxin used was produced by Connaught
Laboratories, Canada. In no instance were more than 40 ml
of antitoxin administered to a single patient. One episode
of anaphylaxis was reported in association with antitoxin
administration; in a second case it was unclear whether
antitoxin or penicillin (which the patient was receiving
simultaineously) was responsible for a skin rash. No

TABLE 2. Number of adult botulism patients requiring
respiratory support, by toxin type, 1979-1980

Toxin type	Required respiratory support (%)		Did not require respiratory support	(%)	Total	(%)
A	21	(84%)	4	(16%)	25	(100%)
B[a]	5	(63%)	3	(37%)	8	(100%)
E	4	(100%)	0	-	4	(100%)
					37	

[a]Type A vs type B, p=.32, Fisher exact test, 2-tail

reactions to antitoxin were reported among an additional 6
patients who received antitoxin, but in whom the diagnosis
of botulism was not subsequently confirmed. The percentage
of persons receiving antitoxin did not differ significantly
by disease category (foodborne, classification undetermined,
or wound) or by toxin type.

For foodborne botulism patients, antitoxin was administered a median of 2 days after onset of symptoms (range
0-10 days), compared with a median of 3.5 days (range 3-12
days) for patients with cases of undetermined classification
and 6 days (range 2-7 days) for wound cases; the difference
between foodborne and wound cases approached statistical
significance (p=.057 Mann-Whitney U Test). For 45% of the
patients with foodborne cases for whom data were available
antitoxin was administered on the same day that respiratory
support was initiated; for patients with wound botulism or
botulism of undetermined classification antitoxin was more
likely to be administered >1 day after respiratory support
was required (66% and 75% of cases for which data were
available, respectively). It was not possible with our data
to show that antitoxin influenced the duration of respiratory
therapy.

For patients with type A foodborne and classification
undetermined botulism who had toxin present in their serum
the median time between onset of symptoms and collection of
serum samples was 2 days. Toxin was significantly more
likely to be present in serum in the first three days than
in the period four or more days after onset of illness
(p=.01, Fisher's exact test, 2-tail); however, type A toxin
was detected in the serum of 2 patients more than a week
after onset of symptoms (Fig. 1). For patients with type B
botulism who had toxin detected in their serum the median
time between onset of symptoms and collection of serum
samples was 5 days, which did not differ significantly from
type A cases (p=.075, Mann-Whitney U Test).

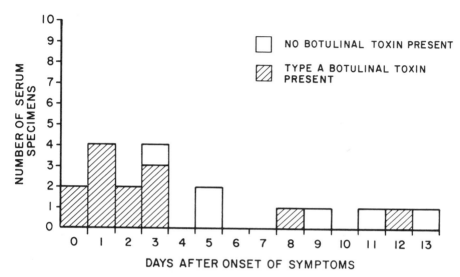

FIGURE 1. Detection of botulinal toxin in serum of
adult patients with Type A botulism, 1979-1980.

Guanidine was administered to 3 (13%) of 24 adult botulism patients for whom data on guanidine use were available.
The percentage of individuals receiving therapy with guanidine did not vary between the various disease categories
(Table 1) or by toxin types. For 1 of the 3 patients given
guanidine the drug was thought to be efficacious. The
patient was treated for 6 weeks at a dosage of 38 mg per
kilogram per day in 4 divided doses; attending physicians
felt that the patient's respiratory parameters and muscle
strength improved with the drug, and noted that on two
occasions when the medication was withdrawn there was a
prompt deterioration of muscle function. For the other 2
patients guanidine was not felt to be efficacious, including
1 patient who received up to 9 grams of guanidine per 24
hours in divided doses.
    Data were not available on antibiotic use for patients
with foodborne botulism or botulism of undetermined classification. In 4 of the 5 wound botulism cases patients were
known to have been receiving antibiotics at the time of onset
of symptoms. All 4 patients were receiving cephalosporins;
in one case the drug was being administered intravenously.
    Five (14%) of the 37 adults diagnosed as having botulism
during 1979-1980 died; this includes 3 patients with foodborne botulism and 2 with botulism of undetermined classification. One patient suffered severe anoxia during a

difficult intubation, while a second patient's death was
attributed to mechanical respirator failure. One patient
had a cardiac arrest while on the respirator; another
developed pulmonary emboli. A fifth patient died of renal
failure (in association with *Pseudomonas sepsis*) approximately 2 months after onset of symptoms; the patient still
required respiratory support at the time of death.

B. *Infant Botulism*

In 20 (48%) of 42 non-California infant botulism cases
patients were known to have required respiratory support.
In 46% of type A cases respiratory support was required,
compared to 44% of type B cases. Duration of respiratory
support was reported in 12 cases; median duration was 23
days (range 2-68 days). In our small sample there was no
significant difference in duration of respiratory support by
toxin type, nor was there a significant difference in
duration between infant and adult cases. No infants are
known to have received antitoxin.

Of the 43 infants for whom surveillance questionnaires
were completed, 23 are known to have received antibiotics at
the time of admission to the hospital and for at least a day
thereafter. All received a penicillin, with 10 receiving
both a penicillin and an aminoglycoside (Table 3). Twenty-
seven percent of those receiving penicillin alone required
respiratory support, compared with 60% of those receiving

TABLE 3. *Number of infant botulism patients requiring
respiratory support, by antibiotic therapy received on
admission, 1979-80 (excluding California patients)*

Antibiotics administered	Required respiratory support	Did not require respiratory support	Total
Penicillins alone	3	8	11
Penicillins and Aminoglycosides[a]	6	4	10
Penicillins and Chloramphenicol	2	0	2
			23

[a]*Penicillins alone vs. penicillins and aminoglycosides
p=.14, Fisher's exact test, 1-tailed.*

both penicillin and an aminoglycoside; with our small sample
this difference was not statistically significant (p=.14,
Fisher's exact test, 2 tail). It was not possible to show a
significant difference between these 2 groups with regard to
duration of hospitalization or duration of respiratory
therapy.

No deaths occurred among the 51 non-California infant
botulism cases reported in 1979-1980. One death was reported
in California during this time period; death was associated
with a transfusion reaction.

IV. DISCUSSION

The decrease in the case-fatality ratio for botulism may
be attributed largely to improvements in mechanical ventilatory support; if they had had botulism in 1910, for example,
the 30 adult botulism patients in 1979-1980 who required
respiratory support would almost certainly have died. As
can be seen in this study, deaths associated with botulism
can generally be attributed to problems inherent in initia-
ting and providing long-term respiratory support. It is
unlikely that the number of fatalities can be reduced substantially without the introduction of some mode of therapy
to shorten the time patients are dependent on mechanical
ventilators.

Antitoxin remains a common component in therapy of botulism in adults. While the efficacy of antitoxin (when
administered early in the course of the disease) has been
demonstrated in animal studies (5), reports of its efficacy
in man deal only with type E botulism and are largely
anecdotal in nature (6,7). Part of the difficulty in
collecting data on antitoxin efficacy is that antitoxin is
often administered late in the course of the disease, as
shown in this study; as antitoxin does not affect already
bound toxin (8), its use in such cases cannot be expected to
be dramatic. Our data do indicate that toxin may be present
in serum of a few patients for over a week after onset of
symptoms, which raises the question of whether antitoxin
should be administered "to neutralize any remaining toxin"
even for patients whose illness is far advanced at the time
of diagnosis. Data were inadequate in our study to show
that antitoxin use had any influence on the duration of
respiratory support; while admittedly difficult, further
studies of this question are needed.

Besides the questions of efficacy, use of antitoxin is
limited by concern about possible side-effects associated
with its being a horse-serum product. One case of anaphy-

laxis was reported in our study, in agreement with the
observation by Black and Gunn (9) that approximately 2% of
individuals who receive equine botulinal antitoxin have an
anaphylactic reaction. No cases of serum sickness were
reported. This does not represent a significant decrease
from the rate of 2.8% reported by Black and Gunn for
Connaught antitoxin; the present rate, however, may
ultimately prove to be somewhat lower due to the current
emphasis on use of <40 ml of antitoxin per patient. It is
possible that the rate may be reduced by use of more highly
purified equine antitoxin preparations; in Japan, where such
preparations have been used, it has been claimed that
virtually no cases of serum sickness occur (10). Use of
human derived immune globulins, which is currently under
study (11), should further reduce the rate of reactions.

Guanidine is still used by some physicians to treat
patients with botulism, with our study providing 1
additional anecdotal report of benefit from such therapy.
In the 1 controlled trial which has been reported (12),
however, it was not possible to show that treatment with
guanidine enhanced recovery from botulism; until it is
possible in a blind, controlled study to show a clear
benefit to guanidine use it is difficult to support routine
administration of the drug to botulism patients. It has
been suggested that the aminopyridines may be of benefit in
treating botulism. 4-Aminopyridine was used in treating
botulism patients in Great Britian, but the observed side
effects were felt to be too severe to permit general use of
the drug (13). Animal studies in the United States have
suggested that 3,4-diaminopyridine may be effective in
botulism (14); further studies of the drug are indicated.

Use of antibiotics for wound botulism patients is widely
accepted, but remains of unproven benefit. The patients
with wound botulism in this study were almost all receiving
cephalosporin antibiotics (to which most *C. botulinum*
strains are sensitive (15)) at the time symptoms of botulism
were first noted; this apparent lack of efficacy may be due
to difficulties in obtaining adequate antibiotic levels in
deep, avascular wounds. For infants, penicillins have not
been shown to have an effect on the clinical course of the
disease, nor has it been possible to show that the drug
eradicates either *C. botulinum* organisms or botulinal toxin
from the intestine (16,17). Both clinical and animal
studies have suggested that aminoglycosides (which are not
active against *C. botulinum* in vitro (15)) may cause
potentiation of neuromuscular blockade and thus increase the
possibility of respiratory failure (18,19). While our study

suggests that the rate of respiratory failure may be higher in infants receiving aminoglycosides, the study was too small to demonstrate a statistical difference.

ACKNOWLEDGMENTS

We thank the physicians and state epidemiologists and their staffs who supplied data included in this report as part of the botulism surveillance program of the Centers for Disease Control.

REFERENCES

1. Centers for Disease Control. Botulism in the United States, 1899-1977. Handbook for Epidemiologists, Clinicians, and Laboratory Workers. CDC, Atlanta, Georgia (issued May 1979).
2. Feldman, R. A., and Morris, J. G. *Proceedings of Biomedical Aspects of Botulism*, Frederick, Maryland, March 16-18, 1981.
3. Centers for Disease Control. *Morbidity and Mortality Weekly Rep. 28*, 73-75, (1979).
4. Morris, J. G., and Hatheway, C. L. *J. Infect. Dis. 142*, 302-5 (1980).
5. Oberst, F. W., Crook, J. W., Cresthull, P., and House, M. J. *Clin. Pharmacol. Therapeutics 9*, 209-14 (1968).
6. Dolman, C. E., and Iida, H. *Can. J. Public Health 54*, 293-308 (1963).
7. Whittaker, R. L., Gilbertson, R. B., and Garrett, A. S. *Ann. Intern. Med. 61*, 448-54 (1964).
8. Simpson, L. L. *Rev. Infect. Dis. 1*, 656-9 (1979).
9. Black, R. E., and Gunn, R. A. *Am. J. Med. 69*, 567-70 (1980).
10. Layton, L. L., Arimoto, L., Lamanna, C., Olson, R., Sharp, D., Kondo, H., and Sakaguchi, G. *Jap. J. Med. Sci. Biol. 25*, 309-19 (1972).
11. Metzger, J. F., and Lewis, G. E. *Rev. Infect. Dis. 1*, 689-90 (1980).
12. Kaplan, J. E., Davis, L.E., Narayan, V., Koster, J., and Katzenstein, D. *Ann. Neurol. 6*, 69-73 (1979).
13. Ball, A. P., Hopkinson, R. B., Farrell, I.D., Hutchison, J. G. P., Paul, R., Watson, R. D. S., Page, A. J. F., Parker, R. G. F., Edwards, C. W., Snow, M., Scott, D. K., Leone-Ganado, A., Hastings, A., Ghosh, A. C., and Gilbert, R. J. *Q. J. Med. 48*, 473-91 (1979).

14. Lewis, G. E., Metzger, J. F., and Wood, R. M. *20th Interscience Conference on Antimicrobial Agents and Chemotherapy,* New Orleans, Louisiana, September 22-24, 1980. Abstract #449.
15. Swenson, J. M., Thornsberry, C., McCroskey, L. M., Hatheway, C. L., and Dowell, V. R. *Antimicrob. Agent Chemother. 18,* 13-19 (1980).
16. Arnon, S. S. *Ann. Rev. Med. 31,* 541-60 (1980).
17. Arnon, S. S., Midura, T. F., Clay, S. A., Wood, P. M., and Chin, J. *J. Am. Med. Assoc. 237,* 1946-51 (1977).
18. L'Hommedieu, C., Stough, R., Brown, L., Kettrick, R., and Polin, R. *J. Pediatr. 95,* 1065-70 (1979).
19. Burr, D. H., Korthals, G. J., and Sugiyama, H. *Annual Meeting of the American Society for Microbiology,* Dallas, Texas, March 1-6, 1981. Abstract #B-33.

BOTULISM: CLINICAL, ELECTRICAL AND
THERAPEUTIC CONSIDERATIONS

M. Cherington

University of Colorado Medical Center
Denver, Colorado

INTRODUCTION

Botulism is a paralyzing disease caused by the most toxic
substance known to man. The toxin is produced by the bacterium, Clostridium botulinum. The toxin has been estimated to
cause death in man in doses as small as 0.1-1.0 µg (1, 2).
Eight immunologically distinct toxins have been identified (A,
B, C_1, C_2, D, E, F and G). Human cases are almost always due
to type A, B or E. When contaminated sea food is found to be
the responsible food, the toxin present is often type E.
Types C and D toxins may not be absorbed by the human gastrointestinal tract (3).
Botulism toxin is heat-labile and thus is often destroyed
by the cooking process. By contrast, the spores of C. botulinum are heat-resistant. When spores are present in food, actively multiplying bacilli produce the toxin at room temperature under anaerobic conditions at a pH of 6 or above (4).
The toxin causes paralysis of skeletal muscles by interfering
with release of acetylcholine.
The reduction of acetylcholine release may be due to the
action of the toxin on the intracellular calcium mechanism (5).

SYMPTOMS AND TREATMENT

The clinical symptoms of botulism usually occur within 12-
36 hours after ingestion of contaminated food. The signs and

symptoms begin in the cranial nerve territory (blurred vision,
dysarthria, dysphagia) and then descend (6, 7). This distinguishes botulism from the Guillain-Barré syndrome, which is
characterized by ascending paralysis.

In botulism, respiratory paralysis can follow quickly and
is often fatal, unless treated. Alertness, mentation and the
sensory system remain normal. The pupils are usually normal,
particularly early in the disease. Patients with severe botulism almost always have marked extraocular muscle weakness,
including ptosis. Weakness of the face, tongue, pharynx, neck
and sometimes, to a lesser degree, the limbs occurs. Weakness
progresses until it reaches a plateau at about 4-5 days. Although the weakness is bilateral, it is often asymmetric.
Severe respiratory paralysis can occur within the first day.
Symptoms of parasympathetic dysfunction may include dryness of
the mouth and eyes, and gastrointestinal ileus. Deep tendon
reflexes are reduced in proportion to the degree of muscular
weakness.

Recovery, it it occurs, is prolonged, but nearly total (8).
Laboratory confirmation usually requires the detection of
toxin in the patient's serum, stool or in the contaminated
food. Mouse toxicity tests with antiserum neutralization are
most useful. Specimens that should be examined include serum,
gastric contents, feces, exudates from wounds and contents of
the suspected jars or cans. Radioimmunoassay tests may be
practical in the future.

The major treatment of botulism is good medical care.
This consists of providing artificial ventilation for patients
with respiratory paralysis. Tracheotomy and a positive pressure support are usually required. Mechanical assistance to
respiration may be needed for as long as weeks or months.
Early administration of antitoxin may be of value in cases of
type E botulism. The literature and our experience suggest
that antitoxin is less effective in types A and B botulism.
Corticosteroid treatment has not been beneficial (9).

The role of guanidine in the treatment of botulism remains
that of an adjunct to therapy and not that of a cure. It has
helped some, but not all, patients. Guanidine was introduced
in the treatment of botulism in 1968. Since that time, it has
been beneficial in 43 cases (39 previously reported plus four
recent cases) and of little or no benefit in 19 cases (10, 11).
In the cases of treatment failure, 18 of 19 patients recovered
anyway. So far, no serious side-effect has occurred with
short-term therapy, although there have been serious side-effects when guanidine has been given for long periods in disorders, such as the Lambert-Eaton syndrome.

Although guanidine therapy results in notable eye and limb
muscle improvement, there often is minimal improvement in
vital capacity or pulmonary function. Increasing the dose of

guanidine may result in considerable epigastric distress and nausea. This is a problem, because guanidine has not been approved for parenteral administration and must be given orally. Another problem in treatment with guanidine is failure of its absorption because of the ileus.

Recently another drug, 4-aminopyridine, has been reported to be effective in reversing the neuromuscular block of botulism. Unfortunately, the drug had little or no benefit in reversing the paralysis of respiratory muscles. In this, it is similar to the action of guanidine (12).

The expected electrophysiological findings in botulism may be summarized as follows: (a) There is almost always a small evoked muscle action potential in response to single supramaximal nerve stimulation. (b) Post-tetanic facilitation is similar to, but less notable than, that seen in the Lambert-Eaton syndrome (13, 14). (c) Postactivation exhaustion is not prominent. (d) The decremented response of muscle action potential to slow rate of stimulation is absent, or not notable. (e) Evoked action potential to single-nerve stimulation is increased after guanidine therapy. (f) Single-fiber EMG studies reveal increased jitter and blocking. Jitter is frequency-dependent and decreases with higher innervation frequency. Fiber density values are lowered (15, 16).

REFERENCES

1. Schantz, E. J., and Sugiyama, H., *J. Agric. Food Chem.*, *22*, 26 (1974).
2. Smith, L. DS., "Botulism," p. 113. Charles C. Thomas, Springfield, Ill. (1977).
3. Bradley, W. G., Ferrucci, J. T., Jr., Shahani, B. T., and Hyslop, N. E., Jr., *N. Engl. J. Med. 303*, 1347 (1980).
4. Finegold, S. F., "Anaerobic Bacteria in Human Disease," p. 472. Academic Press, New York (1977).
5. Messina, C., Dattola, R., and Girlanda, P., *Acta Neurol. (Napoli) 34*, 459 (1979).
6. Cherington, M., *in* "Handbook of Clinical Neurology," vol. 41 (H. Klawans and S. Ringel, eds.), in press (1981).
7. Cherington, M., *in* "Natural Toxins" (D. Eaker, and T. Wadström, eds.), p. 589. Pergamon Press, Oxford (1980).
8. Cherington, M., *Arch. Neurol. 30*, 432 (1974).
9. Cherington, M., and Schultz, D., *Clin. Toxicol. 11*, 19 (1977).
10. Puggliari, M., and Cherington, M., *JAMA 240*, 2276 (1978).
11. Kaplan, J. E., Davis, L. E., Narayan, V., Koster, J., and Katzenstein, D., *Ann. Neurol. 6*, 69 (1979).

12. Ball, A. P., Hopkinson, R. B., Farrell, I. D., Hutchin-
     son, J. G. P., Paul, R., Watson, R. D. S., Page, A. J.
     F., Parker, R. G. F., Edwards, C. W., Snow, M., Scott, D.
     K., Leone-Ganado, A., Hastings, A., Ghosh, A. C., and
     Gilbert, R. J., *Q. J. Med.* *48*, 473 (1979).
13. Cherington, M., *in* "New Developments in Electromyography
     and Clinical Neurophysiology," vol. 1 (J. E. Desmedt,
     ed.), p. 375. S. Karger, Basel (1971).
14. Gutman, L., and Pratt, L., *Arch. Neurol.* *33*, 175 (1976).
15. Schiller, H. H., and Stålberg, E., *Arch. Neurol.* *35*, 346
     (1978).
16. Stålberg, E., and Trontelj, J. V., "Single-fiber Electro-
     myography," p. 131. The Mirvalle Press, Surrey, U.K.
     (1979).

INFANT BOTULISM: PATHOGENESIS, CLINICAL ASPECTS
AND RELATION TO CRIB DEATH[1]

Stephen S. Arnon

Infant Botulism Research Project
California Department of Health Services
Berkeley, California

I. INTRODUCTION

Infant botulism is the recently recognized form of botulism
in which ingested spores of *Clostridium botulinum* germinate,
multiply and produce botulinal toxin in the intestinal lumen of
the patient (1). Infant botulism is not a new disease, only a
newly recognized one. The first clinical cases of botulism in
infants were described in 1976 (2). Soon thereafter, as shown
in Table 1, evidence was obtained that infant botulism, unlike
botulism from food poisoning at other ages, is an infectious
disease (3,4). Bacteriologically-proven cases occurred in 1931
and in 1975, but they were misdiagnosed at the time (5,6).

Clinically, infant botulism is an acute, flaccid paralysis
which manifests as weakness of head, face and throat muscula-
ture that then extends symmetrically to involve the muscles of
the trunk and extremities. Death results either from paralyzed
tongue or pharyngeal muscles occluding the airway, or from
paralysis of diaphragm and intercostal muscles or from secondary complications. Recovery from botulism occurs as terminal
motoneurons regenerate and induce formation of new motor-end
plates, a process that generally takes several weeks (7).

Like other infectious diseases, infant botulism has a spectrum in its clinical severity. Patients with infant botulism

[1]*Supported by the California Department of Health Services
and by grants (HD-12530 and AI-16354) from the National
Institutes of Health.*

TABLE 1. Evidence That Infant Botulism Is an Infectious Disease and Not a Common Source, Food-Borne Intoxication

Epidemiological	Laboratory
1. Of the first 6 cases, 3 were type A and 3 were type B.	1. C. botulinum type B organisms (but no preformed toxin) were found in honey fed to a baby who then developed type B infant botulism.
2. No common food, canned or otherwise, linked these 6 cases.	2. All other ingested food items available for testing were negative for C. botulinum toxin and organisms.
3. These 6 cases occurred in 1975 and 1976, on both the Pacific and Atlantic Coasts.	3. Excretion of toxin and organisms in feces was present at onset of illness and for as long as 20 weeks thereafter.
4. Some of the 6 patients had not yet been born when others of them had already become ill.	4. Neither C. botulinum toxin nor organisms were found in the feces of 24 age-matched healthy control infants.
5. All other family members remained well.	5. Fecal specimens from family members were negative for C. botulinum toxin and organisms.

(Source: Arnon et al. J.A.M.A. 1977; 237:1946)

can be divided into four groups: *i*) mild paralysis, often diagnosed as "failure to thrive," in which hospitalization is not required, *ii*) moderate to severe paralysis, in which the need for hospitalization is clear, *iii*) fulminant paralysis, in which death occurs without warning and without opportunity for hospitalization, and which at autopsy is indistinguishable from Sudden Infant Death Syndrome (SIDS, crib death), and *iv*) a few asymptomatic, transient fecal "carriers" of *C. botulinum* (8-11).

II. CLINICAL EXPERIENCE

A. *Descriptive Features*

Since 1976, 90 patients with infant botulism have been hospitalized and studied in California (Table 2). Unexpected differences were found between hospitalized illness caused by type A toxin and by type B toxin. Patients with type A illness tended to be more severely paralyzed and had a higher frequency of respiratory arrest, a greater need for tracheostomy, and a longer mean hospital stay than did patients with type B illness. The weakness of type B illness appeared to evolve more gradually, as 8% of type B patients were placed on respirators without first having had a frank respiratory arrest. The mean cost of hospitalization for all patients exceeded $10,000.

As occurs in other bacterial infections of the gut (e.g., salmonellosis), excretion of *C. botulinum* persisted for weeks to months after the episode of acute illness had resolved (Figure 1). Surprisingly, botulinal toxin remained detectable in feces long after patients had recovered sufficient strength to leave the hospital.

B. *Aminoglycoside Antibiotics in the Treatment of Infant Botulism*

In a recent report L'Hommedieu et al. questioned whether the paralysis of infant botulism was exacerbated by use of gentamicin or other aminoglycoside antibiotics (12). They observed that 11 patients who received ampicillin and gentamicin appeared to stop breathing more often than did five patients who had not received these antibiotics. Furthermore, the apnea seemed temporally related to the administration of gentamicin, as some patients had a respiratory arrest within hours of their first dose of gentamicin. The association of respiratory

TABLE 2. Clinical Experience of Patients Hospitalized with Infant Botulism in California, 1976–1980

Patients[a]	Length of hospital stay (weeks) Mean	Length of hospital stay (weeks) Median	Respiratory arrest before or after admission N (%)	Needed mechanical ventilation N (%)	Tracheostomy N (%)	Gastrostomy N (%)	Deaths	Case fatality rate, %
Type A (N=50)	5.6	4.2	13 (26%)	13 (26%)	3 (6%)	1 (2%)	1[b]	2%
Type B (N=35)	3.1	2.9	8 (23%)	11 (31%)	0	0	1[b]	3%
Total (N=85)[a]	4.6	3.3	21 (25%)	24 (28%)	3 (4%)	1 (1%)	2	2%

[a]Information unavailable on five patients (4 type A, 1 type B).
[b]The type A patient died 31 days after admission from complications of nosocomial pneumonia, and the type B patient died 13 days after admission from a possible transfusion reaction.

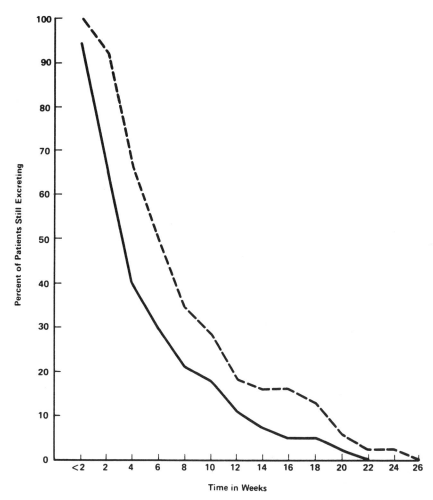

FIGURE 1. Duration of excretion in feces of C. botulinum *toxin and organisms after onset of illness. N = 38 patients, 24 type A, 14 type B.*━━━━━━ *Botulinal Toxin;*━━━━━ C. botulinum *organisms.*

arrest and antibiotic treatment with aminoglycosides was not seen in patients who received only penicillin-class antibiotic drugs. Because gentamicin, like other aminoglycoside antibiotics, can in the setting of general anesthesia enhance blockade of acetylcholine release at the neuromuscular junction,

L'Hommedieu et al. postulated a causal association between
gentamicin exposure and the subsequent respiratory arrest of
their patients.[2]

To determine whether aminoglycoside antibiotics -- or other
antibiotics -- might have a deleterious effect on the course of
infant botulism, several possibilities were examined with information from the California patient population, which was
five times as large as that studied by L'Hommedieu et al.
First, could a significant association be found between treatment with any antibiotic drug and a subsequent respiratory
arrest? Alternatively, could use of antibiotics have increased
the patient's weakness such that, in anticipation of a respiratory arrest, the ill infant was prophylactically placed on a
ventilator? These same questions were then asked specifically
of aminoglycoside (i.e., gentamicin or kanamycin) usage.
Finally, patients who received at least one dose of an aminoglycoside or of another antibiotic were compared for the occurrence of a subsequent respiratory arrest.

With information from 85 California patients, 50 with type
A illness and 35 with type B illness, no association was found
between gentamicin usage and respiratory arrest, nor between
gentamicin usage and subsequent need for a respirator. These
conclusions held for illness caused either by type A toxin or
by type B toxin. When compared to other antibiotics, use of
aminoglycoside antibiotics was not significantly associated
with subsequent respiratory arrest.

It is possible that the apparent association observed by
L'Hommedieu et al. between gentamicin exposure and respiratory
arrest may simply reflect the fact that the most acutely ill
infant botulism patients presented at hospital admission an appearance indistinguishable from that of overwhelming infection -- and so standard antibiotic therapy for this possibility
was started, and a respiratory arrest later occurred from the
continuing effects of botulinal toxin. In contrast, infant
botulism patients who had less severe illness would not have

---

[2]*It is generally agreed that antibiotics should be used
in infant botulism only to treat secondary infections. These
patients were not given gentamicin and ampicillin to treat
their infant botulism. Instead, they received this antibiotic
regimen because at hospital admission their physicians suspected an occult, life-threatening bacterial infection, rather
than infant botulism, to be the cause of their acute lethargy
and weakness. The antibiotic combination of gentamicin and
ampicillin is presently considered to give the broadest spectrum of antimicrobial activity during the days that diagnostic
bacterial cultures are incubating.*

been given aminoglycoside or other antibiotics, and because
their paralysis was less extensive, respiratory arrests did
not occur.

In summary, from experience in California and elsewhere to
date, the preferred management of patients hospitalized with
infant botulism presently consists of meticulous supportive
care (mainly respiratory and nutritional), no equine antitoxin,
use of antibiotics only to treat secondary infections, tracheostomy as a last resort, and no cathartics or enemas. It is
to be hoped that human botulism immune globulin and the aminopyridine derivatives fulfill their therapeutic promise, which
will need to be determined by clinical trials.

III. MILK AND THE PATHOGENESIS AND SEVERITY OF INFANT BOTULISM

With the recognition that infant botulism resulted from the
colonization of the gut microflora by *C. botulinum*, it was
anticipated that different diets would have varying effects on
the intestinal milieu in which *C. botulinum* must establish itself in order to cause illness (1,4,5). Experimental studies
in mice and chickens subsequently identified the importance of
the resident microflora and of normal gut anatomy in permitting
or blocking intestinal *C. botulinum* spore germination (13-15).
Because milk is the central element of the infant's diet, and
because the composition of the intestinal flora differs in
breast- and formula-fed infants (16), the influence of human
milk and formula milk diets on illness was studied (for details
of study design and data analysis see refs. 17 and 18).

Before discussing the results of this study, a brief review
of the recent knowledge of breast milk immunology may help to
place the findings in physiological context. Among the several
immunological constituents found in human milk (but not in formula milk) are leukocytes, lactoferrin, lysozyme, complement
and perhaps most important for enteric infections, secretory
IgA. As a consequence of the recently described "enteromammary
immunological system" (19), lymphocytes in a lactating woman's
intestinal lymphoid tissue become sensitized to bacterial antigens in her gut and then migrate to the breast. Once there,
these sensitized lymphocytes contribute antigen-specific secretory IgA to her milk. When ingested by the breast-fed infant,
these immunological components, particularly secretory IgA, may
prevent transepithelial penetration of intestinal bacteria and
their products. Parenthetically, mother's milk might be expected to contain antibody against somatic antigens of *C.
botulinum* because adults regularly ingest these spores on fresh

agricultural products and because *C. botulinum* antigens cross-react with those of other clostridia commonly found in the adult intestine. The differences in intestinal microflora, pH and buffering capacity between breast- and formula-fed infants may be an important influence on the ability of *C. botulinum* spores to germinate, colonize the infant gut and produce toxin in it.

Investigation of the influence of diet on infant botulism yielded results that might have appeared paradoxical, were it not for the recent advances in knowledge of breast milk immunology. Significantly more hospitalized patients were primarily breast-fed (two-thirds or more milk intake) in the month before onset than were their healthy controls (64.0% vs. 40.8%, respectively, 0.001 < P < 0.01) (Table 3). The disparity in

TABLE 3. *Milk Feeding History in the Month before*
Onset of Patients with Infant Botulism

Group	Primarily breast-fed (%)[a]	Primarily formula-fed (%)[a]	P
Hospitalized patients (N=50)	64.0	36.0	<.01
Controls for hospitalized patients (N=125)[b]	40.8	49.2	<.01
C. botulinum-positive SIDS cases (N=10)[b]	0	100.0	0.02
Controls for C. botulinum-positive SIDS cases (N=20)[b]	40.0	60.0	0.02
Hospitalized patients (N=67)[c]	68.7	31.3	—

[a]*Two-thirds or more of milk intake from the indicated source*
[b]*California*
[c]*Remaining U.S. and world, 1976-1979*
   Source: modified with permission from (18)

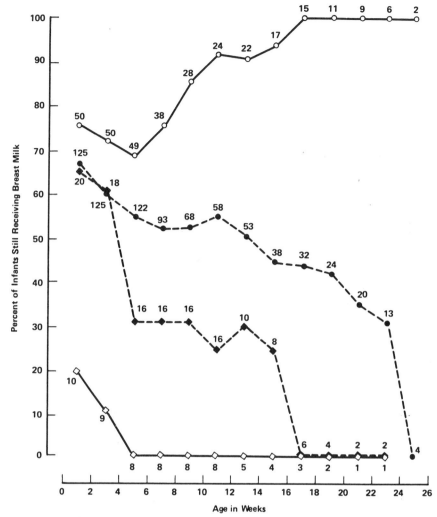

FIGURE 2. The percent of California infants still receiving breast milk by age, 1976-1978. The number of infants
constituting the denominator either of cases or of controls
is above each point. This number changes with time because
each patient and his or her matched controls were excluded
from their respective denominators once illness or death
had occurred.

⚬⎯⎯⎯⚬ Hospitalized infant botulism patients;
●⎯⎯⎯● Healthy control infants for hospitalized cases of
infant botulism; ◆⎯⎯⎯◆ Healthy control infants for SIDS
infants positive for C. botulinum; ◇⎯⎯⎯◇ SIDS infants
positive for C. botulinum.

Source: reproduced from (17) with permission. Copy-
righted by the C. V. Mosby Company, St. Louis, Missouri.

breast-feeding between hospitalized patients and their age-
matched controls became even more apparent when viewed in the
context of age at onset (Figure 2). After 10 weeks of age,
almost every patient hospitalized with infant botulism was
still being nursed (17,18).

In contrast to the experience of hospitalized infant botulism patients, all 10 California infants whose sudden deaths
were attributed to *C. botulinum* infection were primarily
formula-fed (two-thirds or more of milk intake) in the month
before death, a dietary history significantly different
(P = 0.02) from that of their healthy control infants. No
California infant who died suddenly from infant botulism had
been breast-fed within 10 weeks of death (17,18).

To control for the possibility that the milk ingestion
histories obtained in California (64% primarily breast-fed)
represented only local preferences, the same information was
obtained about all patients hospitalized elsewhere with infant
botulism during 1976-1979. A similarly high proportion (71.4%,
55/77) of these patients were primarily breast-fed in the month
before onset of illness. This confirmatory finding suggests
that the association of breast-feeding and the more gradual onset form of infant botulism is real, as is the association between formula-feeding and sudden infant death attributable to
C. botulinum infection (17,18).

It is of course possible that formula-feeding may simply be
one additional confounding variable so closely associated with
sudden infant death that it obscures some still unrecognized
physiological disturbance or environmental factor that causes
the infant's death.

In summary, human milk appears to provide partial protection against fulminant paralysis from infant botulism, thereby
permitting time for hospitalization to be arranged. Formula
milk is associated with the most fulminant form of the disease,
i.e., sudden death. Thus, infant botulism may be added to the
list of other enteric bacterial infections of infancy against
which breast-feeding provides relative protection (20-23).
Finally, the type of milk diet that an infant is fed may be a
key determinant of the composition of the intestinal flora,
which then regulates outgrowth and subsequent toxin production
by *C. botulinum* spores.

IV. INFANT BOTULISM AS A PROTOTYPE CAUSE OF CRIB DEATH

In the developed countries, SIDS is the leading cause of
death of children between one and 12 months of age. In the
United States alone it claims 6-8,000 infants annually. At

present, the generally accepted hypothesis to explain SIDS is "infant apnea," i.e., for unexplained reasons the brainstem respiratory center suddenly fails to signal the respiratory muscles to contract. However, it is also generally agreed that SIDS is a conglomerate of different etiologic entities.

The known potency and mechanism of action of botulinal toxin suggested that its production in the intestine could lead to rapid paralysis of airway and respiratory muscles that in turn might result in sudden, unexpected death (3,4,8). The production or absorption of botulinal toxin which results in characteristic SIDS fatalities may occur so rapidly that the signs and symptoms of illness seen in the typical hospitalized case (constipation, listlessness, poor feeding, weak cry, etc.) do not have time to become apparent.

Present information on the role of infant botulism in SIDS principally derives from a 1977 California study of infant death that found C. botulinum in 4.3% (9/211) of SIDS cases and in none (0/68) of control infants who died of identified causes (8). As discussed elsewhere, for technical and logistical reasons this percentage may represent a minimum estimate of the amount of SIDS attributable to fulminant infant botulism (18).

The association of C. botulinum and sudden infant death was significant (P = 0.02, Fisher's exact test). Subsequently and independently, C. botulinum type A was isolated from a SIDS case in Utah and from another in Washington State (9-11). In Switzerland (24), C. botulinum type G was found in a SIDS case.[3]

One special feature, its age distribution, distinguishes SIDS from all other diseases. As described by Peterson (25):

> "The SIDS age distribution curve rises
> abruptly, peaking at age two or three
> months, and gradually subsides with only a
> small percentage of cases occurring beyond
> six months.... This pattern has been docu-
> mented time after time *and constitutes the
> single most consistent, provocative and
> unique characteristic of SIDS yet identified*."
> [emphasis added]

Figure 3 compares the age distribution of SIDS to the most recent determination of the age distribution of infant botulism. A similarity is evident. The pattern of these two curves may also be found in the infant portion of the age distribution of

[3]*Recently it was suggested that* C. botulinum *may be part of the normal fecal flora of infants and children. As reviewed elsewhere, this report is at variance with all similar studies (18).*

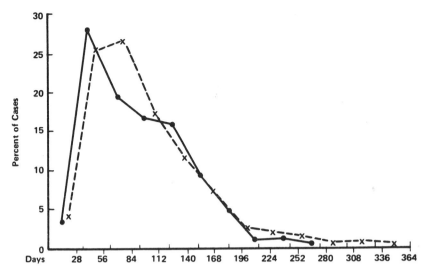

FIGURE 3. Age distribution of all United States hospitalized cases of infant botulism, 1976-1980, compared to a typical
age distribution of SIDS. ●————● 181 infant botulism cases,
age at onset in days; x——————x 425 SIDS cases, age at death
reported in monthly intervals (26).
    Source: redrawn from (18) with permission.

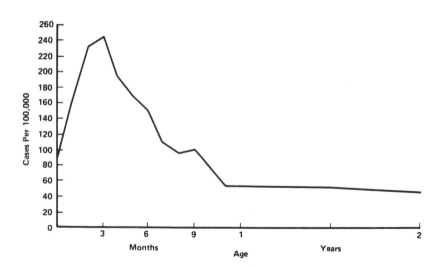

FIGURE 4. Age distribution of reported United States cases
of salmonellosis, 1977, in children aged 0-2 years. (Source:
Centers for Disease Control: Salmonella surveillance annual
summary 1977, issued March, 1979.)

salmonellosis (Figure 4). The virtual identity of the age distributions of infant botulism and of SIDS is probably not a
coincidence, and it suggests that the two entities share a common underlying intestinal pathophysiology.

Thus, infant botulism may represent the prototype of an entire class of toxin-mediated infections of the infant intestine,
heretofore unrecognized, in which toxigenic spore-forming bacteria exploit the unique ecologic conditions found therein
(18). There appears to be no reason to believe that *C.
botulinum* is unique among such pathogenic bacteria in possessing the ability to colonize the infant gut. The extensive
array of potent toxins produced by some species of *Bacillus* and
Clostridium suggests that like *C. botulinum*, these species may
colonize the infant intestine and cause illness, including
sudden death. In addition to the neuromuscular junction, many
potential vital target organs for such toxins exist (e.g.,
brainstem, heart, liver).

Collectively, this class of toxin-mediated enteric infections of infancy may account for a larger number of SIDS cases
than is presently suspected. The search for other etiological
agents in this class, the characterization of their toxin(s)
and resultant syndrome(s), and the identification of host susceptibility factors and methods of prevention, collectively
constitute a considerable challenge for future research.

REFERENCES

1. Arnon, S. S. Infant botulism. *Ann. Rev. Med. 31*, 541-560
   (1980).
2. Pickett, J., Berg, B., Chaplin, E., Brunstetter-Shafer, M.
   Syndrome of botulism in infancy: clinical and electrophysiologic study. *N. Engl. J. Med. 295*, 770-772 (1976).
3. Midura, T. F., Arnon, S. S. Infant botulism: identification of *Clostridium botulinum* and its toxin in faeces.
   Lancet 2, 934-936 (1976).
4. Arnon, S. S., Midura, T. F., Clay, S. A., Wood, R. M.,
   Chin, J. Infant botulism: epidemiological, clinical, and
   laboratory aspects. *J.A.M.A. 237*, 1946-1951 (1977).
5. Arnon, S. S., Werner, S. B., Faber, H. K., Farr, W. H.
   Infant botulism in 1931: discovery of a misclassified
   case. *Am. J. Dis. Child. 133*, 580-582 (1979).
6. Anonymous. Botulism in 1975 - United States. *Morbid.
   Mortal. Wkly. Rept. 25*, 75 (1975).
7. Duchen, L. S. Motor nerve growth induced by botulinum
   toxin as a regeneration phenomenon. *Proc. R. Soc. Med.
   65*, 196-197 (1972).

8. Arnon, S. S., Midura, T. F., Damus, K., Wood, R. M.,
    Chin, J. Intestinal infection and toxin production by
    Clostridium botulinum as one cause of Sudden Infant Death
    Syndrome. *Lancet 1*, 1273-1277 (1978).
9. Arnon, S. S., Chin, J. The clinical spectrum of infant
    botulism. *Reviews Infect. Dis. 1*, 614-621 (1979).
10. Peterson, D. R., Eklund, M. W., Chinn, N. M. The sudden
    infant death syndrome and infant botulism. *Reviews Infect.
    Dis. 1*, 630-634 (1979).
11. Thompson, J. A., Glasgow, L. A., Warpinski, J. R.,
    Olson, C. Infant botulism: clinical spectrum and epi-
    demiology. *Pediatrics 66*, 936-942 (1980).
12. L'Hommedieu, C., Stough, R., Brown, L., Kettrick, R.,
    Polin, R. Potentiation of neuromuscular weakness in
    infant botulism by aminoglycosides. *J. Pediatr. 95*,
    1065-1070 (1979).
13. Sugiyama, H., Mills, D. C. Intraintestinal toxin in
    infant mice challenged intragastrically with *Clostridium
    botulinum* spores. *Infect. Immun. 21*, 59-63 (1978).
14. Moberg, L. J., Sugiyama, H. Microbial ecologic basis of
    infant botulism as studied with germfree mice. *Infect.
    Immun. 25*, 653-657 (1979).
15. Miyazaki, S., Sakaguchi, G. Experimental botulism in
    chickens: the cecum as the site of production and
    absorption of botulinum toxin. *Jpn. J. Med. Sci. Biol.
    31*, 1-15 (1978).
16. Bullen, C. L., Tearle, P. V., Stewart, M. G. The effect
    of "humanised" milks and supplemented breast-feeding on
    the faecal flora. *J. Med. Microbiol. 10*, 403-413 (1977).
17. Arnon, S. S., Damus, K., Thompson, B., Midura, T. F.,
    Chin, J. Protective role of human milk against sudden
    death from infant botulism. *J. Pediatr. (in press)*.
18. Arnon, S. S., Damus, K., Chin, J. Infant botulism:
    epidemiology and relation to Sudden Infant Death Syndrome.
    Epidemiol. Reviews 3, 45-66 (1981).
19. Kleinman, R. E., Walker, W. A. The enteromammary immune
    system: an important new concept in breast milk host
    defense. *Digest. Dis. Sci. 24*, 876-882 (1979).
20. Gunn, R. A., Kimball, A. M., Pollard, R. A., Feeley, J. C.,
    Feldman, R. A., Dutta, S. R., Matthew, P. P.,
    Mahmood, R. A., Levine, M. M. Bottle feeding as a risk
    factor for cholera in infants. *Lancet 2*, 730-732 (1979).
21. France, G. L., Marmer, D. J., Steele, R. W. Breast-
    feeding and *Salmonella* infection. *Am. J. Dis. Child. 134*,
    147-152 (1980).

22. Larson, S. A., Homer, D. R. Relation of breast versus bottle feeding to hospitalization for gastroenteritis in a middle-class U.S. population. *J. Pediatr.* *92*, 417-418 (1978).
23. Bullen, C. L., Willis, A. T. Resistance of the breast-fed infant to gastroenteritis. *Brit. Med. J.* *1*, 338-343 (1971).
24. Sonnabend, O., Sonnabend, W., Heinzle, R., Sigrist, T., Dirnhofer, R., Krech, U. Isolation of *Clostridium botulinum* type G and identification of type G botulinal toxin in humans: report of five sudden unexpected deaths. *J. Infect. Dis.* *143*, 22-27 (1981).
25. Peterson, D. R. Evolution of the epidemiology of Sudden Infant Death Syndrome. *Epidemiol. Reviews 2*, 97-112 (1980).
26. Beckwith, J. B. The sudden infant death syndrome. *Curr. Probl. Pediatr. 3*, 1-34 (1973).

CURRENT CONTROVERSIES IN THE MANAGEMENT
AND TREATMENT OF INFANT BOTULISM

Lawrence W. Brown

Departments of Pediatrics and Neurology
Temple University School of Medicine
Philadelphia, Pennsylvania

INTRODUCTION

Infant botulism is a recently-described disorder in which intestinal colonization with *Clostridium botulinum* leads to systemic absorption of toxin. (1) Affected infants demonstrate a clinical syndrome of constipation, hypotonia, weakness, multiple cranial neuropathies and respiratory depression. (2) Similar to the adult syndromes of food-borne and wound botulism, accepted management and treatment of infant botulism consists of supportive care with particular attention to ventilation and nutrition. Unlike other botulinal syndromes there is no clear indication for specific antitoxin. Cholinergic agonists have never been evaluated in the infant and their efficacy in adult human disease remains debatable.

This paper will address the scientific basis for various therapeutic modalities even though there may be little direct evidence in affected infants. Successful conservative management in the first reported cases led to a lack of enthusiasm for additional invasive or potentially hazardous intervention. Occasional deaths and severe morbidity should warn clinicians that the need persists for more effective early diagnosis and treatment of infant botulism.

RAPID DIAGNOSIS

The clinical syndrome of infant botulism in the hospitalized patient begins with a previously well infant under six months of age who has constipation for several days followed by irritability, poor sucking ability, and progressive weakness. This stereotyped presentation led to a presumptive diagnosis of infant botulism on admission in each of the last ten Philadelphia infants eventually proven to have botulism. However, all of the clinical features are non-specific and other diagnoses must be considered. Meningitis, sepsis, electrolyte disturbance, metabolic encephalopathy, congenital myasthenia gravis, and tick paralysis comprise only a partial list of conditions with similar findings. Initial laboratory studies must be directed at these treatable disorders. Routine laboratory tests including hemogram, electrolytes, calcium, magnesium, blood urea nitrogen, hepatic enzymes, lumbar puncture, and chest x-ray are usually normal. Edrophonium or neostigmine rarely produces a favorable response.

Electrodiagnostic studies demonstrate the most specific abnormalities in infant botulism and can strongly support the clinical diagnosis. Electromyography demonstrates a characteristic finding of brief, small amplitude, abundant motor unit potentials. This myopathic pattern was found in ten of the first 11 Philadelphia infants tested. (3) The "staircase phenomenon" is a marked augmentation of the amplitude of the evoked muscle action potential at rapid rates of stimulation. This is the most characteristic electrophysiologic abnormality in botulism and was seen in all of the 11 individuals tested.

Clinical experience has led to several precautions in the interpretation of the laboratory data. Electrolyte imbalances from poor intake, dehydration, or other metabolic abnormalities may develop secondary to generalized weakness. Poor ventilatory effort can lead to atelectasis which can be radiologically indistinguishable from pneumonia. Follow-up films after institution of appropriate ventilatory support may clarify this dilemma. The edrophonium test is sometimes equivocal early in in the course of infant botulism because the neuromuscular block is still incomplete. Enhancement of neurotransmitter action by anticholinesterases is always less dramatic than the response seen in myasthenia gravis, and positive responses are usually lost on subsequent testing. Some clinicians prefer to use neostigmine because of its longer duration of action; every attempt should be made to obtain a stool specimen prior to administration since anticholinesterase drugs can produce confusing laboratory findings. (4) Electrodiagnostic studies are extremely valuable, but the most critically ill infants cannot be easily transported for such tests.

LAXATIVES AND ENEMAS

Constipation has been the initial manfestation of infant botulism in the vast majority of cases. It is still unclear whether this represents a local effect of the toxin or the first sign of generalized autonomic dysfunction. Abnormalities of the autonomic nervous system including tachycardia, urinary retention, and pupillary dilatation are sometimes overlooked. In either case, the delayed transit time produced by constipation favors further growth of the organism.

Quantitative analysis of fecal flora in infant botulism has demonstrated up to 6×10^8 colony forming units of *Clostridium botulinum* per gram of stool. (5) One anecdotal report documented an eightfold increase in fecal excretion of toxin following laxative administration early in the course of infant botulism. (6) That single bowel movement yielded over 350,000 mouse lethal units of toxin, far more than required for human lethality.

Enemas, cathartic agents, or laxatives are recommended to reduce the enteric burden of toxin as yet unabsorbed. Cathartics and laxatives may be administered cautiously, but saline enemas are probably safer. It is advisable to perform high colonic administration since the cecum and proximal colon are the usual sites of botulinal colonization. Even saline enemas are not entirely without potential risk, and a recent infant became hyponatremic secondary to preferential absorption of free water following such treatment. Unfortunately, purgatives are not always successful in the severely affected, obstipated infant. Repeated treatments are potentially dangerous and unlikely to produce dramatic results if initial attempts are unsuccessful.

MECHANICAL FACTORS

The critical management of these hospitalized infants involves supportive respiratory and nutritional care to prevent upper airway obstruction, hypoventilation and inadequate caloric intake. Generalized weakness and hypotonia are compounded by absent gag and cough reflexes from brain stem involvement to produce pooling of oral secretions, laryngeal obstruction and aspiration of stomach contents.

Endotracheal intubation and mechanical ventilation are frequently necessary to provide good air exchange and insure adequate pulmonary toilet. Some investigators recommend early tracheotomy within one week of intubation, but these hypotonic and weak infants do not usually have enough strength to dislodge the endotracheal tube or cause upper airway irritation. They often tolerate prolonged intubation without subglottic stenosis or other irritative complications. (7)

Maintenance of adequate ventilation in critically ill infants relies on several basic principles. If the infant has intercostal weakness with consequent diaphragmatic breathing, then postures such as tight flexion for lumbar puncture may further compromised an already marginal ventilatory status. Upper airway obstruction can be produced by exaggerated neck flexion. Our only late complication in the past three years occurred in the late recovery phase of infant botulism. At the time, he had been extubated for ten days and strength was improving daily. While rediapering him, his nurse responded to an apnea alarm at an adjacent crib, and within an estimated 30 seconds the infant with resolving botulism developed cyanosis and complete respiratory arrest.

Such potential respiratory hazards have led to local adoption of certain simple techniques. Mild neck extension in the supine position is insured by a rolled diaper. When nasogastric feedings are started the head is immobilized by more rolls added on either side to prevent lateral motion. The infant is always fed in an upright position which is maintained for at least one hour.

Nasogastric feeding has been frequently employed while the infant is too weak to suck effectively or lacking protective gag and cough reflexes. Tube feeding may stimulate peristalsis but there is no evidence demonstrating advantages of breast feeding over proprietary formulas. It can be performed safely even with endotracheal intubation, and there are caloric and other advantages over parenteral hyperalimentation. Recently, most infants with botulism have been discharged from the hospital before complete neuromuscular recovery. The main criterion for discharge is the return of protective respiratory reflexes including gag and cough. Frequently sucking and swallowing are not yet effective at the time of discharge. Such infants frequently require one to two additional weeks of total nasogastric feeding or supplementation after fatigue-limited oral feeding. Full return of muscle strength is usually complete two to four weeks after entirely oral feeding has resumed.

ANTITOXIN

The treatment of adult food-borne botulism has always consisted of supportive care. (8) Type-specific antitoxin has
been generally recommended even though its value is debatable
after the appearance of severe neurologic signs. (9) In the
United States trivalent (ABE) antitoxin is available from the
Center for Disease Control for cases of suspected botulism and
asymptomatic individuals who shared the probable contaminated
meal, but no formal recommendation has been published for infants.
Since botulinal toxin is rapidly and irreversibly bound to
the neuromuscular junction, the finding of measurable toxin
in the serum of affected individuals offers some rationale for
antitoxin administration. (10) Significant amounts of toxin
can conceivably be neutralized before binding to the motor end
plate can occur. Unfortunately, infant botulism is a prolonged
intestinal infection with continual release and systemic absorption of toxin over many weeks. (11) Equine antitoxin is
unlikely to prevent deterioration since it has a short circula-
tory half-life of only several days. (12) Furthermore, most
affected infants have little free toxin in the bloodstream.
Only a single infant has ever been recorded whose serum contained botulinal toxin measurable by currently available techniques. (12) This makes it unlikely that antitoxin will have
a significant impact.
Adverse reactions to equine-derived antitoxin in the adult
population was found in 9% of a recent series of 268 patients
compiled by the Center for Disease Control. (14) Immediate
hypersensitivity reactions included anaphylaxis (2%) and urti-
caria (3%). Several of these nonfatal reactions occurred in
patients who had received only a skin test. Serum sickness was
seen in another 4%. The experience with antitoxin in infant
botulism is limited to two individuals. (1,13) A history of
ingestion of homemade applesauce in one Delaware Valley infant
led to a diagnosis of possible food-borne botulism, and he received trivalent antitoxin shortly after admission. He was
never profoundly weak, and his course was similar to other cases
of mild botulism not treated with antitoxin. The other infant
suffered an anaphylactic reaction despite pretreatment with
epinephrine after receiving only one-tenth of the planned dose.
Human derived hyperimmune globulin is currently under active investigation, but clinical experience is not yet available. Experimental treatment with homologous botulinal antitoxin in guinea pigs prevented signs of botulism for more than
two weeks without adverse reactions or development of measurable antibodies. (15) One can extrapolate from such limited data as well as the experience with other human hyperimmune sera. (16) Human botulinal hyperimmune serum should have similar

advantages of prolonged survival in the circulation and free-
dom from foreign protein reactions.

There are other conceivable immunologic strategies for intervention in infants with botulism. Direct intragastric administration of antitoxin might neutralize intra-intestinal toxin
and could possibly reduce the amount of botulinal toxin absorbed
systemically. However, there is no direct experimental evidence or indirect experience with other enteric toxins. Such
an approach requires prior demonstration that the small infant
does not absorb an equine-derived product which could lead to
anaphylaxis or other hypersensitivity reactions. Furthermore,
there is no reason to suspect that local neutralization of the
toxin would eradicate any ongoing infection or ameliorate effects of toxin already irreversibly bound at the neuromuscular
junction.

PHARMACOLOGIC TREATMENT

There are no reports of infants receiving specific cholinomimetic drugs such as guanidine hydrochloride, germine diacetate, or 4-aminopyridine.

Guanidine was first introduced as an adjunct to botulism
therapy in 1968. (17) Its usage was based upon a demonstrated
enhancement of acetylcholine release, and there had been positive experience in other disorders of the myoneural junction,
including myasthenia gravis and the Eaton-Lambert syndrome.
(18,19) Variable results have been reported in adults with
food-borne botulism. Early enthusiastic case studies demonstrated clinical improvement which appeared to be guanidine-
dependent. (20,21) Other investigators using similar dosage
schedules in affected adults found no improvement. (22) A recent double-blind crossover study demonstrated no objective or
subjective improvement in the rate of recovery from botulism
in guanidine-treated patients compared to the placebo or the
non-treated groups. (23) At doses greater than 50 mg/kg/day
adverse effects clearly outweighed apparent benefits: diarrhea,
paresthesias, and signs of cholinergic poisoning (vomiting,
salivation, bronchospasm, and seizures). Less common toxicity
included bone marrow suppression, hypotension and skin rash.

The mechanism of action of guanidine has been investigated
in animal and human muscle preparations. (24,25) Biochemical
experiments show that guanidine inhibits the binding and uptake
of calcium and other divalent cations to subcellular organelles
such as mitochondria. (26) This evidence suggests that guanidine enhances acetylcholine release by allowing calcium to accumulate at the presynaptic terminal through interference with
intracellular calcium binding. Guanidine increases the release

of acetylcholine quanta most effectively at low frequencies of
nerve stimulation and at the beginning of a tetanus at high
rates of stimulation. (27) This observation explains its potential usefulness in botulism and the Eaton-Lambert syndrome
where the block is most pronounced with individual nerve stimuli and at the beginning of a tetanus.

Germine diacetate is another cholinergic drug which has
been used experimentally in various neuromuscular disorders
with variable success. In animals poisoned with botulinum toxin
germine reverses the neuromuscular block. (28) Human experience with germine is very limited, and not particularly encour-
aging. (28,29)

There is very limited clinical experience with 4-aminopy-
ridine, an extremely interesting cholinomimetic compound which
also enhances transmitter release. (25) Available data suggest that it acts by increasing calcium entry during the release of synaptic vesicles and by inhibiting intracellular binding of free calcium. In rats paralyzed by a potentially lethal
dose of botulinal toxin, 4-aminopyridine was the only drug active in vivo to restore motor tone and strength. (25) Unfortunately, a high incidence of convulsions, transient improvement, and lack of clinical effect on respiratory function make
4-aminopyridine unacceptable for human use. (30) Potentially
less toxic aminopyridine congeners are under active investigation.

ANTIBIOTICS

Clinical and experimental studies have clearly demonstrated that many drugs other than anesthetics interfere with neuromuscular transmission. (31,33) These drugs include antibiotic, cardiovascular, anti-rheumatic, psychotropic, hormonal,
and anticonvulsant agents. Antibiotics are the most important
at all ages. They can unmask or aggravate myasthenia gravis,
produce post-operative respiratory depression, lead to a drug-
induced myasthenic syndrome, or exacerbate the respiratory and
skeletal muscle weakness of botulism. The aminoglycoside antibiotics are the only class of such drugs frequently administered to infants with progressive weakness, irritability, and
lethargy. If sepsis or meningitis is suspected it must be
treated rapidly, and current accepted initial treatment usually includes a penicillin and an aminoglycoside. Serum concentrations of gentamycin and kanamycin achieved at usual dosages
are unlikely to produce discernable weakness in the healthy infant. However, any additional neuromuscular blockade produced
by aminoglycosides may exacerbate weakness in the infant with
botulism by reducing the "margin of safety." (34)

Margin of safety is a useful concept popular with pulmonary and muscle physiologists. By comparing muscle responses to nerve stimulation in the presence of cholinergic antagonists to control responses, one can derive an estimation of availability of acetylcholine receptors left unblocked at the neuromuscular junction. (36,37) These findings correlate well with muscle weakness, as demonstrated in the intact animal, in isolated nerve-muscle preparations, and in limited human studies.

In skeletal muscle there must be occlusion of at least 75% of acetylcholine receptors by tubocurarine before there is any measurable failure of muscle response to a single stimulus or short volley of sub-tetanic stimuli ("train of four"). Diaphragmatic muscle has an even greater protective index of over 90% before diminished contraction can be seen with a single stimulus. Supra-tetanic stimuli at or above 30 hertz will produce neuromuscular failure at lower levels of acetylcholine receptor blockade.

The results of these experiments are summarized in Table 1 which compares levels of neuromuscular function to the degree of receptor blockade. The most vulnerable muscle groups with the least margin of safety are those skeletal muscles requiring sustained effort (i.e. neck flexion and hand grip). The diaphragm is least vulnerable, with a margin of safety of 90 to 95%. Intercostal and accessory muscles of respiration are between these extremes.

Sophisticated measurements of ventilatory function are impossible in the infant, and one must rely on empirical and global parameters such as arterial blood gases. Infants with botulism frequently demonstrate paradoxical respiration with chest collapse on inspiration and chest expansion on expiration produced by intercostal paralysis with preserved diaphragmatic motion. Continued adequate oxygenation depends on the increased margin of safety of the diaphragm.

TABLE 1. Levels of Neuromuscular Block

CLINICAL STATE	RECEPTORS BLOCKED (%)
Diaphragmatic and complete peripheral muscle block	95
Peripheral block almost complete	90
Normal tidal volume, depressed twitch height, minimal peripheral block	75-80
Normal expiratory flow rate and vital capacity	70-75
Normal inspiratory force	50
Normal head lift and hand grip test	33

Peripheral weakness without respiratory failure suggests at least 75% blockade. Any further contribution to neuromuscular blockade by aminoglycosides may produce clinical deterioration as was demonstrated in our recent retrospective analysis. (34) One dramatic example occurred in an infant who presented with weakness, paucity of spontaneous movements, decreased deep tendon reflexes, sluggish pupils, poor suck and weak gag reflex. Chest x-ray showed a unilateral infiltrate versus atelectasis. One hour after the first dose of gentamycin and ampicillin he acutely deteriorated with loss of gag reflex, development of facial diplegia, and requirement for assisted ventilation. Antibiotics were changed to ampicillin, chloramphenicol, and nafcillin with overnight improvement in respiratory function. Admission cultures proved negative, and all antibiotics were discontinued. On the ninth hospital day there was an episode of possible aspiration and he received gentamycin and cephalosporin. Within hours, there was evidence of respiratory compromise requiring prolonged assisted ventilation and subsequent tracheostomy.

Our review led us to the conclusion that clinical deterioration was associated with use of aminoglycosides, although most experienced clinicians have also noted progressive weakness in untreated patients. All five infants in the published series who received aminoglycosides required mechanical ventilation while none of the other four developed respiratory failure. Following these results, a planned prospective study to evaluate aminoglycosides was cancelled since other antibiotics are available without this hazard. Also, further clinical experience has led to avoidance of antibiotics by earlier recognition of the clinical syndrome of infant botulism with unique historical, physical, and laboratory features to distinguish it from meningitis and sepsis.

Penicillin and ampicillin might be expected to modify the course of infant botulism. Theoretically, the effect of clostridiocidal antibiotics could possibly exacerbate or ameliorate botulism. Clear evidence shows that lysis of the baceria leads to release of toxin producing more available toxin for systemic absorption. (38) Alternatively, bacteriocidal antibiotics might be expected to improve a condition involving ongoing intestinal infection, toxin absorption, and neuromuscular blockade. (1) However, there are no reports suggesting any clinical change in infants treated with either drug. There is no experience with more specific clostridiocidal antibiotics such as vancomycin.

CONCLUSION

The management and treatment of infant botulism still consists of supportive care directed at the respiratory and nutritional requirements of the critically ill infant. Such care
includes early purgation by enemas, and meticulous attention
to metabolic and nutritional needs, and prevention of further
respiratory compromise due to mechanically disadvantageous postures. Antibiotics which produce further neuromuscular blockade should be avoided, and clostridiocidal antibiotics are not
indicated. Parenteral equine antitoxin is potentially hazardous and, therefore, not recommended, but human hyperimmune globulin deserves further consideration.

The few reported infant botulism deaths have resulted from
respiratory complications, and the only significant sequellae
in survivors were potentially avoidable respiratory compromise.
(39) Infant botulism is a potentially fatal disorder, but early recognition and conservative treatment should prevent almost
all mortality and long-term morbidity. Better clinical and
laboratory tools for early diagnosis and treatment are still
necessary because of persistent morbidity and mortality in hospitalized cases, as well as the possible relationship of ful-
minating botulism to the sudden infant death syndrome.

Recovery from infant botulism can take many weeks, and factors leading to improvement are poorly understood. Clinical
resolution may occur despite persistence of the enteric infection and ongoing toxin release. Recently developed experimental models for infant botulism may lead to further elucidation
of the pathophysiology of disease and recovery. (40-42) Ongoing research is currently exploring developmental aspects of
the microecology of the infants intestinal bacterial flora,
studying effects of diet on anaerobic bacteria and bile acid
production, developing new techniques in the measurement of
botulinal toxin, and preparing clinical trials with human hyperimmune serum. These are only some of the current approaches which will hopefully lead to improved management and treatment of infant botulism.

REFERENCES

1. Arnon S.S., Midura, T.F., Clay, S.A. et al. *JAMA 237*,
    1946 (1977)
2. Brown, L. *Rev. Infect. Dis. 1,625* (1979).
3. Packer, R.J., Brown, M.J., and Berman, P.H. *Neurol. 30*,
    378 (1980).

4. Horwitz, M.A., Hatheway, C.L., and Dowell, V.R. *Am. J. Clin. Path. 66, 737* (1976).

5. Wilcke, B.W. Jr., Midura, T.F., and Arnon, S.S. *J. Infect. Dis. 141, 419* (1980).

6. Peterson, D.R., Eklund, M.W., and Chinn, N.M. *Rev. Infect. Dis. 1, 630* (1979).

7. Wolfe, J.A., Pasquariello, P., Rowe, L.D. et al. *Ann. Otol. Rhinol. Laryngol. 88, 861* (1979)

8. Donadio, J.A., Gangarosa, E.J. and Faich, G.A. *J. Infect. Dis. 124, 108* (1971).

9. Merson, M.H., Hughes, J.M., Dowell, V.R. et al. *JAMA 229, 1305* (1974).

10. Simpson, L. W. *Rev. Infect. Dis. 2, 656* (1979).

11. Arnon, S.S., and Chin., J. *Rev. Infect. Dis. 1, 614* (1979).

12. Lewis, G.E. Jr., and Metzger, J.F. *Lancet 2, 634* (1978).

13. Alexander, D., Kaplan, A., Lersch, A. et al. *Morbidity Mortality Weekly Rep. 27, 411* (1978).

14. Black, R.E., and Gunn, R.A. *Am. J. Med. 69, 567* (1980).

15. Metzger, J.F. and Lewis, G.E. Jr. *Rev. Infect. Dis. 1, 689* (1979).

16. Stiehm, E.R. *Pediatr. 63, 301* (1979).

17. Cherington, M., and Ryan, D.W. *N. Engl. J. Med. 278, 931* (1968).

18. Scaer, R.C., Tooker, B.S., and Cherington, M. *Neurol. 19, 1107* (1969).

19. Minot, A.N., Dodd, K., and Riven, S.S. *JAMA 113, 553* (1939).

20. Oh, S.J., and Kim, K.W. *Neurol. 23, 1084* (1973).

21. Cherington, M., and Ryan, D.W. *N. Engl. J. Med. 282, 195* (1970).

22. Faich, G.A., Graebner, R.W., and Sato, S. *N. Engl. J. Med. 285, 773* (1971).

23. Kaplan, J.E., Davis, L.W., Narayan, V. et al. *Ann. Neurol. 6, 69* (1979).

24. Kamenskaya, M.A., Elmqvist, D., and Thesleff, S. *Arch. Neurol. 32, 510* (1975).

25. Lundh, H., Leander, S., and Thesleff, S. *J. Neurol. Sci. 32, 29* (1977).

26. Davidhoff, F. *J. Biol. Chem. 249, 6406* (1974).

27. Flacke, W., Caviness, V.S. and Samaha, F.C. *N. Engl. J. Med. 275, 1207* (1966).

28. Cherington, M., and Greenberg, H. *Neurol. 21, 966* (1971).

29. Cherington, M., and Schultz, D. *Clin. Toxicol. 11, 19* (1977).

30. Ball, A.P., Hopkinson, R.B., Farrell, I.D. *Q. J. Med. 48, 473* (1979).

31. Argov, Z., and Mastaglia, F.L. *N. Engl. J. Med. 301, 409* (1979).

32. Pittinger, C.B., Eryasa, Y., and Adamson, R. *Anesthesiol. Analg. 49, 487* (1970).

33. Singh, Y.N., Harvey, A.L., and Marshall, I.G. *Anesthesiol. 48, 418* (1978).

34. L'Hommedieu, C., Stough, R., Brown, L. et al. *J. Pediat. 95, 1065* (1979).

35. Paton, W.D.M., and Waud, D.R. *J. Physiol. 59, 90* (1967).

36. Waud, B.E., and Waud, D.R. *Anesthesiol. 37, 417* (1972)

37. Matteo, R.S., Spector, S., and Horowitz, P.E. *Anesthesiol. 41, 440* (1974).

38. Smith, L.D.S. "Botulism: The Organism, its Toxins, the Disease" (Charles C. Thomas), Springfield, Illinois, (1977).

39. Arnon, S.S. *Ann. Rev. Med. 31, 541* (1980).

40. Sugiyama, H., and Mills, D.C. *Infect. Immun. 21, 59* (1978).

41. Moberg, L.J., and Sugiyama, H. *Infect. Immun. 29, 819* (1980).

42. Swerczek, T.W. *Am. J. Vet. Res. 41, 348* (1980).

SUMMARY

BOTULISM: PERSPECTIVE
ON THE CONFERENCE

William Schaffner

Departments of Medicine and Preventive Medicine
Vanderbilt University School of Medicine
Nashville, Tennessee

I first encountered botulism in the autumn of 1963. As
medical residents on duty in the emergency room, a colleague
and I examined a patient with an unusual neuroparalytic illness. After puzzling a bit, my astute companion thought of
botulism and I consulted a handy reference text. Although
the patient's symptoms and signs were compatible with
botulism, we discarded the diagnosis when a history of eating
home-canned food could not be elicited.

The patient was admitted to the hospital but, I am sad to
say, subsequently died. Later, it was demonstrated that he
had type E botulinal toxin in his serum. He was part of the
tri-state outbreak of type E botulism caused by commercially-
distributed smoked whitefish marketed in pliofilm bags (1).

The late Dr. M. Glenn Koenig directed the Vanderbilt
University investigation of that outbreak (1) (incidentally,
Dr. Lance L. Simpson was then a graduate student at Vanderbilt
and this also was his introduction to botulism). Dr. Koenig
thoroughly reviewed the literature on botulism, including van
Ermengem's classic study and the pioneering work of K. F.
Meyer. He remarked that little new basic information had
been developed since these seminal investigations were published. If you make allowances for Dr. Koenig's customary
hyperbole, there was some truth in his observation.

If he had lived to attend this conference, however, I am
sure Dr. Koenig would have changed his mind. This unique
international convocation of biochemists, physiologists,
pharmacologists, microbiologists, epidemiologists, and clinicians devoted to botulism has encompassed an extraordinary

amount of new information on this disease and the toxins
which produce it.

Dr. Lewis did not ask me to speak at the end of this
conference merely to reiterate what you have heard already.
Rather, I shall mention several reports which attracted my
particular attention and which I have attempted to integrate
into my clinical and epidemiological background. Also, it is
traditional for someone in this location on the program to
look to the future and indicate some of the areas requiring
further investigation.

Dr. Das Gupta began the conference by elegantly describ-
ing structure-function relationships of the botulinum
neurotoxins. I am struck by the role of pancreatic trypsin
in nicking and activation of toxin. This is particularly
apparent for Type E toxin which is released in a form which
is relatively impotent; only after trypsin nicking is its
toxicity fully expressed. In contrast, Types A and B toxin
are released already nicked and activated. These molecular
phenomena may explain the epidemiological observation of
toxin types producing wound botulism. In this disease,
botulinal toxin is released directly from the wound into the
systemic circulation. Thus, the toxin does not encounter
pancreatic trypsin. Wound botulism has been produced only by
Types A and B toxin. There are no reported cases caused by
Type E toxin, the type which requires trypsin activation.

Dr. Sakaguchi has observed that the larger molecular
weight progenitor toxins are associated with greater oral
toxicity. Because these molecules are more stable in the
stomach, they are more readily absorbed. Several participants
and I have speculated whether this finding could explain a
puzzling clinical phenomenon - the rare demonstration of
circulating toxin in the serum of patients with infant botulism. Infants can absorb large molecules and, thus, the
progenitor toxin would be absorbed readily. If only very
small amounts of toxin are required to intoxicate an infant,
perhaps the human infant simply is a more sensitive bioassay
of toxin action than is the standard intra-peritoneal mouse
assay.

Dr. Simpson's conceptual framework helps me understand
the mechanism of action of botulinal toxin. Clinicians
certainly agree with his comment (2) that investigation is
needed into what can reverse the strong third-stage binding
of toxin inside nerve endings. As matters stand, we have
little other than supportive therapy to offer our patients.

Dr. Dolly's belief that botulinal toxin has an effect
within the central nervous system may offer an explanation
for another clinical observation. Perhaps the inhibition of
acetylcholine release in his central nervous system prepara-

tion bears some relationship to the striking somnolence noted in some patients with type B disease (3). Likewise, Dr. Sellin's observation that toxin may produce long-term alterations in the post-synaptic membrane correlates with the increasing reports of prolonged disability among individuals who ostensibly have recovered from botulism.

Professor Thesleff's hypothesis concerning a calcium-independent mechanism of transmitter release from motor nerve terminals is in concert with bedside observations of irregular and fluctuating paralysis, especially during recovery. In addition, the neurophysiologist's use of 3,4 diaminopyridine now has stimulated cautious therapeutic trials with this compound.

Doctors Hatheway, Notermans, and Dowell all addressed an important problem which requires further investigation. Establishing the diagnosis of botulism in a community hospital (or even a university medical center) remains extremely difficult. Dr. Morris' description of often-delayed onset of therapy relates, in part, to the cumbersome laboratory procedures required to identify the toxin and the microorganism in clinical specimens. I can speak to the frustrations inherent in having to refer specimens to distant laboratories, sometimes at night or on weekends. We need a specific, sensitive diagnostic test which can be performed reliably in a clinical laboratory. The diagnosis of botulism must be liberated from the mouse and moved out of the 19th century.

The Doctors Sonnabend presented extremely provocative findings which resulted from their awesome systematic post mortem study. In addition to relating Types D and G to human disease, they raised the possibility that some instances of sudden or unexpected death in adults may be caused by botulinal intoxication. The exciting analogy with the toxico-infection of infant botulism was obvious. This possibility became even more intriguing in the light of Dr. Feldman's description of U. S. cases of adult botulism in which no food vehicle could be identified. Because it is unlikely that other investigations with the scope of the Sonnabend study will be performed, the urgent need for a simple diagnostic test becomes even more apparent.

The recognition of infant botulism and the elucidation of its pathogenesis represent the most important recent events in the history of botulism for clinicians. However, despite the intense interest this "new" disease has engendered, most aspects of its epidemiology remain obscure. Why, for instance, is this disease so focal in its distribution? Some areas of the United States seem to produce large numbers of cases of infant botulism (California, Utah, Pennsylvania, for example) whereas other areas are almost devoid of this

illness. In Tennessee, we have recognized only one case (4),
despite a continuing extensive surveillance mechanism.

I will close by mentioning what may be, for the public,
the highlight of the conference. That would be the report by
Doctors Scott and Schantz that crystalline Type A botulinal
toxin can be used as a therapeutic agent to correct extraocular muscle imbalance. I find it especially apropos that
their report was presented here at Fort Detrick. Just as this
institution has somewhat redirected its concerns, so too,
botulinum toxin (the most potent poison) seems to be useful
in therapy. "They shall beat their swords into plowshares..."
(Isaiah 2:4).

Continuing public support for basic and applied research
into botulism, like research into other biomedical subjects,
requires justification. The therapeutic use of botulinal
toxin, infant botulism and its relation to sudden infant
death, botulism as a possible cause of unexplained death in
adults, the continuing threat of botulinum toxin in commercially distributed food items, and even the economic
consequences of the shaker-foal syndrome (the apparent
counterpart of infant botulism in young horses) together
provide a compelling rationale for supporting investigations
into all aspects of botulinum toxin.

REFERENCES

1. Koenig, M. G., Spickard, A., Cardella, M. A., and Rogers,
    D. E., *Medicine, 43,* 517 (1964).
2. Simpson, L. L., *Rev. Infect. Dis. 1,* 656 (1979).
3. Koenig, M. G., Drutz, D. J., Mushlin, A. L., Schaffner,
    W., and Rogers, D. E., *Am. J. Med. 42,* 208 (1967).
4. McKee, K. T., Kilroy, A. W., Harrison, W. W., and
    Schaffner, W., *Am. J. Dis. Child. 131,* 857 (1977).

INDEX